Preclinical Aspects of Ischemic Stroke

Preclinical Aspects of Ischemic Stroke

Edited by **Robin Deaver**

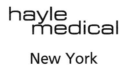

hayle
medical

New York

Published by Hayle Medical,
30 West, 37th Street, Suite 612,
New York, NY 10018, USA
www.haylemedical.com

Preclinical Aspects of Ischemic Stroke
Edited by Robin Deaver

International Standard Book Number: 978-1-63241-323-9 (Hardback)

Contents

Permissions

List of Contributors

Preface

Every book is initially just a concept; it takes months of research and hard work to give it the final shape in which the readers receive it. In its early stages, this book also went through rigorous reviewing. The notable contributions made by experts from across the globe were first molded into patterned chapters and then arranged in a sensibly sequential manner to bring out the best results.

This book presents innovations in the preclinical study of stroke addressing new pathways to neuroprotection. Although hypothermia has been so far the only "neuroprotection" cure that has endured the translation from preclinical to clinical studies, developments in both preclinical studies and in design of clinical trials will hopefully give more and better treatments for ischemic stroke. This book focuses on supplying the preclinical scientists with creative knowledge and instruments to examine new mechanisms of ischemic brain damage and its cure.

It has been my immense pleasure to be a part of this project and to contribute my years of learning in such a meaningful form. I would like to take this opportunity to thank all the people who have been associated with the completion of this book at any step.

Editor

Novel Approaches to Neuroprotection

Neuroprotection in Animal Models of Global Cerebral Ischemia

Miguel Cervantes[1], Ignacio González-Burgos[2], Graciela Letechipía-Vallejo[1], María Esther Olvera-Cortés[3] and Gabriela Moralí[4]
[1]*Laboratorio de Neurociencias. Facultad de Ciencias Médicas y Biológicas "Dr. Ignacio Chávez", Universidad Michoacana de San Nicolás de Hidalgo, Morelia, Michoacán*
[2]*Laboratorio de Psicobiología, División de Neurociencias, Centro de Investigación, Biomédica de Occidente Instituto Mexicano del Seguro Social, Guadalajara, Jalisco*
[3]*Laboratorio de Neurofisiología Experimental, Centro de Investigación Biomédica de Michoacán, Instituto Mexicano del Seguro Social, Morelia, Michoacán*
[4]*Unidad de Investigación Médica en Farmacología, UMAE Hospital de Especialidades, CMN S XXI, Instituto Mexicano del Seguro Social, México, D.F.*
Mexico

1. Introduction

The present chapter deals with some of the main lines of experimental research on global cerebral ischemia, through which a substantial knowledge has been generated, that has contributed in an important measure both to the understanding of the mechanisms of cerebral damage induced by ischemia, and of the subsequent post-ischemic neuroregenerative and cerebral plastic processes taking place in the remaining or newly differentiated neurons. Thus, data obtained from experimental designs in animal models of global cerebral ischemia, on key molecular and cellular events triggered by this condition, have provided a substantial background from which neuroprotection can be rationally approached, in order to develop strategies aimed to antagonize, to interrupt, or to slow the sequence of injurious biochemical and molecular events that would result in irreversible ischemic injury; as well as to promote brain repair and plasticity processes which can favor functional preservation or recovery after global cerebral ischemia.

Transient global cerebral ischemia, which can mainly occur during cardiac arrest and cardiopulmonary resuscitation, but also during asphyxiation, hypotensive shock, or extracorporeal circulation, is a pathophysiological condition that is associated with great morbidity and requires intensive medical treatment (Madl & Holzer, 2004). In certain clinical situations (surgical repair of the thoracic aorta, complex congenital heart lesions, and also during implantable cardiac defibrillator testing in patients with drug-resistant ventricular fibrillation) the possible occurrence of transient global cerebral ischemia, and some neuroprotective procedures, can be anticipated (Hogue et al., 2008); however, this is not the case of cardiac arrest.

Cardiopulmonary arrest remains as one among the most frequent causes of death and disability around the world. Despite quick emergency responses and better techniques of defibrillation, the chances of survival following cardiac arrest are still poor, between 20-50% of patients in whom cardiopulmonary resuscitation is attempted. A complex pathophysiological condition is elicited by cardiac arrest, since it results in whole-body ischemia which compromises systemic circulatory homeostasis and cerebral, pulmonary, renal, and cardiac functions. In the course of cardiac arrest, global cerebral blood flow is severely impaired with the consequent risk of ischemic damage of brain cells, which magnitude seems to be associated with the cumulative time staying in cardiac arrest. Thus, most deaths (60%) during the post-resuscitation period have been attributed to extensive brain injury and neuronal damage that develops as a consequence of alteration of cell processes triggered by cerebral ischemia and reperfusion, during and after cardiac arrest. In addition, it is known that transient interruption or reduction of blood flow in the whole brain, are main causes of permanent brain damage and functional disruptions in human beings, and near around a half of surviving patients show permanent impairment of cognitive functions, such as learning and memory, attention, and executive functioning, and only a small proportion (less than 10%) of those survivors are able to reassume their former usual life styles (Geocardin et al., 2008; Grubb et al., 2000; Krause et al, 1986; Schneider et al., 2009). Thus, development of effective cytoprotective therapies that may be common to the organs more sensitive to cardiac arrest, such as heart or brain, could result in improvement of survival and better outcome following this whole ischemic episode (Karanjia & Geocardin, 2011).

Experimental protocols aimed to gain relevant information regarding those pathophysiological phenomena leading to cerebral damage elicited by ischemia have included, since long time, the use of animal models of cerebral ischemia, in order to support better diagnostic, prophylactic and clinical-therapeutic procedures for ischemic cerebrovascular diseases in human beings (Ginsberg & Busto, 1989; Gupta & Briyal, 2004; Hartman et al., 2005, Hossmann, 2008; Traystman, 2003). Thus, biochemical, electrophysiological, histological, and behavioral parameters of ischemic brain damage have been included in experimental designs to evaluate the efficacy and safety of pharmacological and non pharmacological neuroprotective procedures against brain injury resulting from the significant reduction of blood supply to the whole brain, in several animal models of global cerebral ischemia.

Even though a great number of pharmacological agents have proven to exert effective neuroprotective actions against cellular events leading to ischemic brain injury in experimental models of global cerebral ischemia, unfortunately they have not had enough clinical relevance to date. On the other hand, after evaluation of its effectiveness as a neuroprotective strategy in animal models of global cerebral ischemia, hypothermia has been tested in clinical trials in patients having suffered cardiac arrest, the most frequent cause of global cerebral ischemia in human beings (Castren et al., 2009; Geocardin et al., 2008; Greer, 2006; Inamasu et al., 2010; Knapp et al., 2011; Seder & Jarrah, 2008,). It seems that new and better strategies to translate preclinical data supporting the potential clinical usefulness of neuroprotective drugs to clinical trials, must be developed.

2. Animal models of global cerebral ischemia

Animal models of global cerebral ischemia allow studying, at different levels of biological organization of the central nervous system, the development and temporal course of those processes that may result in irreversible ischemic neuronal damage, as well as in the subsequent cell repair and plasticity underlying either permanent cerebral functional impairment or recovery as a result of intrinsic brain mechanisms or neuroprotective procedures. Thus, animal-related factors (species, strain, age, sex, co-morbidities), animal-model-related factors (choice of ischemic model, anesthetic procedures, duration of ischemia, reperfusion, survival, possibility of monitoring of physiological parameters), selective vulnerability of specific neuron types in several brain structures, outcome assessment (histopathological, biochemical, functional, parameters of brain injury in specific cerebral structures), short- or long-term experimental design, pharmacological characteristics of the presumptive neuroprotective agent itself, timing and dose-response of neuroprotective drug administration with reference to starting and ending of the ischemic episode, may account for the relevance of results from these investigations.

Models of cerebral ischemia have been also developed in *in vitro* models, in particular brain tissue slices and neuronal cultures, allowing to study in detail the cellular phenomena leading either to neuronal damage or to neural recovery and plasticity after ischemia (Benítez-King, 2006; Goldberg & Choi, 1993; Kasai et al., 2003; Whittingham et al., 1984).

Several conditions have to be fulfilled by animal models of global cerebral ischemia in order to become appropriate counterparts of these pathophysiological conditions in human beings, as well as to yield reliable and valid results in supporting clinical therapeutic approaches. Thus, it could be expected that in animal models of global cerebral ischemia the ischemic episode can be induced in a constant and reproducible manner: low variation for the extent, temporal course, and magnitude of the resulting ischemic brain injury under specific experimental conditions, including duration of the ischemic episode; easy control of possible deviations of important physiological variables, feasible neurological, neuropathological, and functional evaluations; lack of influence of anesthetic drugs and surgical procedures on the mechanisms of brain injury, brain recovery and/or neuroprotection; short-, intermediate- and long-term follow up of the outcome; and economical, easily available experimental animals of those species better accepted by public animal welfare concerns to be used in experimental protocols of cerebral ischemia and neuroprotection.

2.1 Main animal models of global cerebral ischemia

Models of global cerebral ischemia have been performed in both large (monkeys, sheep, dogs, pigs, cats, rabbits) and small animals (gerbils, rats, mice). Among these, both advantages and disadvantages can be recognized according to several practical aspects: main objectives of the model; monitoring procedures to be used; nature, number and timing of simultaneous parameters to be recorded in order to evaluate the ischemic brain injury and recovery; degree of similarity of structural and functional characteristics of brains of experimental animals to those of the human brain; and updated ethical outlines for the use of experimental animals in research protocols.

Since the whole brain is exposed to transient ischemia and reperfusion as a result of cardiac arrest and the subsequent cardiorespiratory resuscitation to allow survival in human beings, animal models of global cerebral ischemia have been designed attempting to totally or partially mimic the consequences of this clinical condition on the brain (Ginsberg & Busto, 1989; Gupta & Briyal, 2004; Mc Bean & Kelly, 1998; Traystman, 2003), which are the main cause of neuronal injury to selective vulnerable brain regions, and neurological or cognitive impairment, in human beings.

Cardiac arrest (induced by injection of KCl, electric shock, thoracic compression, asphyxia, and mechanical obstruction of the ascending aorta) followed by cardiopulmonary resuscitation (by artificial ventilation, closed chest massage and electrical defibrillation), both in large experimental animals (formerly a common model, but nowadays rarely used) and also in rodents, has been a technique to produce global cerebral ischemia in an attempt to closely resemble the clinical situation of cardiac arrest, including complete ischemia and reperfusion in renal, splachnic and other peripheral organs. This technique seemed to be an excellent model of global cerebral ischemia, but it is expensive when large experimental animals are used, and intensive care (cardiopulmonary support under unconsciousness, control of blood pressure, pH, body fluids, and temperature) must be provided to the animals, especially during the first 24-48 h after the cardiac arrest. Complete acute global cerebral ischemia during cardiac arrest (8-20 min) and a variable period of incomplete cerebral ischemia during reperfusion, even after a successful cardiopulmonary resuscitation, as well as damage in those brain structures most vulnerable to ischemia, can be expected from this model (Berkowitz, et al., 1991; Bleyaert et al., 1978; Dave et al., 2004; Hossmann, 2008; Katz et al., 1995; Kofler et al., 2004; Radovsky et al., 1995; Safar et al., 1976; Todd et al., 1982). In particular, models of global cerebral ischemia in mice are currently of interest because of the availability of transgenic and knock-out strains for identification of cellular pathways of ischemic damage, and for neuroprotection studies.

Several other animal models of global cerebral ischemia have been designed in cats, monkeys, gerbils, mice, and rats, in order to circumscribe to the brain those harmful effects of the reduced blood flow that follows a cardiac arrest, avoiding affecting other vital organs in a whole body ischemia condition, as can be expected from animal models of cardiac arrest (Ginsberg & Busto, 1989).

Decapitation in small animals has been used as a model of global cerebral ischemia, only allowing the study of the immediate alterations of some biochemical and metabolic parameters elicited by ischemia in the brain contained into the head (Abe et al., 1983; Ikeda et al., 1986; Lowry et al., 1964; Yoshida et al., 1985).

A neck tourniquet or a neck cuff, whether they include or not arterial hypotension, have also been used to produce global cerebral ischemia in rats, cats, dogs, or monkeys. However, these techniques lead to variable ischemic outcomes since the produced ischemia may not be complete because of a remaining cerebral blood flow through the vertebral arteries, as well as complications due to vagal compression and venous congestion (Chopp et al., 1987, 1988; Grenell 1946; Nemoto et al., 1977; Sheller et al., 1992; Siemkowits & Gjedde, 1980; Siemkowitz & Hansen, 1978).

Reduction of cerebral blood flow near to zero has been accomplished in cats and monkeys, by occlusion of the innominate and left subclavian arteries near the aortic arch, and pharmacologically induced hypotension (below 80 mm Hg), without involvement of other organs in the ischemic phenomena. However, these experimental animals require intensive care procedures to their survival, and studies of long-term recovery are difficult to achieve (Bodsch et al., 1986; Clavier et al., 1994; Hossmann, 1971; Hossmann & Grose Ophoff, 1986; Zimmerman & Hossmann, 1975).

Gerbils usually lack of a common posterior communicating artery connecting the carotid and vertebro-basilar arterial system. Thus, the bilateral common carotid artery occlusion results in a reduction of global cerebral blood flow near to zero and injury of the most vulnerable brain structures (hippocampal CA1 pyramidal neurons after 5 min of ischemia) in most animals (Kirino, 1982). This model of forebrain global cerebral ischemia may fail in some animals in which a complete Willis circle persists, and the high susceptibility of gerbils to seizures may influence the ischemic outcome.

The four-vessel occlusion (4-VO) and the two-vessel occlusion with hypotension (2-VO) models in rats became, nowadays, the most widely used animal models that simulate the reduction of blood flow, as it would occur by effect of cardiac arrest, on the forebrain. The 4-VO model (Ginsberg & Busto, 1989; Pulsinelli & Brierley 1979; Pulsinelli & Buchan 1988; Pulsinelli & Duffy 1983; Pulsinelli et al., 1982) provides a method of reversible forebrain ischemia in awake, freely moving rats (but also in anesthetized rats). In a first step of the model procedures, vertebral arteries are permanently occluded and 24 or 48 hours later, the ischemia is produced through transient (10 – 20 min) occlusion of the common carotid arteries under light inhaled anesthesia so that the ischemic episode occurs while the animal is unanesthetized. Loss of the righting reflex, and unconsciousness persisting for at least 20 min after the onset of reperfusion have to occur for each animal to be included in the study. In this way, a reduction in cerebral blood flow to less than 5% of control values, which is followed by hyperemia during 5 to 15 min after reperfusion, and subsequent hypoperfusion lasting for 24 hr result in main ischemic neuronal damage in hippocampus, neocortex and striatum, along hours to days after ischemia, its magnitude relating to the duration of the ischemia. The effects of this insult are, however, quite variable between rat strains, as well as between those individuals surviving (survival rate, 50-75%) after having fulfilled the criteria required to be included in the experimental groups. Similar consequences in selectively vulnerable neurons in specific brain structures result from the 2-VO model of forebrain ischemia, in which bilateral common carotid artery occlusion and systemic hypotension (blood withdrawal and subsequent return with or without pharmacological procedures, leading to arterial blood pressure below 50 mm Hg) are combined to provoke reversible forebrain ischemia (Eklof & Siesjo 1972a, 1972b; Smith et al., 1984a, 1984b).

Mouse models of global cerebral ischemia have been developed through bilateral common carotid occlusion and controlled pulmonary ventilation (Traystman, 2003).

It is known that animal models of global cerebral ischemia require adequate control of certain variables, such as careful control of animal's temperature and blood glucose concentration, in order to achieve consistent pathophysiological effects and brain injury (Colbourne & Corbett, 1994; Lipton, 1999; Siemkowicz, 1981; Siemkowicz.& Gjedde 1980). Hyperthermia and hyperglycemia increase brain injury, while hypothermia results in neuroprotection by itself.

3. Cellular mechanisms of neuronal injury, neuronal repair and plasticity

Models of global cerebral ischemia in experimental animals, as well as *in vitro* models, in particular brain tissue slices and neuronal cultures, have allowed to study in detail the cellular phenomena leading either to neuronal damage, or to neural repair and plasticity after ischemia. From these studies it has been known that mechanisms of cellular damage, repair and plasticity may be the same, in general, both if reduction of blood flow to the brain tissue results from occlusion of one of the main cerebral arteries as would occur in focal ischemia, and if it is the result of reduction of blood flow to the whole brain as it would occur after a cardiorrespiratory arrest.

3.1 Cellular mechanisms of neuronal injury

Interruption of blood flow and hence, of glucose and oxygen supply to the brain, results in an immediate severe energy failure in terms of ATP depletion that leads to alterations of the cell membrane ionic gradients and a severe breakdown in cellular homeostasis. Several mechanisms of neuronal damage are triggered and evolve both in cascade and as parallel pathways (Gwag et al, 2002; Lakhan et al, 2009; Lipton, 1999; Mehta et al, 2007; Schneider et al, 2009; Sugawara et al, 2004; Warner et al., 2004). In particular, a massive accumulation of intracellular calcium and sodium occurs because of failure of their energy-dependent efflux processes, and anoxic depolarization. This further leads to accumulation of lactate and hydrogen ions, and as a consequence, to decreased pH.

As a result of anoxic depolarization, excitatory aminoacids such as glutamate and aspartate are released, activating ligand-gated calcium and sodium channels with a further influx of these ions into the cells. Calcium is also released from intracellular pools, and its excessive, unregulated intracellular overload causes direct Ca^{2+}-dependent activation of lipases, proteases, and endonucleases leading to breakdown of structural and functional proteins, and damage to cytoskeleton and macromolecules including nucleic acids. A result of these phenomena is, among others, cell membrane lipoperoxidation.

Excessive intracellular calcium activate abnormal cell processes promoting functional derangements of mitochondria and an increased production of free radicals, exceeding the neuronal antioxidant reserves, and imposing risks to the structural and functional integrity of neuronal cells. The brain is highly susceptible to oxidative damage as a consequence of its high lipid and metal content, as well as other biochemical characteristics (Margaill et al., 2005; Reiter et al., 2005; Warner el al., 2004). Reperfusion and reoxygenation of the ischemic tissue, which must be reestablished within minutes in an effort to prevent severe neurological damage and favor survival of individuals, also may provide chemical substrates for further increasing cellular alterations, neuronal death and neurological deficits (Margaill et al., 2005).

Free radicals also contribute to the breakdown of the blood-brain barrier and brain edema. Reactive oxygen and nitrogen species including superoxide, hydroxyl free radical, and peroxylnitrite anion are also important mediators of inflammatory tissue damage, of activation and secretion of inflammatory cytokines such as tumor necrosis factor α, interleukin-1, and interleukin-6, and of expression of cyclo-oxigenase (COX)-2, and inducible nitric oxide synthase generating nitric oxide that also contributes to neuronal damage. These changes favor inflammatory reactions soon after cerebral ischemia/reperfusion (Barone & Feuerstein, 1999; Lakhan et al, 2009; Lipton, 1999; Mehta et al, 2007).

Calcium overload may additionally lead to mitochondrial damage and trigger an apoptotic cascade. The pro-apoptotic cascade involves nuclear factor κB- and p53-dependent pathways, changes in the Bcl-2 to Bax ratio, opening of the mitochondrial transition pore, release of cytochrome c, and activation of caspases (Chan, 2001; Chinopoulos & Adam-Vizi, 2006). In addition, caspase-independent pathways may also contribute to neuronal apoptosis.

Several gene families such as immediate early genes, heat-shock proteins, and inflammation-and apoptosis-related genes, are known to be differentially expressed during cerebral ischemia, and some neuropathologic processes triggered by ischemia seem to be mediated in part by alterations of molecular transcriptional and translational activities (Mehta et al, 2007).

Activation of DNA fragmentation enzymes and energy-consuming DNA repair enzymes, finally lead to DNA breakdown, interruption of protein synthesis, and cell death (Iadecola & Alexander, 2001; Leker & Shohami, 2002).

In addition to the above mentioned cellular processes of ischemic damage, brain ischemia/reperfusion may also trigger cellular mechanisms for neuronal repair, and functional recovery through neuronal plasticity involving remaining neurons in vulnerable damaged or undamaged brain structures (Barone & Feuerstein, 1999; Bendel et al., 2005; Crepel et al., 2003; Hurtado et al., 2006; Jourdain et al., 2002; Ruan et al., 2006). The different ischemia/reperfusion induced cellular mechanisms leading either to brain injury and neuronal death, or to neuronal repair, as well as plasticity and brain functional recovery, may occur in a sequential or simultaneous manner. Their latencies and temporal course, from minutes to weeks, are important references in attempting to establish their differential relevance in those critical periods for neuronal damage and death, as well as the "window of opportunity" for specific neuroprotective procedures (Barone & Feuerstein, 1999; Lipton, 1999; Leker & Shohami, 2002; Pulsinelli et al., 1997).

3.2 Differential neuronal vulnerability in animal models of global cerebral ischemia

Brain injury is expected to occur when cerebral blood flow is reduced to less than 10-20% of the normal value; the greater the reduction and/or longer lasting, the worst damage. Under these conditions, damage to specific brain structures due to immediate or delayed death of highly vulnerable neuronal groups, including the pyramidal neurons of the CA1 subfield of the hippocampus, and to a lesser degree those in layers 3 and 5 of the cerebral cortex, the Purkinje cells of the cerebellum, and spiny neurons in the striatum, take place after global cerebral ischemia (Ginsberg & Busto, 1989; Pulsinelli, 1985). Experimental models of global cerebral ischemia have allowed to know some neuronal characteristics that seem to account for selective vulnerability to ischemia, including a high density of excitatory glutamatergic synapses; low antioxidant enzyme reserves; high content of transition metals; increased expression of pro-apoptotic Bax protein; thus leading to differential susceptibility of some cell processes (Ca^{2+} homeostasis, oxidative-antioxidative balance, functional mitochondrial stability) to become out of physiological control under ischemia (Arai et al., 2001; Araki et al., 1989; Chen et al., 1996; Lipton 1999; Schmidt-Kastner et al., 2001; Sugawara et al., 1999). Brain injury after global ischemia/reperfusion is finally evidenced by neuronal death, affecting the neuronal population, circuit connectivity and functioning in specific brain structures involved in the neural integration of cognitive brain functions and behavior.

3.3 Cellular mechanisms of neuronal plasticity and repair

Cellular mechanisms of neuronal repair and plasticity have been observed to occur in vulnerable brain structures in which damage or death of neurons resulted from a sequence of pathophysiological phenomena triggered by global cerebral ischemia and the subsequent reperfusion. Thus, structural and functional characteristics of those neuronal components of circuits in the hippocampus and prefrontal cortex, which are identified, among others, as highly vulnerable to ischemia, and their correlation with the integration of specific cerebral functions (mainly cognitive functions) after global cerebral ischemia, have been analyzed. In this sense, short- and long-term structural alterations have been shown to occur in the remaining pyramidal neurons of the hippocampus after ischemia; thus, axonal degeneration as well as reduction of dendritic length and arborizations, of number and shape of dendritic spines, and of number of synapses, are usually related to impairment of cognitive functions and recognized as degenerative changes. By contrast, cytoarchitectural adjustments such as axonal and dendritic sprouting, increase of number of dendritic spines and synapses, changes in the relative proportion of spine types, are interpreted as compensatory plastic responses of surviving neurons. They contribute to neuronal circuit remodeling and functional recovery, and have been correlated with preservation of cognitive functions after the ischemic insult, even in absence of neuroprotective procedures (Briones et al., 2006; Jourdain et al., 2002; Mudrick & Baimbridge, 1989; Neigh et al., 2004; Onodera et al., 1990; Ruan et al., 2006; Skibo & Nikonenko, 2010; Sorra & Harris, 2000). In addition, neurogenesis and integration of newly differentiated neurons into neuronal circuits in the Ammon's horn may contribute to recovery of hippocampal-dependent cognitive functions (Bendel et al., 2005; Bernabeu & Sharp, 2000).

Similarly, reductions of dendritic length, arborization, and dendritic spine density have also been described, among various cytoarchitectural adjustments, in sensorymotor cortex pyramidal neurons following global cerebral ischemia (Akulinin et al., 1997, 1998, 2004). These cytoarchitectural alterations could be influenced by the extent of neuronal remaining connections; thus, either reduction or increase of afferent connections may result in changes in dendritic arborizations and spine density (Fiala et al., 2002; Johansson & Belinchenko, 2002). It has been emphasized the functional relevance of neuronal connections from the hippocampus to the prefrontal cortex for synaptogenesis and neuronal plasticity accounting for learning and memory (González-Burgos, 2009; Laroche et al., 2000). Thus, a permanent deafferentation of pyramidal neurons at cortical layer V after the extensive reduction of pyramidal neuron population of the CA1 subfield of the Ammon's horn as expected to occur after global ischemia (Letechipía-Vallejo et al., 2007), may lead to changes in neuronal activity, which may in turn affect the cytoarchitectural characteristics of pyramidal prefrontal cortex neurons (García-Chávez et al., 2008; Wellman & Sengelaub, 1991).

These dendritic restructuring (Neigh el al., 2004; Ruan el al., 2006) and reactive synaptogenesis (Briones et al., 2005; Crepel et al., 2003; Jourdain et al., 2002, Kovalenko et al., 2006) among other phenomena including the activation of a variety of potential growth-promoting processes (Arvidsson et al., 2001; Gobbo & O'Mara, 2004; Schmidt-Kastner et al., 2001), that occur in neurons surviving to the ischemic insult in vulnerable brain structures, seem to be a part of mechanisms of adaptive changes, probably accounting for neuronal conditions favoring synaptic plasticity and functional recovery. In fact, a long-term progressive continuous plastic reorganization of the dendritic tree and dendritic spines, initially altered by acute global cerebral ischemia, has been shown to occur in pyramidal neurons at layers 3 and 5 of the sensorymotor cortex of the rat (Akulinin et al., 1997, 1998, 2004).

Thus, preservation or recovery of hippocampal- and pre-frontal cortex- dependent functions after global cerebral ischemia, may involve long-term cytoarchitectural modifications in those remaining hippocampal CA1 and prefronto-cortical (layers 3 and 5) pyramidal neurons, since their morpho-functional organization is critical for normal learning and memory performance (Block, 1999; McDonald & White, 1993; McNamara & Skelton, 1993; Olsen et al., 1994; Olvera-Cortés et al., 2002; Silva et al., 1998), on the basis of the major role played by the CA1 region for the output of information flowing through the hippocampus, via the tri-synaptic circuit (Herreras et al., 1987). It is well known that the prefrontal cortex is directly involved in the organization of sequenced motor actions during working-memory performance (Fuster, 1999; I. Lee & Kesner, 2003), and that hippocampal projections supply of spatial information to the prefrontal cortex allowing suitability of motor responses in the spatial context (Jung et al., 1998). These phenomena may be altered not only by gross lesions of the prefrontal cortex, but fine alterations of its neuronal circuits may also result in impairment of the spatial working memory (Fritts et al., 1998; Lambe et al., 2000; I. Lee & Kesner, 2003; Olvera-Cortés et al., 2001; Taylor et al., 2003). Experimental data have shown that variations in cognitive behavioral performance are related to plastic changes in dendritic spines (Pérez-Vega et al., 2000). In addition, excitatory information flows mostly through dendritic spines-mediated synaptic contacts (Gray, 1959), which are highly sensitive to electrical stimulation and yet to mnemonic activity-related electrical phenomena (Harris, 1999; Hartman et al., 2005; Onodera et al., 1990).

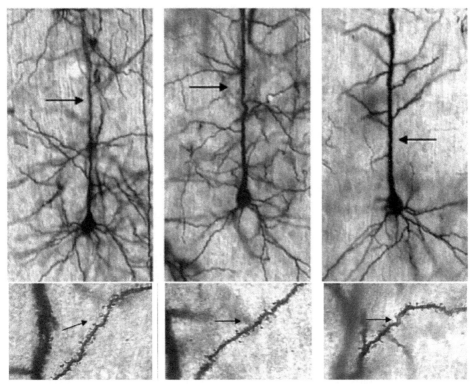

Fig. 1. Photomicrographs of prefrontal third-layer pyramidal neurons of rats: intact (left), after global cerebral ischemia and neuroprotective melatonin (centre) or vehicle (right) treatment. Note the reduction in dendritic arborization protruding from the apical dendrite, and dendritic spine reduction (arrows) in the ischemic and non treated cell in comparison with neurons from intact, and ischemia melatonin treated rats.
(Modified from: García-Chávez et al., 2008).

Since long-term preservation of the neuronal substrate in cerebral vulnerable structures underlying functional recovery after cerebral ischemia has been considered to be a major end point of neuroprotective strategies (STAIR, 1999) it can be expected that experimental designs for neuroprotection studies may lead to reliable interpretations of the efficiency of neuroprotective agents, in view of the proven capability of intrinsic cerebral mechanisms to promote , by themselves, neuronal repair and plasticity after ischemia.

Some neuronal proteins that are involved in structural and functional aspects of synaptic connectivity and neuronal circuits remodeling have been evaluated as parameters of ischemic damage and neuroprotection. In this sense, synaptophysin has been shown to be reduced in the frontal motor and temporal cortex of human beings that have been survived for 1 week to 1 year after a cardiac arrest (Akulinin et al., 1998). Besides, a reduction of synaptophysin 2, Munc-18-interacting proteins, 1-3 days after global cerebral ischemia in mice has been related to delayed neuronal death (Nishimura et al., 2000). On the other hand it has been proposed that progesterone-induced increase (3-35 days after ischemia) in the expression of synaptophysin and growth-associated protein 43, and the effects of venlafaxine preventing the decrease of synaptophysin, in the rat hippocampus are evidences of the neuroprotective effects of these drugs (Fang et al., 2010; Zhao et al., 2011).

4. Approaches to neuroprotection in animal models of global cerebral ischemia

The experimental approach to neuroprotection aimed to influence, through pharmacological and non pharmacological procedures, those early and late neural phenomena accounting either for brain damage or for neuronal repair, plasticity and functional recovery after global cerebral ischemia and reperfusion, has resulted in a considerable amount of reliable information along the last 40 years.

Different strategies of neuroprotection attempting to prevent, reduce, or stop the progress of the ischemic brain damage have been assayed in animal models of global cerebral ischemia, under the premise of an opposition relationship between the mechanism(s) of action of the presumptive neuroprotective drugs or non pharmacological procedures, and the pathophysiological mechanisms of brain damage, which has been maintained as targets of neuroprotective strategies.

Neuroprotection studies in animal models of global cerebral ischemia have maintained the main objective of support proposals of pharmacological and non-pharmacological neuroprotective procedures to be incorporated as a matter for clinical trials aimed to a better management of human beings exposed to global cerebral ischemia, frequently as a consequence of a cardiorespiratory arrest. Translation of knowledge about neuroprotection obtained from models in experimental animals, to clinical practice has not been successful. This situation has been also observed in the case of focal cerebral ischemia, leading to consensus meetings (Fisher et al., 2009; STAIR, 1999) attempting to establish the better conditions for preclinical studies of neuroprotection as to give reliable results to be applied in clinical conditions. If opinion of these consensuses may be recognized as applicable to preclinical studies of global cerebral ischemia, it is apparent that some factors must be taken in account for designing and carrying of the respective experimental protocols. Thus, studies in animal models of global cerebral ischemia should give information on effective neuroprotective doses in the case of drugs being tested; hence, dose-response relationships should be investigated. Routes of drug administration and pharmacokinetic characteristics should also be taken in account as to be compatible with their potential use in human beings.

The time window of opportunity for the effective neuroprotective treatment is an important factor to be considered in preclinical models that may predict the timing of neuroprotective procedures in clinical situations with reference to the onset of global cerebral ischemia and subsequent reperfusion. The initial hypothesis that opportunity window for neuroprotective procedures would be limited to a short period after the ischemic episode has been changed in view of experimental evidence. Thus, different drugs or neuroprotective procedures having predominant mechanisms of action against specific cellular processes of ischemia damage occurring lately within the pathophysiological cascade, may allow to neuroprotection even when administered hours or days after ischemia. Besides, the opportunity time window may be further extended when it is expected that neuroprotective procedures act through promotion of cellular processes of neuronal repair and plasticity.

In view of the multiple pathophysiological processes occurring both in sequence and simultaneously after ischemia and reperfusion, it is considered as an advantage for presumptive neuroprotective drugs to have multiple cellular or molecular mechanisms of action, as occurring with some originally endogenous compounds, namely melatonin, estradiol and progesterone (El-Abhar et al, 2002; Hurn et al, 1995; Jover-Mengual et al, 2010; Lebesgue et al, 2009; Reiter et al, 2005; Wang et al, 2008). By contrast, most synthetic drugs only have one mechanism of action accounting for neuroprotection. Attempting to counteract several mechanisms of ischemic brain injury would require the simultaneous administration of several drugs (Hicks et al, 1999; Matsumoto et al, 1993; Pazos et al, 1999; del Pilar Fernández et al, 1998; Sánchez-Casado et al, 2007; Zapater et al, 1997) (Table 1).

Recommendations arisen from these consensuses of opinion have also highlighted the importance of long-term studies to identify whether functional preservation or recovery may be attributed to effects of the neuroprotective procedures, and/or to intrinsic mechanisms of plasticity and repair triggered by ischemia *per se*. Reliable parameters of long-term structural and functional outcome may allow to evaluate the final result of the neuroprotective procedures on cerebral structures vulnerable to ischemia. Thus, evaluation of neuronal population, cytoarchitectonic characteristics, and connectivity of the neural circuits in these vulnerable structures, as well as different aspects of cognitive functions depending on them should be included as a part of experimental designs of neuroprotection.

It has been described that the neuronal population of remaining neurons in CA1 at survival times of 2-3 weeks may be less than that evaluated 3-4 months after the ischemic episode, suggesting that, without exogenous intervention, CA1 neurons may have been repopulate, became integrated to the hippocampal neuronal circuits, and contribute to functional recovery (Bendel, et al 2005; von Euler et al., 2006, Hartman et al, 2005, Nakatomi et al., 2002). Obviously, the potential repopulation complicates the interpretation of learning and memory studies after global cerebral ischemia, because short-term studies may not give an adequate end point of the cognitive alteration after global cerebral ischemia, which seems to require a long-term follow up.

Experimental designs to evaluate the potential of neuroprotective drugs or hypothermia may have not met all requirements set by these consensuses in a single study, but integration of results of the many experimental studies may give enough information as to support proposals for their clinical usefulness.

Main Mechanism of Action	Neuroprotective Agent	References
PHARMACOLOGICAL AGENTS		
Increase of energy reserve	Creatine	Lensman et al., 2006; Otellin et al., 2003.
Calcium channel blockers	Nimodipine	Cervantes et al., 1992; Choi SK et al., 2011; Haddon et al., 1988; Lazarewicz et al., 1990; Lazarewicz et al., 1993; del Pilar Fernández et al., 1998; Rami & Krieglstein, 1994; Zornow et al, 1996.
	Levemopamil	Block & Schwarz 1998.
	Dantrolene	Nakayama et al, 2002
	Flunarizine	Lee Y.S. et al., 1999.
K⁺ channel activators	Linoleic acid	Blondeau et al., 2002.
Glutamate antagonists	Dizocilpine	Bernabeu, R., & Sharp, 2000; Hicks et al., 1999; Janac et al., 2008; Kwon et al., 2000; Montero et al., 2007; Stevens & Yaksh, 1990; Selakovic et al., 2010; Zhang et al., 2009.
	Dextromethorphan	Block & Schwarz, 1998.
	Lamotrigine	Conroy et al., 1999 ; Crumrine et al., 1997; Lee Y.S. et al., 1999 ; Morimoto et al., 2002 ; Shuaib et al., 1995b ; Wiard et al., 1995.
	Lubeluzole	Koinig et al., 2001; Mueller et al., 2003; Haseldonckx et al., 1997
	$MgSO_4$	Meloni et al., 2009; Miles et al., 2001; Sirin et al., 1998.
	Zinc	Matsushita et al., 1996.
	Antiepileptic agents	Stepień et al., 2005.
GABAergic agents	Clomethiazole	Clarkson et al., 2005; Chaulk et al, 2003; Cross et al, 1995; Liang et al, 1997; Shuaib et al., 1995a; Sydserff et al., 2000.
	Diacepam	Corbett et al, 2008; Dowden et al, 1999; Hall et al, 1998; Johansen FF, Diemer, 1991; Schwartz et al, 1995.
	Thiopental	Kofke et al., 1979; Pappas & Mironovich, 1981; Todd et al, 1982 .
	Propofol	Cai et al., 2011 ; Cervantes et al., 1995 ; Ergün et al, 2002.
	Progesterone, allopregnanolone	Aggarwal et al., 2008 ; Cervantes et al., 2002 ; González-Vidal et al., 1998 ; Moralí et al., 2005 ; Moralí et al., 2011a, 2011b; Ozacmak & Sayan, 2009 ; J.M. Wang et al, 2008 ; Zhao et al, 2011.

Main Mechanism of Action	Neuroprotective Agent	References
Antioxidants	Tirilazad	Li et al., 2010; del Pilar Fernández et al., 2008; Selakovic et al., 2010; Stevens & Yaksh, 1990.
	Pentoxifylline	Sirin et al., 1998; Tuong et al., 1994.
	Edaravone	Kubo et al., 2009 ; Otani et al., 2005.
	Methylene blue	Wiklund et al., 2007.
	Melatonin	Cervantes et al., 2008; Cho et al, 1997; El-Abhar et al., 2002; García-Chávez et al., 2008; González-Burgos et al., 2007; Letechipía-Vallejo et al., 2001; Letechipía-Vallejo et al., 2007; Rennie et al., 2008; Weil et al., 2009.
	Other	Bashkatova et al, 2001; Fang et al, 2010; Gaur & Kumar, 2010; Nanri et al, 1998; Pazos et al., 1999; Sinha et al., 2001; Warner et al, 2004.
	Human albumin	Belayev et al., 1999.
Antiapoptotic agents	Estradiol	Dai et al., 2007 ; He et al., 2002 ; Hurn et al., 1995 ; Jover-Mengual et al, 2010; Koh et al., 2006 ; Lebesgue et al., 2009 ; Littleton-Kearney et al, 2005 ; Lu et al., 2002 ; Wang et al., 2006 ; Wappler et al., 2010.
Other mechanisms	Delta 9-tetrahydro-cannabinol	Zani et al., 2007.
	Linoleic acid and other PUFA's	Blondeau et al., 2002; Fernandes et al., 2008; Lauritzen et al., 2000; Ma et al., 2008; Plamondon & Roberge, 2008.
Cell proliferation stimulants	Erythropoietin	Cotena et al, 2008 ; Givehchian et al., 2010; Incagnioli et al., 2009; Zhang et al, 2007.
Growth Factors	BDNF	D'Cruz et al., 2002; Kiprianova et al., 1999a, 1999b; Larsson et al., 1999; Popp et al., 2004.
NON-PHARMACOLOGICAL AGENTS		
Reduction of: cerebral metabolism and oxygen demands, reactive oxygen species, release of excitatory aminoacids, apoptosis, inflammatory reactions. Enhancement of BDNF	Hypothermia	Asai et al., 2000; Baumann et al, 2009; Chopp et al, 1988; Colbourne & Corbett, 1994; Dong et al, 2001; Noguchi et al., 2011; Silasi & Colbourne, 2011; Webster et al., 2009; Zhang H. et al., 2010; Zhang Z, et al., 2001.

Main Mechanism of Action	Neuroprotective Agent	References
ASSOCIATION OF PHARMACOLOGICAL AND NON-PHARMACOLOGICAL AGENTS		
	Hypothermia + MgSO$_4$	Meloni et al., 2009.
	Hypothermia + MgSO$_4$ + tirilazad	Sánchez Casado et al., 2007

Table 1. Main pharmacological and non-pharmacological agents showing neuroprotective effects through molecular, biochemical , histopathological, behavioral, neurologic, and cognitive parameters.

These strategies have allowed identifying the neuroprotective characteristics of many agents, including non-pharmacological procedures like hypothermia, that have been tested in animal models of global cerebral ischemia from the knowledge of an opposition relationship between their mechanism(s) of action, and the nature of the pathophysiological phenomena of ischemic damage. They may be grouped in relation to their main predominant mechanism of action against ischemic damage: calcium channel blockers, glutamate antagonists, GABAergic drugs, antioxidant agents, anti-inflammatory compounds, etc. Many of these compounds are products of chemical synthesis; but endogenous compounds (melatonin, estradiol, progesterone, allopregnanolone, etc.) playing important physiological roles in mammals, have also been shown to exert potent neuroprotective effects. Table 1 presents some examples of the various groups of neuroprotective agents.

4.1 Outcome assessment of brain injury and neuroprotection in animal models of global cerebral ischemia

Assessment of brain injury and neuroprotection in animal models of global cerebral ischemia can be effected at different levels of biological organization of the central nervous system, from molecular and cellular phenomena to brain functions requiring highly integrated, behavioral expressions. In general, parameters of cellular and molecular processes leading to ischemic brain damage or neuroprotection require obtaining brain tissue samples at a selected time point after ischemia for these phenomena to be evaluated. On the other hand, a follow-up of damage and/or recovery through repeated bioelectrical, behavioral, and cognitive measurements is possible to be done in the same animal along extended periods. Parameters that allow evaluating the presence and magnitude of ischemic brain injury at the different levels of biological organization are also reliable indexes of neuroprotective actions, as they are induced by ischemia and may be counteracted by neuroprotective procedures. A similar consideration can be done regarding cell repair and plasticity mechanisms triggered by the ischemic insult, which are expected to be favored by neuroprotective agents.

Measurements have been done of parameters of each of the various phenomena affected by ischemia which constitute the starting point of ischemic brain injury. These include timely and topographically appropriate evaluation of ionic changes, release of neurotransmitters, modification of receptor molecular structure, excitotoxicy, morphological and functional mitochondrial alterations, reactive oxygen and nitrogen species, antioxidant enzymes and lipoperoxidation, activation of pro- and antiapoptotic cascades, DNA breakdown, pro- and anti-inflammatory processes, among others (Lakhan et al, 2009; Lipton, 1999; Mehta et al, 2007; Schneider et al, 2009).

Neurological, behavioral, electrophysiological and histopathological correlates of the outcome after global cerebral ischemia being end points of cellular processes triggered by ischemia, give information about ischemic brain injury and neuroprotection.

4.1.1 Neurological assessment

Global cerebral ischemia usually does not result in long lasting focal neurological deficits in rats. Thus neurological deficit scores resulting from sensorimotor tests assessing motor-sensory functions in rats, including placement reactions, righting and flexion reflexes, equilibrium, spontaneous motility, among others may be altered shortly after (24 h) global cerebral ischemia, but they appear recovered 7 days after ischemia. These transient neurological deficits have been interpreted as functional alteration of hippocampus and striatum; though correlation between neurological deficit scores and ischemic neuronal damage in these structures, not always were found (Block, 1999; Hartman et al., 2005; Kofler et al, 2004).

4.1.2 Mood and behavioral assessment

Elevated, four (two open and two closed) arms plus maze, and open field tests have been used, among other to evaluate anxiety after global cerebral ischemia especially in rodents. Thus scores of latency to enter to open arms, the number of open and closed arms entries and rears are taken as parameters of anxiety in the elevated plus maze, while in the open field (circular arena 80 cm in diameter, three concentric rings and lines radiating from the center) tests, the number of segments entered with all the four paws, the number of rears, and the number of *faecal boli* are indexes of anxiety (Nelson et al., 1997).

4.1.3 Cognitive functions assessment

Since the clinical consequences of cardiac arrest, as the main cause of global cerebral ischemia, have been consistently described as long-term alterations of cognitive functions, it can be expected that similar cognitive deficits may be elicited by global cerebral ischemia in experimental animals. In fact, the most vulnerable neurons to ischemia are located in brain structures involved in cognitive processes (Ginsberg & Busto, 1989; Gionet et al., 1991; Pulsinelli, 1985); thus, evaluation of cognitive functions mainly dependent on hippocampus, striatum and prefrontal cortex, and its electrophysiological and morphological correlates may be reliable parameters of brain injury and neuroprotection after global cerebral ischemia.

The magnitude and type of cognitive deficits in experimental animals submitted to global cerebral ischemia may vary considerably depending on the animal model, the survival times of testing, and the specific behavioral tests that could have been used. Among these procedures to evaluate cognitive functions, the Morris water maze, the eight-arms radial Olton maze, and the T maze, have been widely used in assessing learning and memory in both 2VO and 4VO models in rats, and its correlation with neuronal loss (Block, 1999; Hartmann et al., 2005; Olsen et al., 1994; Volpe et al., 1984), and functional and morphological characteristics of the neural substrate underlying cognitive functions in brain structures vulnerable to ischemia. Novel object recognition tests have been shown to be a reliable index of cognitive functions since rats or mice normally spend more time exploring novel objects, whereas animals with recognition memory deficits will explore novel and familiar objects equally (Hartman et al., 2005). Cognitive functions have also been assessed in rodents through conditioned avoidance tasks (Block, 1999; Kofler et al., 2004; Langdon et al., 2008).

Several paradigms in the Morris water maze and in the eight-arms radial Olton maze, that have been used in most of neuroprotection studies in which cognitive functions are assessed, have proven to be useful for testing hippocampal, striatum and prefrontal cortex functioning as end points of brain damage or neuroprotection after global cerebral ischemia (Morris, 1984; Olton et al, 1982).

Hippocampal functioning has been evaluated in rats and mice through some behavioral paradigms that require the integrity of this brain structure and related structures in the temporal lobe (Barnes, 1979; Morris et al., 1982, 1990), in order to configure cognitive spatial representations, i.e., a cognitive spatial map (Cassels, 1998; Jarrad, 1993; McDonald and White, 1994; 1995; Moser et al, 1993). Thus parameters of spatial learning training to locate a hidden platform, (escape latency: time spent by the animal to reach the platform; swimming path length: distance swam until reaching the platform; searching strategy: pattern of the swimming path towards the platform) and probe trial to evaluate retention of spatial learning (time spent, or the distance traveled by the animal in each of the four quadrants of the maze; number of crossings over the former platform location) in the Morris water maze including extra maze spatial clues, have been used in testing the morpho-functional state of the hippocampus (Dalm et al 2000; D'Hooge & De Deyn, 2001; Eichenbaum et al, 1990; Morris, 1984; Myhrer, 2003)..

Under these training conditions and since there are no intra maze clues to guide the animal's behavior, it is assumed that, to achieve the goal, the animal has to build the cognitive map and thus, a hippocampal processing of information occurs (Gallagher and Pelleymounter, 1988, O'Keffe & Nadel 1978). For this reason, studies of neuroprotection use the spatial learning in the Morris water maze paradigm, as a reliable index of the hippocampal functioning.

However, in addition to place learning, spatial navigation in the water maze may occur through at least, two additional strategies not depending on the hippocampus but on the striatum: signal learning and egocentric learning (Brandeis et al 1989; Gallagher & Pelleymounter, 1988; O'Keefe & Nadel 1978). Signal learning is displayed when the animal reaches a visible platform, or a visible stimulus indicating (signaling) the location of the platform within the maze. Learning of the association between the stimulus and the response is established and depends on the functioning of the striatum (McDonald & White, 1994). The egocentric learning occurs when the animal develops stereotyped motor patterns to locate the invisible platform on the basis of the proprioceptive information provided by its own movement. It is also an ability that depends on the memory system to which the striatum belongs (McDonald & White, 1994; McDonald & White 1995; Oliveira et al., 1997). Results obtained when evaluating both adult and aged male rats, show that some adult rats may use either place, hippocampal dependent allocentric, or striatum-dependent, egocentric strategies; on the other hand, aged rats use egocentric, as their main swimming strategy to solve the task (Dalm et al., 2000; Olvera-Cortés et al, 2011). Thus, deficits in the performance of this task may indicate an alteration of any of these two abilities, place and egocentric learning, so that different parameters should be evaluated to assess the mechanism underlying the observed deficit (D'Hooge & De Deyn, 2001). A qualitative analysis of the swimming paths both during the training period and the probe trial may allow a better determining of the strategy used by the rat in solving the task in the water maze.

Spatial working memory can be evaluated by using the 8-arms Olton radial maze (Myhrer, 2003; Olton, 1983, 1987; Olton et al., 1982; Shibata et al., 2007). For a daily standard evaluation all eight arms are baited and the rat is allowed to collect food from each arm; the number of errors, defined as a re-entry into an arm that had already been visited, is recorded in order to evaluate withholding and updating of information about each arm visited and rewarding obtained. An alternative maze configuration in which only some of the eight arms are baited allows to evaluate reference memory besides working memory through recording of the number of reference memory errors (number of entries into unbaited arms) and working memory errors (re-entry into an already visited arm). Performance in the Olton maze requires an adequate functioning of hippocampal-prefrontocortical neuronal circuits, and is a reliable parameter of morpho-functional integrity of these brain structures after ischemia and neuroprotection (Cassel et al., 1998; Fritts et al., 1998; Izaki et al., 2008; Kolb, 1990, Kolb et al 1982; Laroche et al., 2000; Olton et al., 1982; Seamans et al., 1995; Winocur, 1982). An aquatic version of the 8-arm radial maze has also been described (Kolb et al, 1982), and used to correlate hippocampal pyramidal neurons damage and working memory performance (Nelson et al. 1997).

4.1.4 Histopathological assessment
Neuronal population of different neuron types in brain vulnerable structures has been considered as a reliable parameter of ischemia brain damage and neuroprotection. Thus, pyramidal neuron population in the Ammon´s horn of the hippocampus and in the neocortex (Bleayert et al, 1978; Colbourne & Corbett, 1994; García-Chávez et al., 2008; Hartman et al, 2005; Johansen & Diemer, 1991; Kirino, 1982; Letechipía-Vallejo et al., 2007; Moralí et al., 2011b; Pulsinelli, 1985; Schmidt-Kastner & Freund, 1991; Shuaib et al, 1995), or different neuron types in other brain vulnerable structures (Block & Schwartz, 1998; Cervantes et al., 2002), have been evaluated through the number and proportion of surviving neurons. However, most of these studies deal with histopathological assessment of the hippocampus, the highest vulnerable brain region to global cerebral ischemia. Usually four separate counts of surviving neurons in selected areas of the Ammon´s horn are obtained from each of five coronal sections of the hippocampus per rat, stained with cresyl violet for a total of 20 counts per animal, under the different experimental conditions (Hartman et al., 2005). Similar procedures are followed for neuronal counting in other brain structures vulnerable to ischemia.

Immunohistochemical staining techniques have been also used in animal models of global cerebral ischemia and neuroprotection in order to identify specific proteins or fluorescent DNA labels that may selectively mark cells undergoing an acute necrotic or apoptotic process, as well as the activation of specific cellular processes involved in neuronal damage or repair and survival. Immunohistochemical marks (c-fos/c-jun, heat shock proteins, Bcl-2/Bax immunoreactivity, among others) allow to identify neuron types and neuroanatomical regions where ischemia-induced phenomena take place. Besides, immunohistochemical markers of glial fibrillary acidic protein (GFAP) as well as microglia cell surface components lead to identification of reactive gliosis in the hippocampus, as a consequence of global cerebral ischemia and ischemic neuronal death, which elicited activation of microglial cells and interleukine 1 release that may trigger an astrocyte reaction mainly located in the *stratum lacunosum-moleculare, stratum moleculare*, and *hilus*, and persisting for weeks after ischemia (Buffo et al., 2010; Choi JS et al, 2008; Mori et al, 2008; Morioka et al., 1991, 1992; Nikonenko et al., 2009; Petito & Halaby, 1993). The efficacy of neuroprotective agents can also be determined on the basis of the success in preventing the occurrence of necrosis, apoptosis, heat shock expression, gliosis, etc., as indicated by the immunohistochemical biomarkers (Scallet, 1995). Different parameters of the glial reaction elicited by global cerebral ischemia have been used as indexes of brain damage or neuroprotection (Cervantes et al., 2002; de Yebra et al., 2006; Duan et al., 2011; Korzhevskii et al., 2005; Piao et al., 2002; Soltys et al., 2003).

Neuronal cytoarchitecture and fine structure parameters of synaptic connectivity have also been used for histopathological assessment after brain damage and neuroprotection (Briones et al., 2006; García-Chávez et al., 2008; González-Burgos et al., 2007; Johansson & Belichenko, 2002; Kovalenko et al., 2006, Moralí et al., 2011a; Nikonenko et al., 2009; Ruan et al., 2006).

4.2 Therapeutic opportunity window in animal models of global cerebral ischemia

In any case, recognition of a "therapeutic opportunity window" or "therapeutic time window" in relation to the timing of the ischemic episode, the temporal course of the mechanisms of brain damage and/or repair, and the exerting of actions of presumptive pharmacological or non pharmacological neuroprotective agents, has been a relevant aspect in the approach to neuroprotection in experimental models of global cerebral ischemia (Pulsinelli et al., 1997; Barone & Feuerstein, 1999). In these, the beginning and the extent of this therapeutic window can be expected to be different according to the actions of neuroprotective procedures against immediate or late cellular mechanisms of brain damage, or in favor of later long-lasting cerebral processes of repair and plasticity.

Thus optimal neuroprotective effectiveness may require a schedule of drug administration in which drug actions are coincident with the therapeutic opportunity window, that have to be established for different drugs according to their specific mechanisms of action and pharmacokinetic characteristics. In this sense, counteracting of immediate cell mechanisms of neuronal damage may require the administration of neuroprotective drugs before the ischemic episode, though its administration has to be continued afterwards for variable periods. By contrast, drug-promoting repair or plasticity processes admit the starting of neuroprotective treatment hours or days after ischemia.

Accordingly, designs of neuroprotective studies in experimental animals in supporting proposals of neuroprotection for patients exposed to global cerebral ischemia due to cardiorespiratory arrest, should take in account that this clinical condition usually occurs unexpectedly, and requires cardiorespiratory resuscitation maneuvers; thus neuroprotection procedures have to be installed soon, but after the ischemic episode. Experimental designs of neuroprotection studies assessing neuroprotective procedures against late neuronal damage processes or promoting neuronal repair and plasticity, favoring functional preservation and recovery, may lead supporting to a wideness of the therapeutic opportunity window, for neuroprotection in human beings.

4.2.1 Prophylactic neuroprotection

Transient global cerebral ischemia can occur during certain clinical situations which can either be anticipated, occur during intraoperative emergencies, or even induced, like extracorporeal circulation for cardiac surgery. Under these conditions, prophylactic neuroprotection as that provided by intraoperative hypothermia and pharmacological neuroprotection are possible alternatives to prevent or reduce the risk of ischemic neuronal damage (Savitz & Fisher, 2007; Weigl et al, 2005). This has stimulated designing of experimental studies on prophylactic neuroprotection to assess the effectiveness of several agents and their clinical potential. Some neuroprotective agents have proven to be more effective when applied before the ischemic insult than when given later in time, in particular those agents affecting the early cellular phenomena induced by ischemia, such as calcium channel blockers, GABAergic and anti-excitotoxic agents, as well as antioxidant drugs (Weigl et al, 2005). Pharmacological treatments (antihypertensive, antidiabetic, antithrombotic, antiatherogenic drugs) effective in modifying in the long term the risk for cardiac arrest or cardiac infarct which may result in global cerebral ischemia or in severe hypoperfusion have also been proposed as prophylactic neuroprotection procedures (Savitz & Fisher, 2007).

5. Conclusion

Though an increasing number of drugs have proven to be effective neuroprotective agents in experimental models of global cerebral ischemia, data supporting proposals for their clinical use have not been enough to influence clinical management and outcome of patients exposed to global cerebral ischemia in clinical trials. However, after its evaluation in animal models of global cerebral ischemia, special interest has been paid to carry out clinical trials with a non-pharmacological procedure, hypothermia, as a part of the intensive care of patients after a cardiorespiratory arrest. Nevertheless, the wide perspectives to gain information on neuroprotection through experimental designs including animal models of global cerebral ischemia are maintained to date, despite the tendency to preferentially conduct studies on rodents; in particular if differences between experimental animals and human beings are taken into account, and attention is paid to reproduce those components mainly accounting for brain damage after global cerebral ischemia.

6. Acknowledgement

Partially supported by Instituto Mexicano del Seguro Social, MEXICO (2006/1A/I/029; FIS/IMSS/PROT/196).

7. References

Abe, K.; Yoshida, S.; Watson, B.D.; Busto, R.; Kogure, K. & Ginsberg, M.D. (1983). Alpha-Tocopherol and Ubiquinones in Rat Brain Subjected to Decapitation Ischemia. *Brain Research*,Vol.273, No.1, (August 1983), pp. 166-169, ISSN 0006-8993

Aggarwal, R.; Medhi, B.; Pathak, A.; Dhawan, V. & Chakrabarti, A. (2008). Neuroprotective Effect of Progesterone on Acute Phase Changes Induced by Partial Global Cerebral Ischaemia in Mice. *Journal of Pharmacy and Pharmacology*,Vol.60, No.6, (May 2008), pp. 731-737, ISSN 0022-3573

Akulinin, V.A.; Belichenko, P.V. & Dahlstrom, A. (1998). Quantitative Analysis of Synaptophysin Immunoreactivity in Human Neocortex after Cardiac Arrest: Confocal Laser Scanning Microscopy Study. *Resuscitation*,Vol.39, No.3, (March 1999), pp. 207-213, ISSN 0300-9572

Akulinin, V.A.; Semchenko, V.V.; Stepanov, S.S. & Belichenko, P.V. (2004). Structural Changes in the Dendritic Spines of Pyramidal Neurons in Layer III of the Sensorimotor Cortex of the Rat Cerebral Cortex in the Late Post-Ischemic Period. *Neuroscience and Behavioral Physiology,* Vol.34, No.3, (May 2004), pp. 221-227, ISSN 0097-0549

Akulinin, V.A.; Stepanov, S.S.; Semchenko, V.V. & Belichenko, P.V. (1997). Dendritic Changes of the Pyramidal Neurons in Layer V of Sensory-motor Cortex of the Rat Brain During the Postresuscitation Period. *Resuscitation,* Vol.35, No.2, (October 1997), pp. 157-164, ISSN 0300-9572

Arai, K.; Ikegaya, Y.; Nakatani, Y.; Kudo, I.; Nishiyama, N. & Matsuki, N. (2001). Phospholipase A2 Mediates Ischemic Injury in the Hippocampus: a Regional Difference of Neuronal Vulnerability. *European Journal of Neuroscience*, Vol.13, No.12, (June 2001), pp. 2319-2323, ISSN 1460-9568

Araki, T.; Kato, H. & Kogure, K. (1989). Selective Neuronal Vulnerability Following Transient Cerebral Ischemia in the Gerbil: Distribution and Time Course. *Acta Neurologica Scandinavica,* Vol.80, No.6, (December 1989), pp. 548-553, ISSN 0001-6314

Asai, S.; Zhao, H.; Kohno, T.; Takahashi, Y.; Nagata, T. & Ishikawa, K. (2000). Quantitative Evaluation of Extracellular Glutamate Concentration in Postischemic Glutamate Re-uptake, Dependent on Brain Temperature, in the Rat Following Severe Global Brain Ischemia. *Brain Research*, Vol.864, No.1, (May 2000), pp. 60-68, ISSN 0006-8993

Arvidsson, A.; Kokaia, Z.; Airaksinen, M.S.; Saarma, M. & Lindvall, O. (2001). Stroke Induces Widespread Changes of Gene Expression for Glial Cell Line-derived Neurotrophic Factor Family Receptors in the Adult Rat Brain. *Neuroscience,* Vol.106, No.1, (September 2001), pp. 27-41, ISSN 0306-4522

Barnes, C.A. (1979). Memory Deficits Associated With Senescence: A Neurophysiological and Behavioral Study in the Rat. *Journal of Comparative & Physiological Psychology,* Vol.93, No.1, (February 1979), pp. 74-104, ISSN 0021-9940

Barone, F.C. & Feuerstein, G.Z. (1999). Inflammatory Mediators and Stroke: New Opportunities for Novel Therapeutics. *Journal of Cerebral Blood Flow & Metabolism,* Vol.19, No.8, (August 1999), pp. 819-834, ISSN 0271-678X

Bashkatova, V.G.; Koshelev, V.B.; Fadyukova, O.E.; Alexeev, A.A.; Vanin, A.F.; Rayevsky, K.S.; Ashmarin, I.P. & Armstrong, D.M. (2001). Novel Synthetic Analogue of ACTH 4-10 (Semax) but not Glycine Prevents the Enhanced Nitric Oxide Generation in Cerebral Cortex of Rats with Incomplete Global Ischemia. *Brain Research,* Vol.894, No.1, (March 2001), pp. 145-149, ISSN 0006-8993

Baumann, E.; Preston, E.; Slinn, J. & Stanimirovic, D. (2009). Post-ischemic Hypothermia Attenuates Loss of the Vascular Basement Membrane Proteins, Agrin and SPARC, and the Blood-brain Barrier Disruption After Global Cerebral Ischemia. *Brain Research*, Vol.1269, No.1, (May 2009), pp. 185-97, ISSN 0006-8993

Belayev, L.; Saul, I.; Huh, P.W.; Finotti, N.; Zhao, W.; Busto, R. & Ginsberg, M.D. (1999). Neuroprotective Effect of High-dose Albumin Therapy Against Global Ischemic Brain Injury in Rats. *Brain Research*, Vol.845, No.1, (October n 1999), pp. 107-111, ISSN 0006-8993

Bendel, O.; Bueters, T.; von Euler, M.; Ove Ogren, S.; Sandin, J. & von Euler, G. (2005). Reappearance of Hippocampal CA1 Neurons after Ischemia is Associated with

Recovery of Learning and Memory. *Journal of Cerebral Blood Flow and Metabolism,* Vol.25, No.12, (December 2005), pp. 1586-1595, ISSN 0271-678X

Benítez-King, G. (2006). Melatonin as a Cytoskeletal Modulator: Implications for Cell Physiology and Disease. *Journal of Pineal Research,*Vol.40, No.1, (November 2005), pp. 1-9, ISSN 0742-3098

Berkowitz, I.D.; Gervais, H.; Schleien, C.L.; Koehler, R.C.; Dean, J.M. & Traystman, R.J. (1991). Epinephrine Dosage Effects on Cerebral and Myocardial Blood Flow in an Infant Swine Model of Cardiopulmonary Resuscitation. *Anesthesiology,*Vol.75, No.6, (December 1991), pp. 1041-1050, ISSN 0003-3022

Bernabeu, R. & Sharp, F.R. (2000). NMDA and AMPA/Kainate Glutamate Receptors Modulate Dentate Neurogenesis and CA3 Synapsin-I in Normal and Ischemic Hippocampus. *Journal of Cerebral Blood Flow & Metabolism,*Vol.20, No.12, (December 2000), pp. 1669-1680, ISSN 0271-678X

Bleyaert, A.L.; Nemoto, E.M.; Safar, P.; Stezoski, S.M.; Mickell, J.J.; Moossy, J. & Rao, G.R. (1978). Thiopental Amelioration of Brain Damage After Global Ischemia in Monkeys. *Anesthesiology,*Vol.49, No.6, (December 1978), pp. 390-398, ISSN 0003-3022

Block, F. (1999). Global Ischemia and Behavioural Deficits. *Progress in Neurobiology,*Vol.58, No.3, (May 1999), pp. 279-295, ISSN 0301-0082

Block, F. & Schwarz, M. (1998). Global Ischemic Neuronal Damage Relates to Behavioural Deficits: A Pharmacological Approach. *Neuroscience,*Vol.82, No.3, (March 1998), pp. 791-803, ISSN 0306-4522

Blondeau, N.; Widmann, C.; Lazdunski, M. & Heurteaux, C. (2002). Polyunsaturated Fatty Acids Induce Ischemic and Epileptic Tolerance. *Neuroscience,*Vol.109, No.2, (January 2002), pp. 231-241, ISSN 0306-4522

Bodsch, W.; Barbier, A.; Oehmichen, M.; Grosse Ophoff, B. & Hossmann, K.A. (1986). Recovery of Monkey Brain After Prolonged Ischemia. II. Protein Synthesis and Morphological Alterations. *Journal of Cerebral Blood Flow & Metabolism,*Vol.6, No.1, (February 1986), pp. 22-33, ISSN 0271-678X

Bortolotto, Z.A.; Collett, V.J.; Conquet, F.; Jia, Z.; van der Putten, H. & Collingridge, G.L. (2005). The Regulation of Hippocampal LTP by the Molecular Switch, a Form of Metaplasticity, Requires mGlu5 Receptors. *Neuropharmacology,*Vol.49, Suppl 1, (July 2005), pp. 13-25, ISSN 0028-3908

Briones, T.L.; Suh, E.; Jozsa, L.; Rogozinska, M.; Woods, J. & Wadowska, M. (2005). Changes in Number of Synapses and Mitochondria in Presynaptic Terminals in the Dentate Gyrus Following Cerebral Ischemia and Rehabilitation Training. *Brain Research,*Vol.1033, No.1, (February 2005), pp. 51-57, ISSN 0006-8993

Briones, T.L.; Suh, E.; Jozsa, L. & Woods, J. (2006). Behaviorally Induced Synaptogenesis and Dendritic Growth in the Hippocampal Region Following Transient Global Cerebral Ischemia are Accompanied by Improvement in Spatial Learning. *Experimental Neurology,*Vol.198, No.2, (February 2006), pp. 530-538, ISSN 0014-4886

Buffo, A.; Rolando, C. & Ceruti, S. (2010). Astrocytes in the Damaged Brain: Molecular and Cellular Insights into their Reactive Response and Healing Potential. *Biochemical Pharmacology,* Vol.79, No.2, (January 2010), pp. 77-89, ISSN 0006-2952

Cai, J.; Hu, Y.; Li, W.; Li, L.; Li, S.; Zhang, M. & Li, Q. (2011). The Neuroprotective Effect of Propofol against Brain Ischemia is Mediated by the Glutamatergic Signaling

Pathway in Rats. *Neurochemical Research,* Vol.36, No.10, (October 2011), pp. 1724-1731, ISSN 0364-3190

Cassel, J.C.; Cassel, S.; Galani, R.; Kelche, C.; Will, B. & Jarrard, L. (1998). Fimbria-Fornix vs Selective Hippocampal Lesions in Rats: Effects on Locomotor Activity and Spatial Learning and Memory. *Neurobiology of Learning and Memory,* Vol.69, No.1, (June 1998), pp. 22-45, ISSN 1074-7427

Castren, M.; Silfvast, T.; Rubertsson, S.; Niskanen, M.; Valsson, F.; Wanscher, M. & Sunde, K. (2009). Scandinavian Clinical Practice Guidelines for Therapeutic Hypothermia and Post-resuscitation Care After Cardiac Arrest. *Acta Anaesthesiologica Scandinavica,* Vol.53, No.3, (February 2009), pp. 280-288, ISSN 1399-6576

Cervantes, M.; Chávez-Carrillo, I. & Antonio-Ocampo, A. (1992). Effects of Nimodipine on Multiunit Activity of Several Brain Structures Following Acute Global Cerebral Ischemia-anoxia in Cats. *Boletín de Estudios Médicos y Biológicos* Vol.40, No.1-4, (January-December 1992), pp. 21-30, ISSN 0067-9666

Cervantes, M.; González-Vidal, M.D.; Ruelas, R.; Escobar, A. & Moralí, G. (2002). Neuroprotective Effects of Progesterone on Damage Elicited by Acute Global Cerebral Ischemia in Neurons of the Caudate Nucleus. *Archives of Medical Research,* Vol.33, No.1, (February 2002), pp. 6-14, ISSN 0188-4409

Cervantes, M.; Moralí, G. & Letechipía-Vallejo, G. (2008). Melatonin and Ischemia-reperfusion Injury of the Brain. *Journal of Pineal Research,* Vol.45, No.1, (January 2008), pp. 1-7, ISSN 1600-079X

Cervantes, M.; Ruelas, R.; Chávez-Carrillo, I.; Contreras-Gómez, A. & Antonio-Ocampo, A. (1995). Effects of Propofol on Alterations of Multineuronal Activity of Limbic and Mesencephalic Structures and Neurological Deficit Elicited by Acute Global Cerebral Ischemia. *Archives of Medical Research,* Vol.26, No.4, (January 1995), pp. 385-395, ISSN 0188-4409

Chan, P.H. (2001), Reactive Oxygen Radicals in Signalling and Damage in the Ischemic Brain. *Journal of Cerebral Blood Flow & Metabolism* Vol. 21, No. 1, (January 2001), pp. 2-14, ISSN 0271-678X

Chaulk, D.; Wells, J.; Evans, S.; Jackson, D. & Corbett, D. (2003). Long-term Effects of Clomethiazole in a Model of Global Ischemia. *Experimental Neurology,* Vol.182, No.2, (August 2003), pp. 476-482, ISSN 0014-4886

Chen, J.; Zhu, R.L.; Nakayama, M.; Kawaguchi, K.; Jin, K.; Stetler, R.A.; Simon, R.P. & Graham, S.H. (1996). Expression of the Apoptosis-effector Gene, Bax, is Up-regulated in Vulnerable Hippocampal CA1 Neurons Following Global Ischemia. *Journal of Neurochemistry,* Vol.67, No.1, (July 1996), pp. 64-71, ISSN 0022-3042

Chinopoulos, C. & Adam-Vizi, V. (2006). Calcium, mitochondria and Oxidative Stress in Neuronal Pathology. Novel Aspects of an Enduring Theme. *FEBS Journal,* Vol. 273, No. 3, (February 2006), pp. 433-450, ISSN

Cho, S.; Joh, T.H.; Baik, H.H.; Dibinis, C. & Volpe, B.T. (1997). Melatonin Administration Protects CA1 Hippocampal Neurons After Transient Forebrain Ischemia in Rats. *Brain Research,* Vol.755, No.2, (May 1997), pp. 335-338, ISSN 0006-8993

Choi, S.K.; Lee, G.J.; Choi, S.; Kim, Y.J.; Park, H.K. & Park, B.J. (2011). Neuroprotective Effects by Nimodipine Treatment in the Experimental Global Ischemic Rat Model: Real Time Estimation of Glutamate. *Journal of Korean Neurosurgical Society* Vol.49, No.1, (April 2011), pp. 1-7, ISSN 1598-7876

Choi, J.S.; Shin, Y.J.; Cha, J.H.; Kim, H.Y.; Choi, J.Y.; Chun, M.H. & Lee, M.Y. (2008). Induction of Suppressor of Cytokine Signaling-3 in Astrocytes of the Rat Hippocampus Following Transient Forebrain Ischemia. *Neuroscience Letters*, Vol.441, No.3, (August 2008), pp. 323-327, ISSN 0304-3940

Chopp, M.; Frinak, S.; Walton, D.R.; Smith, M.B. & Welch, K.M. (1987). Intracellular Acidosis During and After Cerebral Ischemia: in Vivo Nuclear Magnetic Resonance Study of Hyperglycemia in Cats. *Stroke,*Vol.18, No.5, (September 1987), pp. 919-923, ISSN 0039-2499

Chopp, M.; Welch, K.M.; Tidwell, C.D.; Knight, R. & Helpern, J.A. (1988). Effect of Mild Hyperthermia on Recovery of Metabolic Function After Global Cerebral Ischemia in Cats. *Stroke,*Vol.19, No.12, (December 1988), pp. 1521-1525, ISSN 0039-2499

Clarkson, A.N.; Liu, H.; Rahman, R.; Jackson, D.M.; Appleton, I. & Kerr, D.S. (2005). Clomethiazole: Mechanisms Underlying Lasting Neuroprotection Following Hypoxia-ischemia. *FASEB Journal,*Vol.19, No.8, (April 2005), pp. 1036-1038, ISSN 1530-6860

Clavier, N.; Kirsch, J. R.; Hurn, P.D. & Traystman, R.J. (1994). Effect of Postischemic Hypoperfusion on Vasodilatory Mechanisms in Cats. *American Journal of Physiology,*Vol.267, No.5 Pt 2, (November 1994), pp. H2012-2018, ISSN 0002-9513

Colbourne, F. & Corbett, D. (1994). Delayed and Prolonged Post-ischemic Hypothermia is Neuroprotective in the Gerbil. *Brain Research,*Vol.654, No.2, (August 1994), pp. 265-272, ISNN 0006-8993

Conroy, B.P.; Black, D.; Lin, C.Y.; Jenkins, L.W.; Crumrine, R.C.; DeWitt, D.S. & Johnston, W.E. (1999). Lamotrigine Attenuates Cortical Glutamate Release during Global Cerebral Ischemia in Pigs on Cardiopulmonary Bypass. *Anesthesiology,*Vol.90, No.3, (March 1999), pp. 844-854, ISSN 0003-3022

Corbett, D.; Larsen, J. & Langdon, K.D. (2008) Diazepam Delays the Death of Hippocampal CA1 Neurons Following Global Ischemia. *Experimental Neurology*, Vol.214, No.2, (December 2008), pp. 309-14, ISSN

Cotena, S.; Piazza, O. & Tufano, R. (2008). The Use of Erythtropoietin in Cerebral Diseases. *Panminerva Medica,*Vol.50, No.2, (July 2008), pp. 185-192, ISSN 0031-0808

Crepel, V.; Epsztein, J. & Ben-Ari, Y. (2003). Ischemia Induces Short- and Long-Term Remodeling of Synaptic Activity in the Hippocampus. *Journal of Cellular and Molecular Medicine,*Vol.7, No.4, (February 2004), pp. 401-407, ISSN 1582-1838

Cross, A.J.; Jones, J.A.; Snares, M.; Jostell, K.G.; Bredberg, U. & Green, A.R. (1995). The Protective Action of Chlormethiazole against Ischaemia-induced Neurodegeneration in Gerbils when Infused at Doses Having Little Sedative or Anticonvulsant Activity. *British Journal of Pharmacology* Vol.114, No.8, (April 1995), pp. 1625-1630, ISSN 0007-1188

Crumrine, R.C.; Bergstrand, K.; Cooper, A.T.; Faison, W.L. & Cooper, B.R. (1997). Lamotrigine Protects Hippocampal CA1 Neurons from Ischemic Damage after Cardiac Arrest. *Stroke,*Vol.28, No.11, (November 1997), pp. 2230-2236, ISSN 0039-2499

D'Cruz, B.J.; Fertig, K.C.; Filiano, A.J.; Hicks, S.D.; DeFranco, D.B. & Callaway, C.W. (2002). Hypothermic Reperfusion After Cardiac Arrest Augments Brain-Derived Neurotrophic Factor Activation. *Journal of Cerebral Blood Flow & Metabolism*, (July 2002), Vol.22, No.7, pp. 843-851, ISSN 0271-678X

D'Hooge, R. & De Deyn, P.P. (2001). Applications of the Morris Water Maze in the Study of Learning and Memory. *Brain Research Brain Research Reviews,*Vol.36, No.1, (August 2001), pp. 60-90, ISSN 0006-8993

Dai, X.; Chen, L. & Sokabe, M. (2007). Neurosteroid Estradiol Rescues Ischemia-induced Deficit in the Long-term Potentiation of Rat Hippocampal CA1 Neurons. *Neuropharmacology,*Vol.52, No.4, (January 2007), pp. 1124-1138, ISSN 0028-3908

Dalm, S.; Grootendorst, J.; de Kloet, E.R. & Oitzl, M.S. (2000). Quantification of Swim Patterns in the Morris Water Maze. *Behavior Research Methods, Instruments, & Computers,*Vol.32, No.1, (April 2000), pp. 134-139, ISSN 0743-3808

Dave, K.R.; Raval, A.P.; Prado, R.; Katz, L.M.; Sick, T.J.; Ginsberg, M.D.; Busto, R. & Perez-Pinzon, M.A. (2004). Mild Cardiopulmonary Arrest Promotes Synaptic Dysfunction in Rat Hippocampus. *Brain Research,*Vol.1024, No.1-2, (September 2004), pp. 89-96, ISSN 0006-8993

De Yebra, L.; Malpesa, Y.; Ursu, G.; Pugliese, M.; Lievéns, J.C.; Goff, L.K. & Mahy, N. (2006). Dissociation Between Hippocampal Neuronal Loss, Astroglial and Microglial Reactivity after Pharmacologically Induced Reverse Glutamate Transport. *Neurochemistry International,* Vol.49, No.7, (December 2006), pp. 691-697, ISSN 0197-0186

Dong, H.; Moody-Corbett, F.; Colbourne, F.; Pittman, Q. & Corbett, D. (2001). Electrophysiological Properties of CA1 Neurons Protected by Postischemic Hypothermia in Gerbils. *Stroke,* Vol.32, No.3, (March 2001), pp. 788-95, ISSN 0039-2499

Dowden, J.; Reid, C.; Dooley, P. & Corbett, D. (1999). Diazepam-Induced Neuroprotection: Dissociating the Effects of Hypothermia Following Global Ischemia. *Brain Research,* Vol.829, No.1-2, (May 1999), pp. 1-6, ISSN 0006-8993

Duan, Y.L.; Wang, S.Y.; Zeng, Q.W.; Su, D.S.; Li, W.; Wang, X.R. & Zhao, Z. (2011). Astroglial Reaction to Delta Opioid Peptide [D-Ala2, D-Leu5] Enkephalin Confers Neuroprotection Against Global Ischemia in the Adult Rat Hippocampus. *Neuroscience,* Vol.192, (September 2011), pp. 81-90, ISSN 0306-4522

Eichenbaum, H.; Stewart, C. & Morris, R. G. (1990). Hippocampal Representation in Place Learning. *Journal of Neuroscience,* Vol.10, No.11, (November 1990), pp. 3531-3542, ISSN 0270-6474

Eklof, B. & Siesjo, B.K. (1972a). The Effect of Bilateral Carotid Artery Ligation Upon Acid-base Parameters and Substrate Levels in the Rat Brain. *Acta Physiologica Scandinavica,*Vol.86, No.4, (December 1972), pp. 528-538, ISSN 0001-6772

Eklof, B. & Siesjo, B.K. (1972b). The Effect of Bilateral Carotid Artery Ligation Upon the Blood Flow and the Energy State of the Rat Brain. *Acta Physiologica Scandinavica,*Vol.86, No.2, (October 1972), pp. 155-165, ISSN 0001-6772

El-Abhar, H.S.; Shaalan, M.; Barakat, M. & El-Denshary, E.S. (2002). Effect of Melatonin and Nifedipine on some Antioxidant Enzymes and Different Energy Fuels in the Blood and Brain of Global Ischemic Rats. *Journal of Pineal Research,*Vol.33, No.2, (August 2002), pp. 87-94, ISSN 0742-3098

Ergün, R.; Akdemir, G.; Sen, S.; Taşçi, A. & Ergüngör. F. (2002). Neuroprotective Effects of Propofol Following Global Cerebral Ischemia in Rats. *Neurosurgical Review,* Vol.25, No.1-2, (March 2002), pp. 95-98, ISSN 0344-5607 von Euler, M.; Bendel, O.; Bueters, T.; Sandin, J. & von Euler, G. (2006).Profound but Transient Deficits in Learning and memory after Global Cerebral Ischemia Using a Novel Water Maze Test. *Behavioral Brain research*, Vol.166, No.2, (January 2006), pp. 204-210, ISSN 0166-4328

Fang, S.; Yan, B.; Wang, D.; Bi, X.; Zhang, Y.; He, J.; Xu, H.; Yang, Y.; Kong, J.; Wu, J. & Li, X.M. (2010). Chronic Effects of Venlafaxine on Synaptophysin and Neuronal Cell Adhesion Molecule in the Hippocampus of Cerebral Ischemic Mice. *Biochemistry and Cell Biology* Vol.88, No.4, (July 2010), pp. 655-663, ISSN 1208-6002

Fernandes, J.S.; Mori, M.A.; Ekuni, R.; Oliveira, R.M. & Milani, H. (2008). Long-term Treatment with Fish Oil Prevents Memory Impairments but not Hippocampal Damage in Rats Subjected to Transient, Global Cerebral Ischemia. *Nutrition Research* Vol.28, No.11, (December 2008), pp. 798-808, 1879-0739

Fiala, J.C.; Spacek, J. & Harris, K.M. (2002). Dendritic Spine Pathology: Cause or Consequence of Neurological Disorders? *Brain Research Reviews*, Vol.39, No.1, (June 2002), pp. 29-54, ISSN 0165-0173

Fisher, M.; Feuerstein, G.; Howells, D.W.; Hurn, P.D.; Kent, T.A.; Savitz, S.I. & Lo, E.H. (2009). Update of the Stroke Therapy Academic Industry Roundtable Preclinical Recommendations. *Stroke*, Vol.40, No.6, (February 2009), pp. 2244-2250, ISSN 0039-2499

Fritts, M.E.; Asbury, E.T.; Horton, J.E. & Isaac, W.L. (1998). Medial Prefrontal Lesion Deficits Involving or Sparing the Prelimbic Area in the Rat. *Physiology & Behavior*, Vol.64, No.3, (September 1998), pp. 373-380, ISSN 0031-9384

Fuster, J.M. (1997). *The Prefrontal Cortex. Anatomy, Physiology, and Neuropsychology of the Frontal Lobe*, Lippincott-Raven, ISBN 978-0881674668, New York, USA

Fuster, J.M. (1999). Synopsis of Function and Dysfunction of the Frontal Lobe. *Acta Psychiatrica Scandinavica*, Vol.395, Supplementum, (May 1999), pp. 51-57, ISSN 0065-159

Gallagher, M. & Pelleymounter, M.A. (1988). Spatial Learning Deficits in Old Rats: a Model for Memory Decline in the Aged. *Neurobiology of Aging*, Vol.9, No.5-6, (September 1988), pp. 549-556, ISSN 0197-4580

García-Chávez, D.; González-Burgos, I.; Letechipía-Vallejo, G.; López-Loeza, E.; Moralí, G. & Cervantes, M. (2008). Long-term Evaluation of Cytoarchitectonic Characteristics of Prefrontal Cortex Pyramidal Neurons, Following Global Cerebral Ischemia and Neuroprotective Melatonin Treatment, in Rats. *Neuroscience Letters*, Vol.448, No.1, (October 2008), pp. 148-152, ISSN 0304-3940

Gaur, V. & Kumar, A. (2010). Protective Effect of Desipramine, Venlafaxine and Trazodone against Experimental Animal Model of Transient Global Ischemia: Possible Involvement of NO-cGMP Pathway. *Brain Research*, Vol.1353, (July 2010), pp. 204-212, ISSN 0006-8993

Geocadin, R.G.; Koenig, M.A.; Jia, X.; Stevens, R.D. & Peberdy, M.A. (2008). Management of Brain Injury After Resuscitation from Cardiac Arrest. *Neurologic Clinics*, Vol.26, No.2, (June 2008), pp. 487-506, ix, ISSN 0733-8619

Ginsberg, M.D. & Busto, R. (1989). Rodent Models of Cerebral Ischemia. *Stroke*, Vol.20, No.12, (December 1989), pp. 1627-1642, ISSN 0039-2499

Gionet, T.X.; Thomas, J.D.; Warner, D.S.; Goodlett, C.R.; Wasserman, E.A. & West, J.R. (1991). Forebrain Ischemia Induces Selective Behavioral Impairments Associated with Hippocampal Injury in Rats. *Stroke*,Vol.22, No.8, (August 1991), pp. 1040-1047, ISSN 0039-2499

Givehchian, M.; Beschorner, R.; Ehmann, C.; Frauenlob, L.; Morgalla, M.; Hashemi, B.; Ziemer, G. & Scheule, A.M. (2010). Neuroprotective Effects of Erythropoietin During Deep Hypothermic Circulatory Arrest. *European Journal of Cardio-thoracic Surgery*,Vol.37, No.3, (September 2009), pp. 662-668, ISSN 1873-734X

Gobbo, O.L. & O'Mara, S.M. (2004). Impact of Enriched-environment Housing on Brain-derived Neurotrophic Factor and on Cognitive Performance After a Transient Global Ischemia. *Behavioral Brain Research*,Vol.152, No.2, (June 2004), pp. 231-241, ISSN 0166-4328

Goldberg, M.P. & Choi, D.W. (1993). Combined Oxygen and Glucose Deprivation in Cortical Cell Culture: Calcium-dependent and Calcium-independent Mechanisms of Neuronal Injury. *Journal of Neuroscience*,Vol.13, No.8, (August 1993), pp. 3510-3524, ISSN 0270-6474

González-Burgos, I. (2009). Dendritic Spines Plasticity and Learning/Memory Processes: Theory, Evidence and Prospectives, In: *Dendritic Spines. Biochemistry, Modelling and Properties*. L.R. Baylon, (Ed.), pp. 163-186. Nova Science Publishers, Inc, ISBN 978-1607414605, New York, USA

González-Burgos, I.; Letechipía-Vallejo, G.; López-Loeza, E.; Moralí, G. & Cervantes, M. (2007). Long-term Study of Dendritic Spines from Hippocampal CA1 Pyramidal Cells, After Neuroprotective Melatonin Treatment Following Global Cerebral Ischemia in Rats. *Neuroscience Letters*,Vol.423, No.2, (August 2007), pp. 162-166, ISSN 0304-3940

González-Vidal, M.D.; Cervera-Gaviria, M.; Ruelas, R.; Escobar, A.; Moralí, G. & Cervantes, M. (1998). Progesterone: Protective Effects on the Cat Hippocampal Neuronal Damage Due to Acute Global Cerebral Ischemia. *Archives of Medical Research*,Vol.29, No.2, (July 1998), pp. 117-124, ISSN 0188-4409

Gray, E.G. (1959). Electron Microscopy of Synaptic Contacts on Dendrite Spines of the Cerebral Cortex. *Nature*,Vol.183, No.4675, (June 1959), pp. 1592-1593, ISSN 0028-0836

Greer, D.M. (2006). Hypothermia for Cardiac Arrest. *Current Neurology and Neuroscience Reports*,Vol.6, No.6, (November 2006), pp. 518-524, ISSN 1528-4042

Grenell, R.G. (1946). Central Nervous System Resistance; the Effects of Temporary Arrest of Cerebral Circulation for Periods of Two to Ten Minutes. *Journal of Neuropathology & Experimental Neurology*,Vol.5, (April 1946), pp. 131-154, ISSN 0022-3069

Grubb, N.R.; Fox, K.A.; Smith, K.; Best, J.; Blane, A.; Ebmeier, K.P.; Glabus, M.F. & O'Carroll, R.E. (2000). Memory Impairment in Out-of-Hospital Cardiac Arrest Survivors is Associated with Global Reduction in Brain Volume, not Focal Hippocampal Injury. *Stroke*,Vol.31, No.7, (July 2000), pp. 1509-1514, ISSN 0039-2499

Gupta, Y.K. & Briyal, S. (2004). Animal Models of Cerebral Ischemia for Evaluation of Drugs. *Indian Journal of Physiology and Pharmacology*,Vol.48, No.4, (May 2005), pp. 379-394, ISSN 0019-5499

Gwag, B.J.; Won, S.J. & Kim, D.Y. (2002). Excitotoxicity, Oxidative Stress, and Apoptosis in Ischemic Neuronal Death, In: *New Concepts in Cerebral Ischemia. Methods and New Frontiers In Neuroscience*, R.C.S. Lin, (Ed.), 79-112, CRC Press, ISBN 0-8493-0119-X, Boca Raton, USA

Haddon, W.S.; Prough, D.S.; Kong, D. & Petrozza, P. (1988). Effects of Nimodipine on the Production of Thromboxane A2 Following Total Global Cerebral Ischemia. *Journal of Neurosurgery*,Vol.69, No.3, (September 1988), pp. 416-420, ISSN 0022-3085

Hall, E.D.; Fleck, T.J. & Oostveen, J.A. (1998). Comparative Neuroprotective Properties of the Benzodiazepine Receptor Full Agonist Diazepam and the Partial Agonist PNU-101017 in the Gerbil Forebrain Ischemia Model. *Brain Research*, Vol.798, No.1-2, (July 1998), pp. 325-329, ISSN 0006-8993

Harris, K.M. (1999). Calcium From Internal Stores Modifies Dendritic Spine Shape. *Proceedings of the National Academy of Sciences of the United States of America*,Vol.96, No.22, (October 1999), pp. 12213-12215, ISSN 0027-8424

Hartman, R.E.; Lee, J.M.; Zipfel, G.J. & Wozniak, D.F. (2005). Characterizing Learning Deficits and Hippocampal Neuron Loss Following Transient Global Cerebral Ischemia in Rats. *Brain Research*,Vol.1043, No.1-2, (May 2005), pp. 48-56, ISSN 0006-8993

Haseldonckx, M.; Van Reempts, J.; Van de Ven, M.; Wouters, L. & Borgers, M. (1997). Protection with Lubeluzole Against Delayed Ischemic Brain Damage in Rats. A Quantitative Histopathologic Study. *Stroke*,Vol.28, No.2, (February 1997), pp. 428-432, ISSN 0039-2499

He, Z.; He, Y.J.; Day, A.L. & Simpkins, J.W. (2002). Proestrus Levels of Estradiol During Transient Global Cerebral Ischemia Improves the Histological Outcome of the Hippocampal CA1 Region: Perfusion-dependent and-independent Mechanisms. *Journal of the Neurological Sciences*,Vol.193, No.2, (January 2002), pp. 79-87, ISSN 0022-510X

Herreras, O.; Solıs, J.M.; Martin del Rio, R. & Lerma, J. (1987). Characteristics of CA1 Activation Through the Hippocampal Trisynaptic Pathway in the Unanaesthetized Rat. *Brain Research*,Vol.413, No.1, (June 1987), pp. 75-86, ISSN 0006-8993

Hicks, C.A.; Ward, M.A.; Swettenham, J.B. & O'Neill, M.J. (1999). Synergistic Neuroprotective Effects by Combining an NMDA or AMPA Receptor Antagonist with Nitric Oxide Synthase Inhibitors in Global Cerebral Ischaemia. *European Journal of Pharmacology*,Vol.381, No.2-3, (November 1999), pp. 113-119, ISSN 0014-2999

Hogue, C.W.; Gottesman, R.F. & Stearns, J. (2008). Mechanisms of Cerebral Injury from Cardiac Surgery. *Critical Care Clinics*,Vol.24, No.1, (February 2008), pp. 83-98, viii-ix, ISSN 0749-0704

Hossmann, K.A. (1971). Cortical Steady Potential, Impedance and Excitability Changes During and After Total Ischemia of Cat Brain. *Experimental Neurology*,Vol.32, No.2, (August 1971), pp. 163-175, ISSN 0014-4886

Hossmann, K.A. (2008). Cerebral Ischemia: Models, Methods and Outcomes. *Neuropharmacology*,Vol.55, No.3, (January 2008), pp. 257-270, ISSN 0028-3908

Hossmann, K.A. & Grosse Ophoff, B. (1986). Recovery of Monkey Brain After Prolonged Ischemia. I. Electrophysiology and Brain Electrolytes. *Journal of Cerebral Blood Flow & Metabolism*,Vol.6, No.1, (February 1986), pp. 15-21, ISSN 0271-678X

Hurn, P.D.; Littleton-Kearney, M.T.; Kirsch, J.R.; Dharmarajan, A.M. & Traystman, R.J. (1995). Postischemic Cerebral Blood Flow Recovery in the Female: Effect of 17 Beta-Estradiol. *Journal of Cerebral Blood Flow & Metabolism*,Vol.15, No.4, (July 1995), pp. 666-672, ISSN 0271-678X

Hurtado, O.; Pradillo, J.M.; Alonso-Escolano, D.; Lorenzo, P.; Sobrino, T.; Castillo, J.; Lizasoain, I. & Moro M.A. (2006). Neurorepair versus Neuroprotection in Stroke. *Cerebrovascular Diseases,* Vol. 21, (Suppl. 2), pp. 54-63, ISSN 1015-9770

Iadecola, C. & Alexander, M. (2001) Cerebral Ischemia and Inflammation. *Current Opinion in Neurology,* Vol. 14, No.1 , (February 2001), pp. 89-94, ISSN 0959-4388

Ikeda, M.; Yoshida, S.; Busto, R.; Santiso, M. & Ginsberg, M.D. (1986). Polyphosphoinositides as a Probable Source of Brain Free Fatty Acids Accumulated at the Onset of Ischemia. *Journal of Neurochemistry,* Vol.47, No.1, (July 1986), pp. 123-132, ISSN 0022-3042

Inamasu, J.; Nakatsukasa, M.; Suzuki, M. & Miyatake, S. (2010). Therapeutic Hypothermia for Out-of-Hospital Cardiac Arrest: An Update for Neurosurgeons. *World Neurosurgery,* Vol. 74, No. 1, (July 2010), pp. 120-128, ISSN 1878-8750

Incagnoli, P.; Ramond, A.; Joyeux-Faure, M.; Pepin, J.L.; Levy, P. & Ribuot, C. (2009). Erythropoietin Improved Initial Resuscitation and Increased Survival After Cardiac Arrest in Rats. *Resuscitation,* Vol.80, No.6, (May 2009), pp. 696-700, ISSN 1873-1570

Izaki, Y.; Takita, M. & Akema, T. (2008). Specific Role of the Posterior Dorsal Hippocampus-Prefrontal Cortex in Short-Term Working Memory. *European Journal of Neuroscience,* Vol.27, No.11, (June 2008), pp. 3029-3034, ISSN 1460-9568

Janac, B.; Selakovic, V. & Radenovic, L. (2008). Temporal Patterns of Motor Behavioural Improvements by MK-801 in Mongolian Gerbils Submitted to Different Duration of Global Cerebral Ischemia. *Behavioural Brain Research,* Vol.194, No.1, (July 2008), pp. 72-78, ISSN 0166-4328

Jarrard, L.E. (1993). On the Role of the Hippocampus in Learning and Memory in the Rat. *Behavioral and Neural Biology,* Vol.60, No.1, (July 1993), pp. 9-26, ISSN 0163-1047

Johansen, F.F. & Diemer, N.H. (1991). Enhancement of GABA Neurotransmission After Cerebral Ischemia in the Rat Reduces Loss of Hippocampal CA1 Pyramidal Cells. *Acta Neurologica Scandinavica,* Vol.84, No.1, (July 1991), pp. 1-6. ISSN

Johansson, B.B. & Belichenko, P.V. (2002). Neuronal Plasticity and Dendritic Spines: Effect of Environmental Enrichment on Intact and Postischemic Rat Brain. *Journal of Cerebral Blood Flow & Metabolism,* Vol.22, No.1, (January 2002), pp. 89-96, ISSN 0271-678X

Jourdain, P.; Nikonenko, I.; Alberi, S. & Muller, D. (2002). Remodeling of Hippocampal Synaptic Networks by a Brief Anoxia-hypoglycemia. *Journal of Neuroscience,* Vol.22, No.8, (April 2002), pp. 3108-3116, ISSN 1529-2401

Jover-Mengual, T.; Miyawaki, T.; Latuszek, A.; Alborch, E.; Zukin, R.S. & Etgen, A.M. (2010). Acute Estradiol Protects CA1 Neurons from Ischemia-induced Apoptotic Cell Death Via the PI3K/Akt Pathway. *Brain Research,* Vol.1321, (February 2010), pp. 1-12, ISSN 1872-6240

Jung, M.W.; Qin, Y.; McNaughton, B.L. & Barnes, C.A. (1998). Firing Characteristics of Deep Layer Neurons in Prefrontal Cortex in Rats Performing Spatial Working Memory Tasks. *Cerebral Cortex,* Vol.8, No.5, (August 1998), pp. 437-450, ISSN 1047-3211

Karanjia, N. & Geocadin, R.G. (2011). Post-cardiac Arrest Syndrome: Update on Brain Injury Management and Prognostication. *Current Treatment Options in Neurology,* Vol.13, No.2, (January 2011), pp. 191-203, ISSN 1534-3138

Kasai, H.; Matsuzaki, M.; Noguchi, J.; Yasumatsu, N. & Nakahara, H. (2003). Structure-Stability-Function Relationships of Dendritic Spines. *Trends in Neurosciences,* Vol.26, No.7, (July 2003), pp. 360-368, ISSN 0166-2236

Katz, L.; Ebmeyer, U.; Safar, P.; Radovsky, A. & Neumar, R. (1995). Outcome Model of Asphyxial Cardiac Arrest in Rats. *Journal of Cerebral Blood Flow & Metabolism*,Vol.15, No.6, (November 1995), pp. 1032-1039, ISSN 0271-678X

Kiprianova, I.; Freiman, T.M.; Desiderato, S.; Schwab, S.; Galmbacher, R.; Gillardon, F. & Spranger, M. (1999a). Brain-Derived Neurotrophic Factor Prevents Neuronal Death and Glial Activation After Global Ischemia in the Rat. *Journal of Neuroscience Research*, Vol.56, No.1, (April 1999), pp. 21-27, ISSN 0270-6474

Kiprianova, I.; Sandkühler, J.; Schwab, S.; Hoyer, S. & Spranger, M. (1999b). Brain-Derived Neurotrophic Factor Improves Long-Term Potentiation and Cognitive Functions After Transient Forebrain Ischemia in the Rat. *Experimentsal Neurology*, (October 1999), Vol.159, No.2, pp. 511-519, ISSN

Kirino, T. (1982). Delayed Neuronal Death in the Gerbil Hippocampus Following Ischemia. *Brain Research*, Vol.239, No.1, (May 1982), pp. 57-69, ISSN 0006-8993

Knapp, J.; Heinzmann, A.; Schneider, A.; Padosch, S.A.; Böttiger, B.W.; Teschendorf, P. & Popp, E. (2011). Hypothermia and Neuroprotection by Sulfide After Cardiac Arrest and Cardiopulmonary Resuscitation. *Resuscitation*, Vol.82, No.8, (August 2011) pp. 1076-1080, ISSN

Kofke, W.A.: Nemoto, E.M.; Hossmann, K.A.; Taylor, F.; Kessler, P.D. & Stezoski, S.W. (1979). Brain Blood Flow and Metabolism after Global Ischemia and Post-Insult Thiopental Therapy in Monkeys. *Stroke*, (September-October 1979), Vol.10, No.5, pp. 554-560, ISSN 0039-2499

Kofler, J.; Hattori, K.; Sawada, M.; DeVries, A.C.; Martin, L.J.; Hurn, P.D. & Traystman, R.J. (2004). Histopathological and Behavioral Characterization of a Novel Model of Cardiac Arrest and Cardiopulmonary Resuscitation in Mice. *Journal of Neuroscience Methods*,Vol.136, No.1, (May 2004), pp. 33-44, ISSN 0165-0270

Koh, P.O.; Cho, G.J. & Choi, W.S. (2006). 17beta-Estradiol Pretreatment Prevents the Global Ischemic Injury-Induced Decrease of Akt Activation and Bad Phosphorylation in Gerbils. *Journal of Veterinary Medical Science*,Vol.68, No.10, (November 2006), pp. 1019-1022, ISSN 0916-7250

Koinig, H.; Vornik, V.; Rueda, C. & Zornow, M. H. (2001). Lubeluzole Inhibits Accumulation of Extracellular Glutamate in the Hippocampus During Transient Global Cerebral Ischemia. *Brain Research*, Vol.898, No.2, (April 2001), pp. 297-302, ISSN 0006-8993

Kolb, B. (1990) In: *The Cerebral Cortex of the Rat*. B. Kolb & R.C. Tees, (Eds.), 437-458, MIT Press, ISBN: 978-026-2610-64-3, Cambridge, Massachussetts, USA

Kolb, B.; Pittman, K.; Sutherland, R.J. & Whishaw, I.Q. (1982). Dissociation of the Contributions of the Prefrontal Cortex and Dorsomedial Thalamic Nucleus to Spatially Guided Behavior in the Rat. *Behavioural Brain Research*, Vol.6, No.4, (December 1982), pp. 365-378, ISSN 0166-4328

Kolb, B.; Teskey, G.C. & Gibb, R. (2010). Factors Influencing Cerebral Plasticity in the Normal and Injured Brain. *Frontiers in Human Neuroscience*, Vol.4, (November 2010), pp. 1-12, ISSN 1662-5161

Korzhevskii, D.E.; Otellin, V.A.; Grigor'ev, I.P.; Kostkin, V.B.; Polenov, S.A.; Lentsman, M.V. & Balestrino, M. (2005). Structural Organization of Astrocytes in the Rat Hippocampus in the Post-ischemic Period. *Neuroscience & Behavioral Physiology*, Vol.35, No.4, (May 2005), pp. 389-392, ISSN 0097-0549

Kovalenko, T.; Osadchenko, I.; Nikonenko, A.; Lushnikova, I.; Voronin, K.; Nikonenko, I.; Muller, D. & Skibo, G. (2006). Ischemia-Induced Modifications in Hippocampal CA1 Stratum Radiatum Excitatory Synapses. *Hippocampus,* Vol.16, No.10, (August 2006), pp. 814-825, ISSN 1050-9631

Krause, G.S.; Kumar, K.; White, B.C.; Aust, S.D. & Wiegenstein, J.G. (1986). Ischemia, Resuscitation, and Reperfusion: Mechanisms of Tissue Injury and Prospects for Protection. *American Heart Journal*, Vol.111, No.4, (April 1986), pp. 768-780, ISSN 0002-8703

Kubo, K.; Nakao, S.; Jomura, S.; Sakamoto, S.; Miyamoto, E.; Xu, Y.; Tomimoto, H.; Inada, T. & Shingu, K. (2009). Edaravone, a Free Radical Scavenger, Mitigates Both Gray and White Matter Damages After Global Cerebral Ischemia in Rats. *Brain Research*, Vol. 1279, No. 3, (July 2009), pp. 139-46, ISSN ISSN 0006-8993

Kwon, Y.B.; Yang, I.S.; Kang, K.S.; Han, H.J.; Lee, Y.S. & Lee, J.H. (2000). Effects of Dizocilpine Pretreatment on Parvalbumin Immunoreactivity and Fos Expression after Cerebral Ischemia in the Hippocampus of the Mongolian Gerbil. *Journal of Veterinary Medical Science,*Vol.62, No.2, (March 2000), pp. 141-146, ISSN 0916-7250

Lakhan, S.E.; Kirchgessner, A. & Hofer, M. (2009). Inflammatory Mechanisms in Ischemic Stroke: Therapeutic Approaches. *Journal of Translational Medicine,*Vol.7, (November 2009), pp. 97, ISSN 1479-5876

Lambe, E.K.; Goldman-Rakic, P.S. & Aghajanian, G.K. (2000). Serotonin Induces EPSCs Preferentially in Layer V Pyramidal Neurons of the Frontal Cortex in the Rat. *Cerebral Cortex,*Vol.10, No.10, (September 2000), pp. 974-980, ISSN 1047-3211

Langdon, K.D.; Granter-Button, S. & Corbett, D. (2008). Persistent Behavioral Impairments and Neuroinflammation Following Global Ischemia in the Rat. *European Journal of Neuroscience,*Vol.28, No.11, (November 2008), pp. 2310-2318, ISSN 1460-9568

Laroche, S.; Davis, S. & Jay, T. M. (2000). Plasticity at Hippocampal to Prefrontal Cortex Synapses: Dual Roles in Working Memory and Consolidation. *Hippocampus,*Vol.10, No.4, (September 2000), pp. 438-446, ISSN 1050-9631

Larsson, E.; Nanobashvili, A.; Kokaia, Z & Lindvall, O. (1999) Evidence for Neuroprotective Effects of Endogenous Brain-Derived Neurotrophic Factor After Global Forebrain Ischemia in Rats. *Journal of Cerebral Blood Flow & Metab*, Vol.19, No.11, (November 1999), pp. 1220-1228, ISSN

Lauritzen, I.; Blondeau, N.; Heurteaux, C.; Widmann, C.; Romey, G. & Lazdunski, M. (2000). Polyunsaturated Fatty Acids are Potent Neuroprotectors. *EMBO Journal,*Vol.19, No.8, (April 2000), pp. 1784-1793, ISSN 0261-4189

Lazarewicz, J.W.; Pluta, R.; Puka, M. & Salinska, E. (1990). Diverse Mechanisms of Neuronal Protection by Nimodipine in Experimental Rabbit Brain Ischemia. *Stroke*, Vol.21, (12 Supplement), (December 1990), pp. IV108-110, ISSN 0039-2499

Lazarewicz, J.W.; Pluta, R.; Puka, M. & Salinska, E. (1993). Local Nimodipine Application Improves Early Functional Recovery in the Rabbit Hippocampus After 15-min Global Cerebral Ischemia. *Acta Neurobiologiae Experimentalis* Vol.53, No.4, (January 1993), pp. 499-510, ISSN 0065-1400

Lebesgue, D.; Chevaleyre, V.; Zukin, R.S. & Etgen, A.M. (2009). Estradiol Rescues Neurons from Global Ischemia-Induced Cell Death: Multiple Cellular Pathways of Neuroprotection. *Steroids*, Vol.74, No.7, (May 2009), pp. 555-561, ISSN 0039-128X

Lee, I. & Kesner, R. P. (2003). Time-dependent Relationship between the Dorsal Hippocampus and the Prefrontal Cortex in Spatial Memory. *Journal of Neuroscience*, Vol.23, No.4, (February 2003), pp. 1517-1523, ISSN 1529-2401

Lee, Y.S.; Yoon, B.W. & Roh, J.K. (1999). Neuroprotective Effects of Lamotrigine Enhanced by Flunarizine in Gerbil Global Ischemia. *Neuroscience Letters*, Vol.265, No.3, (May 1999), pp. 215-217, ISSN 0304-3940

Leker, R.R. & Shohami, E. (2002). Cerebral Ischemia and Trauma – Different Ethiologies yet Similar Mechanisms: Neuroprotective Opportunities. *Brain Research Brain Research Reviews*, Vol. 39, No. 1, (January 2002), pp. 55-73, ISSN 0165-0173

Lensman, M.; Korzhevskii, D.E.; Mourovets, V.O.; Kostkin, V.B.; Izvarina, N.; Perasso L.; Gandolfo C.; Otellin, V.A.; Polenov, S.A. & Balestrino, M. (2006). Intracerebroventricular Administration of Creatine Protects against Damage by Global Cerebral Ischemia in Rat. *Brain Research*. Vol. 1114, No. 1, (October 2006), pp. 187-194, ISSN 0006-8993

Letechipía-Vallejo, G.; González-Burgos, I. & Cervantes, M. (2001). Neuroprotective Effect of Melatonin on Brain Damage Induced by Acute Global Cerebral Ischemia in Cats. *Archives of Medical Research*, Vol.32, No.3, (June 2001), pp. 186-192, ISSN 0188-4409

Letechipía-Vallejo, G.; López-Loeza, E.; Espinoza-González, V.; González-Burgos, I.; Olvera-Cortés, M. E.; Moralí, G. & Cervantes, M. (2007). Long-term Morphological and Functional Evaluation of the Neuroprotective Effects of Post-ischemic Treatment with Melatonin in Rats. *Journal of Pineal Research*, Vol.42, No.2, (February 2007), pp. 138-146, ISSN 0742-3098

Li, R.C.; Guo, S.Z.; Lee, S.K. & Gozal, D. (2010). Neuroglobin Protects Neurons Against Oxidative Stress in Global Ischemia. *Journal of Cerebral Blood Flow & Metabolism*, Vol.30, No.11, (June 2010), pp. 1874-1882, ISSN 1559-7016

Liang, S.P.; Kanthan, R.; Shuaib, A., & Wishart, T. (1997). Effects of Clomethiazole on Radial-arm Maze Performance Following Global Forebrain Ischemia in Gerbils. *Brain Research*, Vol.751, No.2, (March 1997), pp. 189-195, ISSN 0006-8993

Lipton, P. (1999). Ischemic Cell Death in Brain Neurons. *Physiology Reviews*, Vol.79, No.4, (October 1999), pp. 1431-1568, ISSN 0031-9333

Littleton-Kearney, M.T.; Gaines, J.M.; Callahan, K.P.; Murphy, S.J. & Hurn, P.D. (2005). Effects of Estrogen on Platelet Reactivity after Transient Forebrain Ischemia in Rats. *Biological Research for Nursing*, Vol.7, No.2, (November 2005), pp. 135-145, ISSN 1099-8004

Lowry, O.H.; Passonneau, J.V.; Hasselberger, F.X. & Schulz, D.W. (1964). Effect of Ischemia on Known Substrates and Cofactors of the Glycolytic Pathway in Brain. *Journal of Biological Chemistry*, Vol.239, (January 1964), pp. 18-30, ISSN 0021-9258

Lu, A.; Ran, R.Q.; Clark, J.; Reilly, M.; Nee, A. & Sharp, F.R. (2002). 17-beta-Estradiol Induces Heat Shock Proteins in Brain Arteries and Potentiates Ischemic Heat Shock Protein Induction in Glia and Neurons. *Journal of Cerebral Blood Flow & Metabolism*, Vol.22, No.2, (February 2002), pp. 183-195, ISSN 0271-678X

Ma, D.; Lu, L.; Boneva, N.B.; Warashina, S.; Kaplamadzhiev, D.B.; Mori, Y.; Nakaya, M.A.; Kikuchi, M.; Tonchev, A.B.,; Okano, H. & Yamashima, T. (2008). Expression of Free Fatty Acid Receptor GPR40 in the Neurogenic Niche of Adult Monkey Hippocampus. *Hippocampus*, Vol.18, No.3, (December 2007), pp. 326-333, ISSN 1098-1063

Madl, C. & Holzer, M. (2004). Brain Function after Resuscitation from Cardiac Arrest. *Current Opinion in Critical Care*, Vol.10, No.3, (May 2004), pp. 213-217, ISSN 1070-5295

Margaill, I.; Plotkine, M. & Lerouet, D. (2005). Antioxidant Strategies in the Treatment of Stroke. *Free Radical Biology & Medicine*, Vol. 39, No.4 , (August 2005), pp. 429-443, ISSN 0891-5849

Matsumoto, M.; Scheller, M.S.; Zornow, M.H. & Strnat, M.A. (1993). Effect of S-emopamil, Nimodipine, and Mild Hypothermia on Hippocampal Glutamate Concentrations after Repeated Cerebral Ischemia in Rabbits. *Stroke*, Vol.24, No.8, (August 1993), pp. 1228-1234, ISSN 0039-2499

Matsushita, K.; Kitagawa, K.; Matsuyama, T.; Ohtsuki, T.; Taguchi, A.; Mandai, K.; Mabuchi, T.; Yagita, Y.; Yanagihara, T. & Matsumoto, M. (1996). Effect of Systemic Zinc Administration on Delayed Neuronal Death in the Gerbil Hippocampus. *Brain Research*, Vol.743, No.1-2, (December 1996), pp. 362-365, ISSN 0006-8993

McBean, D.E. & Kelly, P.A. (1998). Rodent Models of Global Cerebral Ischemia: a Comparison of Two-vessel Occlusion and Four-vessel Occlusion. *General Pharmacology*, Vol.30, No.4, (April 1998), pp. 431-434, ISSN 0306-3623

McDonald, R.J. & White, N.M. (1993). A Triple Dissociation of Memory Systems: Hippocampus, Amygdala, and Dorsal Striatum. *Behavior Neuroscience*, Vol.107, No.1, (February 1993), pp. 3-22, ISSN 0735-7044

McDonald, R.J. & White, N.M. (1994). Parallel Information Processing in the Water Maze: Evidence for Independent Memory Systems Involving Dorsal Striatum and Hippocampus. *Behavioral and Neural Biology*, Vol.61, No.3, (May 1994), pp. 260-270, ISSN 0163-1047

McDonald, R.J. & White, N.M. (1995). Hippocampal and Nonhippocampal Contributions to Place Learning in Rats. *Behavioral Neuroscience*, Vol.109, No.4, (August 1995), pp. 579-593, ISSN 0735-7044

McNamara, R.K. & Skelton, R.W. (1993). The Neuropharmacological and Neurochemical Basis of Place Learning in the Morris Water Maze. *Brain Research Brain Research Reviews*, Vol.18, No.1, (January 1993), pp. 33-49, ISSN 0165-0173

Mehta, S.L.; Manhas, N. & Raghubir, R. (2007). Molecular Targets in Cerebral Ischemia for Developing Novel Therapeutics. *Brain Research Reviews*, Vol.54, No.1, (January 2007), pp. 34-66, ISSN 0165-0173

Meloni, B.P.; Campbell, K.; Zhu, H. & Knuckey, N.W. (2009). In Search of Clinical Neuroprotection after Brain Ischemia: the Case for Mild Hypothermia (35 Degrees C) and Magnesium. *Stroke*, Vol.40, No.6, (April 2009), pp. 2236-2240, ISSN 0039-2499

Miles, A.N.; Majda, B.T.; Meloni, B.P. & Knuckey, N.W. (2001). Postischemic Intravenous Administration of Magnesium Sulfate Inhibits Hippocampal CA1 Neuronal Death after Transient Global Ischemia in Rats. *Neurosurgery*, Vol.49, No.6, (February 2002), pp. 1443-1450, ISSN 0148-396X

Montero, M.; Nielsen, M.; Ronn, L.C.; Moller, A.; Noraberg, J. & Zimmer, J. (2007). Neuroprotective Effects of the AMPA Antagonist PNQX in Oxygen-glucose Deprivation in Mouse Hippocampal Slice Cultures and Global Cerebral Ischemia in Gerbils. *Brain Research*, Vol.1177, (September 2007), pp. 124-135, ISSN 0006-8993

Moralí, G.; Letechipía-Vallejo, G.; López-Loeza, E.; Montes, P.; Hernández-Morales, L. & Cervantes, M. (2005). Post-ischemic Administration of Progesterone in Rats Exerts Neuroprotective Effects on the Hippocampus. *Neuroscience Letters*, Vol.382, No.3, (May 2005), pp. 286-290, ISSN 0304-3940

Moralí, G.; Montes, P.; González-Burgos, I.; Velázquez-Zamora, D.A. & Cervantes, M. (2011a). Cytoarchitectural Characteristics of Hippocampal CA1 Pyramidal Neurons of Rats, Four Months After Global Cerebral Ischemia and Progesterone Treatment. *Restorative Neurology and Neuroscience*, (September 2011), ISSN 0922-6028 [Epub ahead of print]

Moralí, G.; Montes, P.; Hernández-Morales, L.; Monfil, T.; Espinosa-García, C. & Cervantes, M. (2011b). Neuroprotective Effects of Progesterone and Allopregnanolone on Long-term Cognitive Outcome after Global Cerebral Ischemia. *Restorative Neurology and Neuroscience*, Vol.29, No.1, (February 2011), pp. 1-15, ISSN 0922-6028

Mori, T.; Tan, J.; Arendash, G.W.; Koyama, N.; Nojima, Y. & Town, T. (2008). Overexpression of Human S100B Exacerbates Brain Damage and Periinfarct Gliosis after Permanent Focal Ischemia. *Stroke*, Vol.39, No.7, (July 2008), pp. 2114-2121, ISSN 0039-2499

Morimoto, Y.; Kwon, J. Y.; Deyo, D. J. & Zornow, M. H. (2002). Effects of Lamotrigine on Conditioned Learning after Global Cerebral Ischemia in Rabbits. *Journal of Anesthesia,*Vol.16, No.4, (October 2003), pp. 349-353, ISSN 0913-8668

Morioka, T.; Kalehua, A.N. & Streit, W.J. (1991). The Microglial Reaction in the Rat Dorsal Hippocampus Following Transient Forebrain Ischemia. *Journal of Cerebral Blood Flow & Metabolism*, Vol.11, No.6, (November 1991), pp. 966-973, ISSN 0271-678X

Morioka, T.; Kalehua, A.N. & Streit, W.J. (1992). Progressive Expression of Immunomolecules on Microglial Cells in Rat Dorsal Hippocampus Following Transient Forebrain Ischemia. *Acta Neuropathologica (Berlin)*, Vol.83, No.2, (February 1992), pp. 149-157, ISSN 0001-6322

Morris, R. (1984). Development of a Water-maze Procedure for Studying Spatial Learning in the Rat. *Journal of Neuroscience Methods*, Vol.11, No.1, (May 1984), pp. 47-60, ISSN 0165-0270

Morris, R.G.; Garrud, P.; Rawlins, J.N. & O'Keefe, J. (1982). Place Navigation Impaired in Rats with Hippocampal Lesions. *Nature*, Vol.297, No.5868, (June 1982), pp. 681-683, ISSN 0028-0836

Morris, R.G.; Schenk, F.; Tweedie, F. & Jarrard, L E. (1990). Ibotenate Lesions of Hippocampus and/or Subiculum: Dissociating Components of Allocentric Spatial Learning. *European Journal of Neuroscience,*Vol.2, No.12, (January 1990), pp. 1016-1028, ISSN 1460-9568

Moser, E.; Moser, M.B. & Andersen, P. (1993). Spatial Learning Impairment Parallels the Magnitude of Dorsal Hippocampal Lesions, but is Hardly Present Following Ventral Lesions. *Journal of Neuroscience*, Vol.13, No.9, (September 1993), pp. 3916-3925, ISSN 0270-6474

Mudrick, L.A. & Baimbridge, K.G. (1989). Long-term Structural Changes in the Rat Hippocampal Formation Following Cerebral Ischemia. *Brain Research*, Vol.493, No.1, (July 1989), pp. 179-184, ISSN 0006-8993

Mueller, R.N.; Deyo, D.J.,; Brantley, D.R.; Disterhoft, J.F. & Zornow, M.H. (2003). Lubeluzole and Conditioned Learning after Cerebral Ischemia. *Experimental Brain Research,*Vol.152, No.3, (August 2003), pp. 329-334, ISSN 0014-4819

Myhrer, T. (2003). Neurotransmitter Systems Involved in Learning and Memory in the Rat: a Meta-analysis Based on Studies of Four Behavioral Tasks. *Brain Research Brain Research Reviews,* Vol.41, No.2-3, (March 2003), pp. 268-287, ISSN 0165-0173

Nakatomi, H.; Kuriu, T.; Okabe, S.; Yamamoto, S.; Hatano, O.; Kawahara, N.; Tamura, A.; Kirino, T. & Nakafuku, M. (2002). Regeneration of Hippocampal Pyramidal Neurons after Ischemic Brain Injury by Recruitment of Endogenous Neural Progenitors. *Cell,* Vol.110, No.4, (August 2002), pp. 429-441, ISSN 0092-8674

Nakayama, R.; Yano, T.; Ushijima, K.; Abe, E. & Terasaki, H. (2002). Effects of Dantrolene on Extracellular Glutamate Concentration and Neuronal Death in the Rat Hippocampal CA1 Region Subjected to Transient Ischemia. *Anesthesiology,* Vol.96, No.3, (March 2002), pp. 705-710, ISSN 0003-3022

Nanri, K.; Montecot, C.; Springhetti, V.; Seylaz, J. & Pinard, E. (1998). The Selective Inhibitor of Neuronal Nitric Oxide Synthase, 7-nitroindazole, Reduces the Delayed Neuronal Damage Due to Forebrain Ischemia in Rats. *Stroke,* Vol.29, No.6, (June 1998), pp. 1248-1253; discussion 1253-1244, ISSN 0039-2499

Neigh, G.N.; Glasper, E.R.; Kofler, J.; Traystman, R.J.; Mervis, R.F.; Bachstetter, A. & DeVries, A.C. (2004). Cardiac Arrest with Cardiopulmonary Resuscitation Reduces Dendritic Spine Density in CA1 Pyramidal Cells and Selectively Alters Acquisition of Spatial Memory. *European Journal of Neuroscience,* Vol.20, No.7, (September 2004), pp. 1865-1872, ISSN 0953-816X

Nelson, A.; Lebessi, A.; Sowinski, P. & Hodges, H. (1997). Comparison of Effects of Global Cerebral Ischaemia on Spatial Learning in the Standard and Radial Water Maze: Relationship of Hippocampal Damage to Performance. *Behavioral Brain Research,* Vol.85, No.1, (April 1997), pp. 93-115, ISSN 0166-4328

Nemoto, E.M.; Bleyaert, A.L.; Stezoski, S.W.; Moossy, J.; Rao, G.R. & Safar, P. (1977). Global Brain Ischemia: a Reproducible Monkey Model. *Stroke,* Vol.8, No.5, (September 1977), pp. 558-564, ISSN 0039-2499

Nikonenko, A.G.; Radenovic, L.; Andjus, P.R. & Skibo, G.G. (2009). Structural Features of Ischemic Damage in the Hippocampus. *The Anatomical Record,* Vol.292, No.12, (December 2009), pp. 1914-1921, ISSN 1932-8486

Nishimura, H.; Matsuyama, T.; Obata, K.; Nakajima, Y.; Kitano, H.; Sugita, M. & Okamoto, M. (2000). Changes in Mint1, a Novel Synaptic Protein, after Transient Global Ischemia in Mouse Hippocampus. *Journal of Cerebral Blood Flow & Metabolism,* Vol.20, No.10, (November 2000), pp. 1437-1445, ISSN 0271-678X

Noguchi, K.; Matsumoto, N.; Shiozaki, T.; Tasaki, O.; Ogura, H.; Kuwagata, Y.; Sugimoto, H. & Seiyama A. (2011). Effects of Timing and Duration of Hypothermia on Survival in an Experimental Gerbil Model of Global Ischaemia. *Resuscitation,* Vol.82, No.4, (April 2011), pp. 481-486, ISSN 0300-9572

O'Keefe, J. & Nadel, L. (1978). *The Hippocampus as a Cognitive Map,* Oxford University Press, ISBN 0-19-857206-9, New York, USA

Oliveira, M.G.; Bueno, O.F.; Pomarico, A.C. & Gugliano, E.B. (1997). Strategies Used by Hippocampal- and Caudate-Putamen-Lesioned Rats in a Learning Task.

Neurobiology of Learning and Memory, Vol.68, No.1, (July 1997), pp. 32-41, ISSN 1074-7427

Olsen, G.M.; Scheel-Kruger, J.; Moller, A. & Jensen, L.H. (1994). Relation of Spatial Learning of Rats in the Morris Water Maze Task to the Number of Viable CA1 Neurons Following Four-vessel Occlusion. *Behavioral Neuroscience,*Vol.108, No.4, (August 1994), pp. 681-690, ISSN 0735-7044

Olton, D.S. (1983). Memory Functions and the Hippocampus, In: *Neurobiology of the Hippocampus*, W. Seifer, (Ed.), 335-373, Academic Press, ISBN 0126348804, New York, USA

Olton, D.S. (1987). The Radial Arm Maze as a Tool in Behavioral Pharmacology. *Physiology & Behavior*, Vol. 40, No. 6, (December 1987), pp. 793-797, ISSN 0031-9384

Olton, D.S.; Walker, J.A. & Wolf, W.A. (1982). A Disconnection Analysis of Hippocampal Function. *Brain Research*, Vol.233, No.2, (February 1982), pp. 241-253, ISSN 0006-8993

Olvera-Cortés, E.; Barajas-Pérez, M.; Morales-Villagrán, A. & González-Burgos, I. (2001). Cerebral Serotonin Depletion Induces Egocentric Learning Improvement in Developing Rats. *Neuroscience Letters*, Vol.313, No.1-2, (October 2001), pp. 29-32, ISSN 0304-3940

Olvera-Cortés, E.; Cervantes, M. & González-Burgos, I. (2002). Place-learning, but not Cue-learning Training, Modifies the Hippocampal Theta Rhythm in Rats. *Brain Research Bulletin*, Vol.58, No.3, (July 2002), pp. 261-270, ISSN 0361-9230.

Olvera-Cortés, M.E.; García-Alcántar, I.; Gutiérrez-Guzmán, B.E.; Hernández-Pérez, J.J.; López-Vázquez, M.A. & Cervantes, M. (2012). Differential Learning-Related Changes in Theta Activity During Place Learning in Young and Old Rats. Behavioural Brain Research, *Behavioural Brain Research*, Vol.226, No.2, (January 2012), pp. 555-562, ISSN 0166-4328 (In Press)

Onodera, H.; Aoki, H.; Yae, T. & Kogure, K. (1990). Post-ischemic Synaptic Plasticity in the Rat Hippocampus After Long-term Survival: Histochemical and Autoradiographic Study. *Neuroscience*, Vol.38, No.1, (January 1990), pp. 125-136, ISSN 0306-4522

Otani, H.; Togashi, H.; Jesmin, S.; Sakuma, I.; Yamaguchi, T.; Matsumoto, M.; Kakehata, H. & Yoshioka, M. (2005). Temporal Effects of Edaravone, a Free Radical Scavenger, on Transient Ischemia-induced Neuronal Dysfunction in the Rat Hippocampus. *European Journal of Pharmacology*, Vol. 512, No. 2-3, (April 2005), pp. 129-37, ISSN 0014-2999

Otellin, V.A.; Korzhevskii, D.E.; Kostkin, V.B.; Balestrino, M.; Lensman, M.V. & Polenov, S.A. (2003). The Neuroprotective Effect of Creatine in Rats with Cerebral Ischemia. *Doklady Biological Sciences*, Vol. 390, No. 3, (May-Jun 2003), pp. 197-199, ISSN 0012-4966

Ozacmak, V.H. & Sayan, H. (2009). The Effects of 17beta Estradiol, 17alpha Estradiol and Progesterone on Oxidative Stress Biomarkers in Ovariectomized Female Rat Brain Subjected to Global Cerebral Ischemia. *Physiological Research*, Vol.58, No.6, (December 2008), pp. 909-912, ISSN 0862-8408

Pappas, T.N. & Mironovich, R.O. (1981). Barbiturate-Induced Comma to Protect Against Cerebral Ischemia and Increased Intracranial Pressure. *American Journal of Hospital Pharmacy*, (April 1981), Vol.38, No.4, pp. 494-498, ISSN 0002-9289

Pazos, A.J.; Green, E.J.; Busto, R.; McCabe, P.M.; Baena, R.C.; Ginsberg, M.D.; Globus, M.Y.; Schneiderman, N. & Dietrich, W.D. (1999). Effects of Combined Postischemic Hypothermia and Delayed N-tert-butyl-alpha-pheylnitrone (PBN) Administration on Histopathological and Behavioral Deficits Associated with Transient Global Ischemia in Rats. *Brain Research*, Vol.846, No.2, (November 1999), pp. 186-195, ISSN 0006-8993

Pérez-Vega, M.I.; Feria-Velasco, A. & González-Burgos, I. (2000). Prefrontocortical Serotonin Depletion Results in Plastic Changes of Prefrontocortical Pyramidal Neurons, Underlying a Greater Efficiency of Short-term Memory. *Brain Research Bulletin*, Vol.53, No.3, (December 2000), pp. 291-300, ISSN 0361-9230

Petito, C.K. & Halaby, I.A. (1993). Relationship Between Ischemia and Ischemic Neuronal Necrosis to Astrocyte Expression of Glial Fibrillary Acidic Protein. *International Journal of Developmental Neuroscience*, Vol.11, No.2, (April 1993), pp. 239-47, ISSN 0736-5748

Piao, C.S.; Che, Y.; Han, P.L. & Lee, J.K. (2002). Delayed and Differential Induction of p38 MAPK Isoforms in Microglia and Astrocytes in the Brain after Transient Global Ischemia. *Brain Research. Molecular Brain Research*, Vol.107, No.2, (November 2002), pp. 137-144, ISSN 0169-328X

del Pilar Fernández, M., Meizoso, M.J., Lodeiro, M.J. & Belmonte, A. (1998). Effect of Desmethyl Tirilazad, Dizocilpine Maleate and Nimodipine on Brain Nitric Oxide Synthase Activity and Cyclic Guanosine Monophosphate During Cerebral Ischemia in Rats. *Pharmacology*,Vol.57, No.4, (September 1998), pp. 174-179, ISSN 0031-7012

Plamondon, H. & Roberge, M.C. (2008). Dietary PUFA Supplements Reduce Memory Deficits But not CA1 Ischemic Injury in Rats. *Physiology & Behavior*,Vol.95, No.3, (August 2008), pp. 492-500, ISSN 0031-9384

Popp, E.; Padosch, S.A.; Vogel, P.; Schäbitz, W.R.; Schwab, S. & Böttiger, B.W. (2004). Effects of Intracerebroventricular Application of Brain-Derived Neurotrophic Factor on Cerebral Recovery After Cardiac Arrest in Rats. *Critical Care Medicine*, (September 2004), Vol.32, (9 Suppl), pp. S359-65, ISSN 0090-3493

Pulsinelli, W.A. (1985). Selective Neuronal Vulnerability: Morphological and Molecular Characteristics. *Progress in Brain Research*, Vol.63, (January 1985), pp. 29-37, ISSN 0079-6123

Pulsinelli, W.A. & Brierley, J.B. (1979). A New Model of Bilateral Hemispheric Ischemia in the Unanesthetized Rat. *Stroke*, Vol.10, No.3, (May 1979), pp. 267-272, ISSN 0039-2499

Pulsinelli, W.A. & Buchan, A.M. (1988). The Four-vessel Occlusion Rat Model: Method for Complete Occlusion of Vertebral Arteries and Control of Collateral Circulation. *Stroke*, Vol.19, No.7, (July 1988), pp. 913-914, ISSN 0039-2499

Pulsinelli, W.A. & Duffy, T.E. (1983). Regional Energy Balance in Rat Brain after Transient Forebrain Ischemia. *Journal of Neurochemistry*, Vol.40, No.5, (May 1983), pp. 1500-1503, ISSN 0022-3042

Pulsinelli, W.A.; Jacewicz, M.; Levy, D.E.; Petito, C.K. & Plum, F. (1997). Ischemic Brain Injury and the Therapeutic Window. *Annals of the New York Academy of Sciences*, Vol.835, (June 1998), pp. 187-193, ISSN 0077-8923

Pulsinelli, W.A.; Levy, D.E. & Duffy, T.E. (1982). Regional Cerebral Blood Flow and Glucose Metabolism Following Transient Forebrain Ischemia. *Annals of Neurology*, Vol.11, No.5, (May 1982), pp. 499-502, ISSN 0364-5134

Radovsky, A.; Safar, P.; Sterz, F.; Leonov, Y.; Reich, H. & Kuboyama, K. (1995). Regional Prevalence and Distribution of Ischemic Neurons in Dog Brains 96 Hours After Cardiac Arrest of 0 to 20 Minutes. *Stroke*, Vol.26, No.11, (November 1995), pp. 2127-2133; discussion 2133-2124, ISSN 0039-2499

Rami, A. & Krieglstein, J. (1994). Neuronal Protective Effects of Calcium Antagonists in Cerebral Ischemia. *Life Sciences*, Vol.55, No.25-26, (January 1994), pp. 2105-2113, ISSN 0024-3205

Reiter, R.J.; Tan, D.X.; Leon, J.; Kilic, U. & Kilic, E. (2005). When Melatonin Gets on your Nerves: Its Beneficial Actions in Experimental Models of Stroke. *Experimental Biology & Medicine (Maywood)*, Vol.230, No.2, (February 2005), pp. 104-117 ISSN 1535-3702

Rennie, K.; de Butte, M.; Frechette, M. & Pappas, B.A. (2008). Chronic and Acute Melatonin Effects in Gerbil Global Forebrain Ischemia: Long-term Neural and Behavioral Outcome. *Journal of Pineal Research*, Vol.44, No.2, (February 2008), pp. 149-156, ISSN 1600-079X

Roberge, M.C.; Hotte-Bernard, J.; Messier, C. & Plamondon, H. (2008). Food Restriction Attenuates Ischemia-induced Spatial Learning and Memory Deficits Despite Extensive CA1 Ischemic Injury. *Behavioral Brain Research*, Vol.187, No.1, (October 2007), pp. 123-132, ISSN 0166-4328

Robinson, T.E. & Kolb, B. (2004). Structural Plasticity Associated with Exposure to Drugs of Abuse. *Neuropharmacology*, Vol.47, Suppl 1, (October 2004), pp. 33-46, ISSN 0028-3908

Ruan, Y.W.; Zou, B.; Fan, Y.; Li, Y.; Lin, N.; Zeng, Y.S.; Gao, T.M.; Yao, Z. & Xu, Z.C. (2006). Dendritic Plasticity of CA1 Pyramidal Neurons After Transient Global Ischemia. *Neuroscience*, Vol.140, No.1, (March 2006), pp. 191-201, ISSN 0306-4522

Safar, P.; Stezoski, W. & Nemoto, E.M. (1976). Amelioration of Brain Damage after 12 Minutes' Cardiac Arrest in Dogs. *Archives of Neurology*, Vol.33, No.2, (February 1976), pp. 91-95, ISSN 0003-9942

Sánchez-Casado, M.; Sánchez-Ledesma, M.J.; Goncalves-Estella, J.M.; Abad-Hernández, M.M.; García-March, G. & Broseta-Rodrigo, J. (2007). Effect of Combination Therapy with Hypothermia, Magnesium and Tirilazad in an Experimental Model of Diffuse Cerebral Ischemia]. *Medicina Intensiva*, Vol.31, No.3, (April 2007), pp. 113-119, ISSN 0210-5691

Savitz, S.I. & Fisher, M. (2007). Prophylactic Neuroprotection. *Current Drug Targets*, Vol.8, No.7, (July 2007), pp. 846-849, ISSN 1389-4501

Scallet, A.C. (1995). Quantitative Histological Evaluation of Neuroprotective Compounds. *Annals of the New York Academy of Sciences*, Vol.765, (September 1995), pp. 47-61, ISSN 0077-8923, Book: ISBN 0-89766-946-0

Scheller, M.S.; Grafe, M.R.; Zornow, M.H. & Fleischer, J.E. (1992). Effects of Ischemia Duration on Neurological Outcome, CA1 Histopathology, and Nonmatching to Sample Learning in Monkeys. *Stroke*,Vol.23, No.10, (October 1992), pp. 1471-1476; discussion 1477-1478, ISSN 0039-2499

Schmidt-Kastner, R. & Freund, T.F. (1991). Selective Vulnerability of the Hippocampus in Brain Ischemia. *Neuroscience*, Vol.40, No.3, (March 1991), pp. 599-636, ISSN 0306-4522

Schmidt-Kastner, R.; Truettner, J.; Lin, B.; Zhao, W.; Saul, J.; Busto, R. & Ginsberg, M.D. (2001). Transient Changes in Brain-Derived Neurotrophic Factor (BDNF) mRNA Expression in Hippocampus During Moderate Ischemia Induced by Chronic Bilateral Common Carotid Artery Occlussion in the Rat. *Molecular Brain Research*, Vol. 92, No.1-2, (August 2001), pp. 157-166, ISSN 0169-328X

Schneider, A.; Bottiger, B.W. & Popp, E. (2009). Cerebral Resuscitation after Cardiocirculatory Arrest. *Anesthesia and Analgesia*, Vol.108, No.3, (February 2009), pp. 971-979, ISSN 1526-7598

Schwartz, R.D.; Yu, X.; Katzman, M.R.; Hayden-Hixson, D.M. & Perry, J.M. (1995). Diazepam, Given Postischemia, Protects Selectively Vulnerable Neurons in the Rat Hippocampus and Striatum. *Journal of Neuroscience*, Vol.15, (1 Pt 2), (January 1995), pp. 529-39, ISSN 0270-6474

Seamans, J.K.; Floresco, S.B. & Phillips, A.G. (1995). Functional Differences Between the Prelimbic and Anterior Cingulate Regions of the Rat Prefrontal Cortex. *Behavioral Neuroscience*, Vol.109, No.6, (December 1995), pp. 1063-1073, ISSN 0735-7044

Seder, D.B. & Jarrah, S. (2008). Therapeutic Hypothermia for Cardiac Arrest: a Practical Approach. *Current Neurology and Neuroscience Reports*, Vol.8, No.6, (October 2008), pp. 508-517, ISSN 1534-6293

Selakovic, V.; Janac, B. & Radenovic, L. (2010). MK-801 Effect on Regional Cerebral Oxidative Stress Rate Induced by Different Duration of Global Ischemia in Gerbils. *Molecular and Cellular Biochemistry*, Vol.342, No.1-2, (April 2010), pp. 35-50, ISSN 1573-4919

Shibata, M.; Yamasaki, N.; Miyakawa, T.; Kalaria, R.N.; Fujita, Y.; Ohtani, R.; Ihara, M.; Takahashi, R. & Tomimoto, H. (2007). Selective Impairment of Working Memory in a Mouse Model of Chronic Cerebral Hypoperfusion. *Stroke*, Vol.38, No.10, (September 2007), pp. 2826-2832, ISSN 0039-2499

Shuaib, A.; Ijaz, S. & Kanthan, R. (1995a). Clomethiazole Protects the Brain in Transient Forebrain Ischemia When Used up to 4 h After the Insult. *Neuroscience Letters*, Vol. 197, No. 2, (September 1995), pp. 109-12, ISSN 0304-3940

Shuaib, A.; Mahmood, R.H.; Wishart, T.; Kanthan, R.; Murabit, M.A.; Ijaz, S.; Miyashita, H. & Howlett, W. (1995b). Neuroprotective Effects of Lamotrigine in Global Ischemia in Gerbils. A Histological, in Vivo Microdialysis and Behavioral Study. *Brain Research*, Vol.702, No.1-2, (December 1995), pp. 199-206, ISSN 0006-8993

Siemkowicz, E. (1981). Hyperglycemia in the Reperfusion Period Hampers Recovery from Cerebral Ischemia. *Acta Neurologica Scandinavica*, Vol.64, No.3, (September 1981), pp. 207-216, ISSN 0001-6314

Siemkowicz, E. & Gjedde, A. (1980). Post-ischemic Coma in Rat: Effect of Different Pre-ischemic Blood Glucose Levels on Cerebral Metabolic Recovery after Ischemia. *Acta Neurologica Scandinavica*,Vol.110, No.3, (November 1980), pp. 225-232, ISSN 0001-6772

Siemkowicz, E. & Hansen, A.J. (1978). Clinical Restitution Following Cerebral Ischemia in Hypo-, Normo- and Hyperglycemic Rats. *Acta Neurologica Scandinavica*,Vol.58, No.1, (July 1978), pp. 1-8, ISSN 0001-6314

Silasi, G. & Colbourne, F. (2011). Therapeutic Hypothermia Influences Cell Genesis and Survival in the Rat Hippocampus Following Global Ischemia. *Journal of Cerebral Blood Flow and Metab*, Vol.31, No.8, (August 2011), pp. 1725-35, ISSN

Silva, A.J.; Giese, K.P.; Fedorov, N.B.; Frankland, P.W. & Kogan, J.H. (1998). Molecular, Cellular, and Neuroanatomical Substrates of Place Learning. *Neurobiology of Learning and Memory*, Vol.70, No.1-2, (October 1998), pp. 44-61, ISSN 1074-7427

Sinha, J.; Das, N. & Basu, M. K. (2001). Liposomal Antioxidants in Combating Ischemia-reperfusion Injury in Rat Brain. *Biomedicine and Pharmacotherapy*, Vol.55, No.5, (June 2001), pp. 264-271, ISSN 0753-3322

Sirin, B.H.; Coskun, E.; Yilik, L.; Ortac, R.; Sirin, H. & Tetik, C. (1998). Neuroprotective Effects of Preischemia Subcutaneous Magnesium Sulfate in Transient Cerebral Ischemia. *European Journal of Cardio-thoracic Surgery*,Vol.14, No.1, (September 1998), pp. 82-88, ISSN 1010-7940

Sirin, B.H.; Yilik, L.; Coskun, E.; Ortac, R. & Sirin, H. (1998). Pentoxifylline Reduces Injury of the Brain in Transient Ischaemia. *Acta Cardiologica*, Vol.53, No.2, (July 1998), pp. 89-95, ISSN 0001-5385

Skibo, G.G. & Nikonenko, A.G. (2010). Brain Plasticity after Ischemic Episode. *Vitamins & Hormones*, Vol.82, (May 2010), pp. 107-127, ISSN 0083-6729

Smith, M.L.; Auer, R.N. & Siesjo, B.K. (1984a). The Density and Distribution of Ischemic Brain Injury in the Rat Following 2-10 min of Forebrain Ischemia. *Acta Neuropathologica*,Vol.64, No.4, (January 1984), pp. 319-332, ISSN 0001-6322

Smith, M.L.; Bendek, G.; Dahlgren, N.; Rosen, I.; Wieloch, T. & Siesjo, B.K. (1984b). Models for Studying Long-term Recovery Following Forebrain Ischemia in the Rat. 2. A 2-Vessel Occlusion Model. *Acta Physiologica Scandinavica*,Vol.69, No.6, (June 1984), pp. 385-401, ISSN 0001-6314

Soltyz, Z.; Janeczko, K.; Orzylowska-Sliwinska, O.; Zaremba, M.; Januszewski, S. & Aderfeld-Nowak, B. (2003). Morphological Ttransformation of Cells Immunopositive to GFAP, TrkA or p75 in CA1 Hippocampal Area Following Transient Global Ischemia in the Rat. A Quantitative Study. *Brain Research*, Vol.987, No.2, (October 2003), pp. 186-193, ISSN 0006-8993

Sorra, K.E. & Harris, K.M. (2000). Overview on the Structure, Composition, Function, Development, and Plasticity of Hippocampal Dendritic Spines. *Hippocampus*, Vol.10, No.5, (November 2000), pp. 501-511, ISSN 1050-9631

STAIR. (1999). Recommendations for Standards Regarding Preclinical Neuroprotective and Restorative Drug Development. *Stroke*, Vol.30, No.12, (December 1999), pp. 2752-2758, ISSN 0039-2499

Stepień, K.; Tomaszewski, M. & Czuczwar, S.J. (2005). Profile of Anticonvulsant Activity and Neuroprotective Effects of Novel and Potential Antiepileptic Drugs -- An Update. *Pharmacological Reports*,Vol.57, No.6, (December 2005), pp. 719-733, ISSN 1734-1140

Stevens, M.K. & Yaksh, T.L. (1990). Systematic Studies on the Effects of the NMDA Receptor Antagonist MK-801 on Cerebral Blood Flow and Responsivity, EEG, and Blood-brain Barrier Following Complete Reversible Cerebral Ischemia. *Journal of Cerebral Blood Flow & Metabolism*, Vol.10, No.1, (January 1990), pp. 77-88, ISSN 0271-678X

Sugawara, T.; Fujimura, M.; Morita-Fujimura, Y.; Kawase, M. & Chan, P.H. (1999). Mitochondrial Release of Cytochrome c Corresponds to the Selective Vulnerability of Hippocampal CA1 Neurons in Rats After Transient Global Cerebral Ischemia. *Journal of Neuroscience*, Vol. 19, No. 22, (November 1999), pp. RC39 1-6. ISSN 1529-2401

Sugawara, T.; Fujimura, M.; Noshita, N.; Kim, G.W.; Saito, A.; Hayashi, T.; Narasimhan, P.; Maier, C.M. & Chan, P.H. (2004). Neuronal Death/Survival Signaling Pathways in Cerebral Ischemia. *NeuroRx*, Vol.1, No.1, (February 2005), pp. 17-25, ISSN 1545-5343

Sydserff, S.G.; Cross, A.J.; Murray, T.K.; Jones, J.A. & Green, A.R. (2000). Clomethiazole is Neuroprotective in Models of Global and Focal Cerebral Ischemia when Infused at Doses Producing Clinically Relevant Plasma Concentrations. *Brain Research*, Vol.862, No.1-2, (May 2000), pp. 59-62, ISSN 0006-8993

Tarelo-Acuna, L.; Olvera-Cortés, E. & González-Burgos, I. (2000). Prenatal and Postnatal Exposure to Ethanol Induces Changes in the Shape of the Dendritic Spines from Hippocampal CA1 Pyramidal Neurons of the Rat. *Neuroscience Letters*, Vol.286, No.1, (May 2000), pp. 13-16, ISSN 0304-3940

Taylor, C.L.; Latimer, M.P. & Winn, P. (2003). Impaired Delayed Spatial Win-shift Behaviour on the Eight Arm Radial Maze Following Excitotoxic Lesions of the Medial Prefrontal Cortex in the Rat. *Behavioral Brain Research*, Vol.147, No.1-2, (December 2003), pp. 107-114, ISSN 0166-4328

Todd, M.M.; Chadwick, H.S.; Shapiro, H.M.; Dunlop, B.J.; Marshall, L.F. & Dueck, R. (1982). The Neurologic Effects of Thiopental Therapy Following Experimental Cardiac Arrest in Cats. *Anesthesiology*, Vol.57, No.2, (August 1982), pp. 76-86, ISSN 0003-3022

Toung, T.J.; Kirsch, J.R.; Maruki, Y. & Traystman, R.J. (1994). Effects of Pentoxifylline on Cerebral Blood Flow, Metabolism, and Evoked Response after Total Cerebral Ischemia in Dogs. *Critical Care Medicine*, Vol.22, No.2, (February 1994), pp. 273-281, ISSN 0090-3493

Traystman, R.J. (2003). Animal Models of Focal and Global Cerebral Ischemia. *Institute for Laboratory Animal Research*, Vol.44, No.2, (March 2003), pp. 85-95, ISSN 1084-2020

Volpe, B.T.; Pulsinelli, W.A.; Tribuna, J. & Davis, H.P. (1984). Behavioral Performance of Rats Following Transient Forebrain Ischemia. *Stroke*, Vol.15, No.3, (May 1984), pp. 558-562, ISSN 0039-2499

Wang, J.M.; Liu, L.; Irwin, R.W.; Chen, S. & Diaz-Brinton, R. (2008). Regenerative Potential of Allopregnanolone. *Brain Research Reviews*, Vol.57, No.2, (March 2008), pp. 398-409, ISSN 0165-0173

Wang, R.; Zhang, Q.G.; Han, D.; Xu, J.; Lu, Q. & Zhang, G. Y. (2006). Inhibition of MLK3-MKK4/7-JNK1/2 Pathway by Akt1 in Exogenous Estrogen-induced Neuroprotection against Transient Global Cerebral Ischemia by a Non-genomic Mechanism in Male Rats. *Journal of Neurochemistry*, Vol.99, No.6, (October 2006), pp. 1543-1554, ISSN 0022-3042

Wappler, E.A.; Felszeghy, K.; Szilagyi, G.; Gal, A.; Skopal, J.; Mehra, R.D.; Nyakas, C. & Nagy, Z. (2010). Neuroprotective Effects of Estrogen Treatment on Ischemia-induced Behavioural Deficits in Ovariectomized Gerbils at Different Ages. *Behavioral Brain Research*, Vol.209, No.1, (January 2010), pp. 42-48, ISSN 1872-7549

Warner, D.S.; Sheng, H. & Batinie-Haberle, I. (2004). Oxidants, Antioxidants and the Ischemic Brain. *Journal of Experimental Biology*, Vol. 207, Pt.18, (August 2004), pp. 3221-3231, ISSN 0022-0949

Webster, C.M.; Kelly, S.; Koike, M.A.; Chock, V.Y.; Giffard, R.G. & Yenari, M.A. (2009). Inflammation and NFkappaB Activation is Decreased by Hypothermia Following Global Cerebral Ischemia. *Neurobiology of Disease*, Vol.33, No.2, (February 2009), pp. 301-312, ISSN 0969-9961

Weigl, M.; Tenze, G.; Steinlechner, B.; Skhirtladze, K.; Reining, G.; Bernardo, M.; Pedicelli, E. & Dworschak, M. (2005). A Systematic Review of Currently Available Pharmacological Neuroprotective Agents as a Sole Intervention before Anticipated or Induced Cardiac Arrest. *Resuscitation*, Vol.65, No.1, (April 2005), pp. 21-39, ISSN 0300-9572

Weil, Z.M.; Karelina, K.; Su, A.J.; Barker, J.M.; Norman, G.J.; Zhang, N.; Devries, A.C. & Nelson, R.J. (2009). Time-of-day Determines Neuronal Damage and Mortality after Cardiac Arrest. *Neurobiology of Disease*, Vol.36, No.2, (August 2009), pp. 352-360, ISSN 0969-9961

Wellman, C.L. & Sengelaub, D.R. (1991). Cortical Neuroanatomical Correlates of Behavioral Deficits Produced by Lesion of the Basal Forebrain in Rats. *Behavioral and Neural Biology*, Vol.56, No.1, (July 1991), pp. 1-24, ISSN 0163-1047

Whittingham, T.S.; Lust, W.D. & Passonneau, J.V. (1984). An in Vitro Model of Ischemia: Metabolic and Electrical Alterations in the Hippocampal Slice. *Journal of Neuroscience*, Vol.4, No.3, (March 1984), pp. 793-802, ISSN 0270-6474

Wiard, R.P.; Dickerson, M.C.; Beek, O.; Norton, R. & Cooper, B.R. (1995). Neuroprotective Properties of the Novel Antiepileptic Lamotrigine in a Gerbil Model of Global Cerebral Ischemia. *Stroke*, Vol.26, No.3, (March 1995), pp. 466-472, ISSN 0039-2499

Wiklund, L.; Basu, S.; Miclescu, A.; Wiklund, P.; Ronquist, G. & Sharma, H.S. (2007). Neuro- and Cardioprotective Effects of Blockade of Nitric Oxide Action by Administration of Methylene Blue. *Annals of the New York Academy of Sciences*, Vol.1122, (December 2007), pp. 231-244, ISSN 0077-8923

Winocur, G. (1982). Radial-arm-maze Behavior by Rats with Dorsal Hippocampal Lesions: Effect of Cuing. *Journal of Comparative and Physiological Psychology*, Vol.96, No.2, (April 1982), pp. 155-169, ISSN 0021-9940

Yoshida, S.; Busto, R.; Watson, B.D.; Santiso, M. & Ginsberg, M.D. (1985). Postischemic Cerebral Lipid Peroxidation in Vitro: Modification by Dietary Vitamin E. *Journal of Neurochemistry*, Vol.44, No.5, (May 1985), pp. 1593-1601, ISSN 0022-3042

Zani, A.; Braida, D.; Capurro, V. & Sala, M. (2007). Delta9-tetrahydrocannabinol (THC) and AM 404 Protect against Cerebral Ischaemia in Gerbils through a Mechanism Involving Cannabinoid and Opioid Receptors. *British Journal of Pharmacology* Vol.152, No.8, (October 2007), pp. 1301-1311, ISSN 0007-1188

Zapater, P.; Moreno, J. & Horga, J.F. (1997). Neuroprotection by the Novel Calcium Antagonist PCA50938, Nimodipine and Flunarizine, in Gerbil Global Brain Ischemia. *Brain Research*, Vol.772, No.1-2, (December 1997), pp. 57-62, ISSN 0006-8993

Zhang, Z.; Sobel, R.A.; Cheng, D.; Steinberg, G.K. & Yenari, M.A. (2001). Mild Hypothermia Increases Bcl-2 Protein Expression Following Global Cerebral Ischemia. *Brain Research Molecular Brain Research*, Vol.95, No.1-2, (November 2001), pp. 75-85, ISSN

Zhang, F.; Wang, S.; Cao, G.; Gao, Y. & Chen, J. (2007). Signal Transducers and Activators of Transcription 5 Contributes to Erythropoietin-mediated Neuroprotection Against

Hippocampal Neuronal Death after Transient Global Cerebral Ischemia. *Neurobiology of Disease*, Vol.25, No.1, (September 2006), pp. 45-53, ISSN 0969-9961

Zhang, Q.G.; Wang, R.M.; Han, D.; Yang, L.C.; Li, J. & Brann, D.W. (2009). Preconditioning Neuroprotection in Gobal Cerebral Ischemia Involves NMDA Receptor-mediated ERK-JNK3 Crosstalk. *Neuroscience Research*, Vol.63, No.3, (April 2009), pp. 205-212, ISSN 0168-0102

Zhang, H.; Xu, G.; Zhang, J.; Murong, S.; Mei, Y. & Tong E. (2010). Mild Hypothermia Reduces Ischemic Neuron Death via Altering the Expression of p53 and bcl-2. *Neurological Research*, Vol.32, No.4, (May 2010), pp. 384-9, ISSN 0161-6412

Zhao, Y.; Wang, J.; Liu, C.; Jiang, C.; Zhao, C. & Zhu, Z. (2011). Progesterone Influences Postischemic Synaptogenesis in the CA1 Region of the Hippocampus in Rats. *Synapse*, Vol.65, No.9, (February 2011), pp. 880-891, ISSN 1098-2396

Zimmermann, V. & Hossmann, K.A. (1975). Resuscitation of the Monkey Brain after One Hour's Complete Ischemia. II. Brain Water and Electrolytes. *Brain Research*, Vol.85, No.1, (February 1975), pp. 1-11, ISSN 0006-8993

Zornow, M.H. & Prough, D.S. (1996). Neuroprotective Properties of Calcium-channel Blockers. *New Horizons*, Vol.4, No.1, (February 1996), pp. 107-114, ISSN 1063-7389

Preconditioning and Postconditioning

Joseph T. McCabe[1], Michael W. Bentley[2] and Joseph C. O'Sullivan[2]
[1]Department of Anatomy, Physiology & Genetics, and
The Center for Neuroscience & Regenerative Medicine,
Uniformed Services University of the Health Sciences, Bethesda, Maryland
[2]U.S. Army Graduate School of Anesthesia Nursing, Graduate School,
AMEDD Center and School, Academy of Health Sciences,
Fort Sam Houston, San Antonio, Texas
USA

1. Introduction

Cerebral ischemic events from trauma, stroke, hemorrhagic shock, or other cerebral perfusion deficit, initiate a cascade of detrimental processes leading to long lasting tissue injury and poor neurological outcome. Correction of the perfusion deficit is vital. However, no interventions have been identified that protect compromised cerebral tissue during the resolution of the ischemic event.

This chapter reviews two emerging concepts: *preconditioning*, which may have therapeutic utility for the protection of patients for *planned* treatments such as surgical intervention, and *postconditioning*, which may have benefits for amelioration of deficits from ischemic events, vascular injury and accidents. Preconditioning (described below) was first described from maneuvers that induced cytoprotection by temporarily occluding vessels serving the tissue or region of interest. There are inherent risks in performing such a maneuver, so that pharmacological agents — particularly for *delayed preconditioning* (described later) — affecting the aforementioned signal transduction and genomic pathways, are a safer, more realistic area of study. Conditioning is still primarily an experimental phenomenon. However, investigators have made considerable strides in uncovering the multiple, albeit complex signal transduction pathways that mediate conditioning effects. This knowledge may help clinicians one day develop schemes for neuroprotection.

2. Ischemic preconditioning: Origins in cardiology

The preconditioning concept has roots in cardiovascular research. Ischemic preconditioning was originally described in a landmark 1986 study by Murry and associates (Murry, et al., 1986). Using a cardiac dog model, these investigators found that multiple, brief ischemic episodes protected the heart from a subsequent sustained ischemic insult. An experimental group of dogs experienced circumflex artery occlusion for 5-minute intervals with 5-minute reperfusions. This cycle was repeated a total of four times — clamping for 5 minutes and unclamping for 5 minutes. The circumflex artery was then clamped for 40 minutes. The control group of dogs had their circumflex artery occluded for 40 minutes. Surprisingly, despite the additional 20 minutes of ischemia in the preconditioned animals, cardiac damage, measured by infarct size, was significantly reduced to just ¼th of the infarct observed in the hearts of dogs in the control group. This paper was the first to demonstrate and coin the term, *ischemic preconditioning*.

2.1 Preconditioning

Preconditioning has been demonstrated in all species studied to date (rat, mouse, rabbit, dog, human, chicken, sheep, pig and including cell lines), and in all organs studied thus far, including skeletal muscle, brain, kidney, small intestine, heart, and liver (Peralta, et al., 1996; Glazier, et al., 1994; Pang, et al., 1995). Other preconditioning manipulations, such as global hypoxia (Emerson, et al., 1999) and thermal injury (Marber, et al., 1993), are also effective in protection from lasting insult. Prior to this 1986 discovery, the best pharmacological treatments (with varying reproducible results) for the protection of cardiac muscle from infarction only preserved 10-20% of tissue compared to the 75% protection afforded by preconditioning (Yellon & Downey, 2003).

Research has determined that ischemic preconditioning can be subdivided into two distinctive types; *classical* and *delayed*. In *classical* preconditioning, the protective effects of ischemia/perfusion cycles are evident within minutes after the insult and persist for 2-3 hours (Ishida, et al., 1997). Classical preconditioning is independent of protein synthesis, and is therefore dependent upon existing cellular pathways. It involves the direct modulation of energy supplies, pH regulation, Na^+ and Ca^{2+} homeostasis and caspase inactivation (Carini, & Albano, 2003). Investigations have shown many triggers can activate classical ischemic preconditioning, including agonists of G protein-coupled receptors [bradykinin (Goto, et al., 1995), opioids (Schultz, et al., 1998), norepinephrine (Hu & Nattel, 1995), adenosine (Liu, et al., 1991), potassium ATP channel (K_{ATP}) openers, such as diazoxide, pinacidil (Legtenberg, et al., 2002), succinate dehydrogenase inhibitors, such as 3-nitropropionic acid (Ockaili, et al., 2001), and volatile anesthetics, such as sevoflurane and isoflurane (Zaugg, et al., 2002)].

With classic preconditioning, a trigger event, such as brief ischemia, activates a number of intracellular pathways that lead to the protected cell phenotype. The actual sequence of these pathways has not been determined, but some components of the cascade have been identified. G-coupled receptors, for example, activate the epsilon (ε) isoform of protein kinase C (PKC-ε; Mitchell, et al., 1995; Kilts, et al., 2005), which has been implicated as the key PKC subtype involved in preconditioning. Also important is the upstream signaling molecule, phosphatidylinositol-3-kinase (PI3K; Tong, et al., 2000), and mitogen-activated protein kinases (MAPKs; Armstrong, 2004). PI3K activates the serine/threonine kinase, Akt, which inactivates the pro-apoptotic kinase glycogen synthase kinase-3 (GSK-3) via phosphorylation (Tong, et al., 2002). Phosphorylation of GSK-3, in turn, inhibits the opening of the mitochondrial permeability transition pore (mPTP). Cell apoptosis or necrosis often occurs during reperfusion due to opening of the mPTP, a large nonselective pore traversing both inner and outer membranes of mitochondria. Cytochrome c and apoptotic-inducing factor (AIF) are both released through the mPTP during ischemic reperfusion, leading to the activation of caspase and caspase-independent apoptotic pathways (Kadenbach, et al., 2011; Penninger, & Kroemer, 2003). K_{ATP} channels are key intracellular triggers of early ischemic preconditioning. This channel will be described in more detail later in this chapter.

Although not as effective as classical preconditioning, *delayed* or *late* preconditioning becomes apparent approximately 24 hours after initial preconditioning and it can persist for up to 72 hours (Ishida, et al., 1997). The most significant difference between classical and delayed preconditioning is the latter's requirement of the manufacture of new proteins needed to obtain protection; inhibition of new protein synthesis attenuates the protection derived from delayed preconditioning (Rizvi, et al., 1999).

The triggers for delayed preconditioning are similar to classical preconditioning. These include cellular stress factors (sub-lethal ischemia, heat stress, cardiac pacing), which release factors such as reactive oxygen species, adenosine, and endogenous nitric oxide (NO). NO has been determined to have no effect on classical preconditioning and is a trigger specific only for delayed preconditioning (Bolli, 2000). Endogenous preconditioning agents also initiate delayed preconditioning and include adenosine agonists, bradykinin, opioids, NO donors, acetylcholine and norepinephrine (Bolli, 2000). Exogenous agents that activate the preconditioning pathways include, diazoxide, nicorandil, some hypercholesterolemic agents, and volatile anesthetics (Gross, 2005).

Kinase intracellular pathways play a central role in delayed preconditioning, with activation of the PKC-ε isoform being particularly essential. Downstream to PKC-ε, tyrosine kinases and other kinases then activate the important transcription factor, NF-κB, which leads to the upregulation of many protective proteins in the nucleus. Some key proteins identified thus far include: inducible NO synthase (iNOS) (Takano, et al., 1998, cyclooxygenase (COX-2) (Shinmura, et al., 2000), the antioxidant enzyme superoxide dismutase (SOD) (Hoshida, et al., 2002), and heat shock proteins, HSP70, HSP25, and HSP32 (Bolli, 2000). Delayed preconditioning also reduces apoptosis by upregulating the anti-apoptotic protein, Bcl-2, which has been shown to inhibit opening of the mPTP, leading to cell survival (Maulik, et al., 1999). Mitochondrial K_{ATP} (mK_{ATP}) channel opening seems to be the final common pathway for these signaling pathways but it is not yet clear how the opening of these channels affords protection. Delayed preconditioning requires the opening of the mK_{ATP} channels during the ischemic event; its role after 24 hours, when delayed preconditioning occurs, is less clear (Takano, et al., 2000).

By 1993, an appreciable number of studies had confirmed that the direct application of various stimuli (hypoxia, ischemia, triggering agents) resulted in tissue and organ protection. In that year, however, Przyklenk and colleagues made a startling discovery. Using a canine model in which the circumflex artery was occluded (as in Murry's 1986 study), Przyklenk and colleagues observed that cardiac muscle supplied by the descending left coronary artery was also protected from ischemic insult, indicating that the preconditioning stimulus offered protection that was not confined to one area of an organ (Przyklenk, et al., 1993). Further experiments have shown *remote* classical ischemic preconditioning also is effective in other organs. A preconditioning trigger in one area of an organ offers protection to a different region of that same organ or to a different organ. For example, one group demonstrated that intermittent tourniquet application to a hind limb (ischemic preconditioning) implemented protection in other skeletal muscles (Addison, et al., 2003). Remote classical preconditioning of the heart was also obtained via transient ischemia of the small intestine (Liem, et al., 2005; Patel, et al., 2002) or the kidney (Gho, et al., 1996). Other studies have demonstrated remote delayed preconditioning. Induction of small intestine ischemia, for example, engenders myocardial protection 24-72 hours later (Wang, et al., 2001; Xiao, et al., 2001).

The precise mechanism of remote ischemic preconditioning is unknown, but putative factors have been identified. Protection from kidney or intestinal preconditioning on cardiac muscle was eliminated with application of the ganglionic blocker, hexamethonium, suggesting involvement of a neuronal pathway (Gho, et al., 1996). However, stronger evidence exists that a humoral factor may play a more important role. Effluent from a preconditioned heart, transferred by whole blood transfusion, protected a non-conditioned heart from ischemic insult (Dickson, et al., 1999a; 1999b). Remote preconditioning was not activated by adenosine or bradykinin, but was found to be attenuated by the opioid antagonist, naloxone, suggesting opioid receptor involvement (Dickson, et al., 2001).

2.2 Postconditioning

One promising approach for neuroprotective therapies may be derived from *postconditioning*, where supportive measures are employed following an injury. Postconditioning is very similar to preconditioning with the exception of the temporal relationship of the protective maneuver in respect to the prolonged period of ischemia. Preconditioning is an intervention that occurs *prior to* injury while postconditioning interventions occur *after* an injury has occurred and thus may be more clinically relevant. The origin of postconditioning stems from the work of Okamoto and colleagues (Okamoto, et al., 1986). Okamoto's group established that post-ischemic damage could be limited by the use of timely low-pressure reperfusion. Following a period of ischemia, dog hearts were reperfused either with the sudden release of a coronary occlusion, or by low-pressure (40 to 50 mm Hg) coronary reperfusion with normal blood for 20 minutes before completely removing the coronary occlusion. This maneuver focused on the initial stage of reperfusion and established the basis for novel postconditioning approaches to resuscitation. Years later, Mizumura et al. (1995) first demonstrated pharmacological postconditioning. Mizumura's group used the K_{ATP} channel opener, bimakalin. Bimakalin markedly reduced cardiac infarct size in dogs when given 10 minutes before and during the 60-minute coronary reperfusion period following a set time of occlusive hypoxia. Collectively, these initial findings firmly established the concept of postconditioning and emphasized a critical factor that altering the initial moments of reperfusion was beneficial.

In 2003, Zhao and colleagues (2003) first used the term *postconditioning*. They found in a model of occlusive hypoxia in dogs that short, repeated (or stuttered) periods of arterial occlusion and release of previously occluded coronary arteries (three occlusions of 30 seconds each) prior to restoration of perfusion reduced infarct area by 44% as compared to controls. This was an example of a mechanical postconditioning intervention and implied that the first minute of reperfusion is critical in thwarting cellular demise. These findings were further validated by Kin et al. (2004). Kin and colleagues stated that the first minute of reperfusion in the rat was crucial for postconditioning. Three cycles of 10 seconds of coronary occlusion and 10 seconds of coronary release, preceding a full coronary occlusion release, decreased cardiac infarct size by 23%. In the broadest sense, the cellular processes activated by postconditioning are analogous to those activated by preconditioning, and the sole difference between the two interventions is the timing related to the prolonged period of ischemia.

3. Signaling processes linked to preconditioning and postconditioning

Many studies have investigated the mechanism of postconditioning with the aspiration to utilize this powerful protective system in the clinical setting. Recent observations from the employment of mechanical and pharmacological postconditioning suggest the activation of mitochondrial K_{ATP} (mK_{ATP}) channels initiates a series of events that close the mitochondrial permeability transition pore (mPTP) and converge onto the Reperfusion Injury Survival Kinase (RISK) Pathway.

3.1 K_{ATP} channels

K_{ATP} channels were first discovered in 1983 by A. Noma in a patch clamp study using cardiac muscle membrane preparations (Noma, 1983). There are cell surface K_{ATP} (sK_{ATP}) and mitochondrial K_{ATP} (mK_{ATP}) forms. Pharmacologically, these are different channels, but their opening (via PKC or pharmacological agents) leads to increased cell survival. One hypothesis is that activation of K_{ATP} channels hyperpolarizes the cell membrane thereby protecting the cell from detrimental depolarization (Kirino, 2002). In 1997, Garlid and coworkers presented evidence that mK_{ATP} channels have a cardioprotectve role in ischemia and reperfusion, and were a component in the mechanism for preconditioning (Garlid, et al., 1997). A prototypical mK_{ATP} channel, as reviewed by Aguilar-Bryan and Bryan (1999), is an octameric structure consisting of four sulfonylurea receptor (SUR1 or SUR2) subunits and four K^+ inward-rectifying (Kir6.1 or Kir6.2) subunits. Attached to the SUR subunits are two nucleotide binding domains (NBD). The mK_{ATP} channel is activated in low energy states by ADP, binding to NBDs, allowing the influx of K^+ into the mitochondrial inner matrix. Conversely, the mK_{ATP} channel is inhibited in high energy states when ATP closes the Kir channel. In the brain, it appears the predominant subtypes are SUR2 and Kir6.2, although the SUR1 and Kir6.1 subunits are present in smaller amounts (Lacza, et al., 2003). The mK_{ATP} channel may trigger preconditioning or postconditioning via mechanisms dependent on matrix volume stabilization, respiratory inhibition, controlled production of reactive oxygen species (ROS), and the closure of the mPTP.

The physiological functions of mK_{ATP} channels have been debated. The activities of the mK_{ATP} channel and the K^+/H^+ exchanger are believed to maintain K^+ homeostasis within mitochondria by controlling mitochondrial volume and moderating the outer-to-inner pH gradient needed to drive ATP synthesis. In the presence of hypoxia, whole cell pH decreases and ATP production declines. This causes a switch to anaerobic metabolism. A decrease in pH combined with an increase in the AMP/ADP ratio secondary to ATP metabolism causes the mK_{ATP} channel to open allowing the influx of K^+ into the inner matrix. This, in turn, activates the K^+(out)/H^+(in) exchanger decreasing the hydrogen gradient between the outer membrane and inner matrix (Szewczyk & Marbán, 1999). By doing so, the proton motive forces driving ATP production are attenuated and mitochondria energetics slow. During this time, the mPTP is closed as membrane stability and electrical potential are better maintained by the simultaneous activity of the mK_{ATP} channel and the K^+/H^+ exchanger. In addition, reactive oxygen species (ROS) generation is proportional to the availability of oxygen and activation of mK_{ATP} channel appears to moderate ROS production (Ferranti, et al., 2003; Saitoh, et al., 2006). However, this effect is only protective to a limited extent. For example, a moderate or controlled production of ROS signals promote prosurvival signaling while excessive ROS production promotes apoptotic signaling.

As anaerobic metabolism continues in response to an extended period of severe hypoxia, ATP hydrolysis exceeds ATP generation causing a dramatic rise in H^+ within the cell and mitochondrial inner matrix. At some point H^+ entry becomes lethal as it exceeds the outward pumping capacity of the mitochondrial electron transport chain already hindered by anaerobic metabolism. This results in a total loss of proton motive force driving ATP production. If prolonged, this loss results in osmotic matrix swelling, mitochondrial degradation, and release of apoptotic proteins such as cytochrome C.

Upon resolution of a perfusion defect, abrupt reperfusion following prolonged ischemia results in a substantial amount of ROS generation. Following restoration of flow to intact but vulnerable cells, ATP levels begin to rise, mK_{ATP} channels close and K^+ transport into the mitochondrial matrix declines. This indirectly decreases the activity of the K^+/H^+ exchanger. As H^+ ions are rapidly removed from the matrix during mitochondrial respiration, the inner matrix quickly alkalinizes, causing the mPTP to open (Vinten-Johansen, et al., 2007). Opening the mPTP rapidly elevates inner matrix osmotic pressure leading to matrix distension and if allowed to remain open, mitochondrial rupture.

In total, mK_{ATP} channel closure associated with abrupt reperfusion cand result in the significant elevation of ROS and increase the mitochondrial inner matrix osmotic pressure, causing the mitochondria to quickly swell or rupture, releasing apoptotic factors such as cytochrome C (Armstrong, 2004). It is reasonable to suggest that maintaining the patency of the mK_{ATP} channel would be beneficial during reperfusion. Allowing the mK_{ATP} channel to remain open during reperfusion could: 1) moderate the generation of ROS, 2) reduce osmotic force within the matrix by promoting ion exchange, and 3) reduce the activity of the mPTP thereby providing a protective effect.

Activation of mK_{ATP} channels have been shown to be protective during reperfusion in cardiac and brain tissue (Obal, et al., 2005; O'Sullivan, et al., 2007; Penna, et al., 2007; Wu, et al., 2006). Obal and colleagues (2005), for example, demonstrated the utility of inhaling volatile anesthetics as a postconditioning trigger through mK_{ATP} channel activation. In rats subjected to cardiac ischemia, postconditioning was invoked by administering 1 minimum alveolar concentration (MAC) of sevoflurane for 2 minutes with the onset of reperfusion. This resulted in a significant decrease in cardiac infarct size. Penna et al. (2007, isolated rat hearts and exposed them to an ischemic period followed by reperfusion. Their results suggested that postconditioning mechanisms are activated by a bradykinin or a diazoxide mechanism resulting in the upregulation of protein kinase G (PKG). This upregulation was dependent on early ROS generation triggered by mK_{ATP} channel activation. They emphasized that their results were different from mechanical manipulations by showing that pharmacological agents, such as bradykinin or diazoxide, administered during the reperfusion period could induce protection. ROS also regulate the activity of heat shock proteins (HSPs). Using an *in vitro* vascular smooth muscle preparation, Madamanchi and colleagues (2001) discovered that the application of H_2O_2 significantly upregulated HSP70.

3.2 mPTPs

As previously mentioned, the mPTP is inhibited with the activation of mK_{ATP}. The existence of the mPTP was confirmed in 1992 in rat liver mitoblast membranes (Szabó & Zoratti, 1992). The primary components of the mPTP are the voltage-dependent anion channel in the outer membrane, the adenine nucleotide translocator, and the cyclophilin D protein within the matrix (Lin & Lechleiter, 2002). In general, it is thought that the opening of the mPTP occurs with a decrease in the inner matrix potential, decreased AMP and ADP levels, increased matrix Ca^{2+}, with alkalinization, or during oxidative stress (Gateau-Roesch, et al., 2006). mPTP opening blocks ATP formation and allows for the equilibration of small molecules (Gateau-Roesch, et al., 2006; Halestrap, 2004). mPTP opening increases osmotic forces within the mitochondria inner matrix and leads to degradation of the matrix membrane, causing the release of apoptotic factors, especially cytochrome C (Honda, et al., 2005). Also, as the mitochondrial membrane potential is perturbed, ATP synthase reverses its primary function and serves as an ATPase; further depleting cellular ATP concentrations and increasing H^+ levels.

Feng and colleagues (2005) determined that volatile anesthesia-induced postconditioning prevented the opening of the mPTP by inhibiting glycogen synthase kinase 3β (GSKβ). This inactivation was a result of PI3K-AKT signaling pathway inactivation with the resulting phosphorylation and inactivation of GSKβ, which protected against reperfusion damage. Argaud et al. (2005) found that mechanical postconditioning decreased cellular Ca^{2+} and protected *in vivo* rabbit hearts, suggesting that the mPTP could be inhibited by the PI3K-AKT-eNOS cascade. Bopassa et al. (2006), using a rat heart preparation undergoing postconditioning, concluded that PI3K signaling regulates the closure of mPTP. In addition, Cohen, Yan, and Downey (2007) observed that postconditioning prevented mPTP opening as a result of inhaled CO_2-induced acidosis during the first minutes of reperfusion. They suggested that low cellular pH inhibits the opening of mPTP in heart tissue, but as the cellular pH normalizes, the inhibition of mPTP is lost. They hypothesized that by maintaining the cellular pH at a lower level while introducing oxygen during reperfusion, it was possible to keep the mPTP closed allowing the redox signaling necessary to trigger preconditioning-like protection. Cohen, Yan, and Downey further suggest that moderate acidosis during reperfusion might be protective. This hypothesis was addressed through the use of sodium bicarbonate ($NaHCO_3$) during postconditioning. In isolated rabbit hearts, acidic CO_2 perfusate at the time of reperfusion mimicked postconditioning while an alkaline $NaHCO_3$ perfusate blocked that effect. They hypothesized that an acidic environment inhibited mPTP opening while an alkaline environment favored mPTP opening. Fujita and colleagues (2007) also hypothesized that $NaHCO_3$ would blunt the protective properties of postconditioning. Using *in vivo* dog hearts that underwent ischemia, the administration of $NaHCO_3$ during four intermittent cycles of one-minute reperfusion with one-minute reocclusion of a coronary vessel completely abolished the postconditioning effects. Their results suggested that postconditioning leads to the opening of mK_{ATP} channels as a result of decreased pH, leading to the attenuation of cardiac infarct size.

3.3 Reperfusion Survival Kinase Pathway

The Reperfusion Injury Survival Kinase (RISK) pathway begins with the activation of PI3K and ERK to promote cell survival. RISK can be activated by insulin, urocortin, atorvastatin, adenosine, bradykinin, opioid agonists, volatile anesthetics, or diazoxide (Bell & Yellon, 2003a,b; Chiari, et al., 2005; Gross, et al., 2004; Jonassen, et al., 2001; Schulman, et al., 2002; Wang, et al., 2004; Yang, et al., 2004). The RISK pathway promotes pro-survival signaling while inhibiting pathways associated with apoptosis. In 2004, Tsang and colleagues (2004) reported that in isolated rat hearts, which had undergone mechanical postconditioning following a period of ischemia, postconditioning is mediated by the PI3K-AKT-eNOS/p70s6K pathway. They also suggested MEK 1/2-ERK 1/2 pathways were indirectly involved. Zhu and coworkers (2006) followed by finding that cardioprotection from postconditioning in the remodeled rat myocardium is regulated through PI3K-AKT signaling. The role of ERK 1/2 was addressed by Darling et al. (2005) and Krolikowski et al. (2006). Darling and colleagues utilized mechanical postconditioning in isolated rabbit hearts and found ERK1/2 but not PI3K activity provided cardiac protection. Krolikowski and colleagues exposed rabbits to isoflurane before and during early reperfusion and suggested a central role of ERK1/2, p70s6k, and eNOS in anesthetic-induced postconditioning.

Downstream in the RISK pathway, phosphorylation of AKT occurs with the subsequent phosphorylation of protein kinase C (PKC) and GSKβ. When PKC is phosphorylated it is stimulated while the phosphorylation of GSKβ inhibits its activity. In a rabbit model, Philipp and colleagues (2006) demonstrated through inhibitor studies that adenosine, PKC, and PI3K mediated the effects of mechanical postconditioning. In their investigation, they concluded that protection was conferred through the activation of adenosine receptors by endogenous adenosine, a cellular metabolite. This, in turn, activated the PI3K component of the RISK pathway resulting in activation of PKC. In regards to GSKβ, Feng and colleagues (2005), using isoflurane as a postconditioning trigger along with an AKT inhibitor, showed that when inhaled early in reperfusion, isoflurane phosphorylated AKT and GSKβ. Phosphorylated GSKβ was inhibited and could not promote the opening of mPTP. They also determined that while the PI3K-AKT signal was strong, the ERK1/2-p38 MAPK was not altered. This suggests a primary role of PI3K-AKT in the RISK pathway and in mPTP closure. Recently, in human tissue, it has been found that the cytoprotective proteins, HSP25 and HSP70, are upregulated by the PI3K-AKT pathway (Dickson, et al., 2001).

3.4 The heat shock response

Both preconditioning and postconditioning upregulate proteins identified as Heat Shock Proteins (HSPs), specifically HSP25 and HSP70. The heat shock response was discovered in 1962. *Drosophilia* larvae, when heated, developed puffing patterns in certain chromosomal regions. This suggested a change in the synthetic activity of the chromosomal bands concerned (Ritossa, 1962). Sixteen years later, the RNA for *Drosophilia* exposed to a thermal stimulus was coded using hybrid-arrested translation and indicated that proteins of 83, 72, 70, 68, 28, 26, 23 and 22 kilodaltons were upregulated (Livak, et al., 1978). Over the following decades, the investigation of the heat shock response has confirmed that a family of highly conserved HSPs is upregulated following a variety of sublethal stressors, possibly as a result of non-native proteins accumulating in a stressed cell (Voellmy & Boellmann, 2007). These proteins are subcategorized by their molecular weight and are either inherently present or can be induced following sublethal stress (O'Sullivan, et al., 2008). In particular, HSP25 and HSP70 have been thoroughly investigated with the consensus being they are protective when upregulated following stress (Beere, et al., 2000; Garrido, et al., 2006; Takayama, et al., 2003).

3.4.1 Heat Shock Protein 25/27

HSP25 is the rodent equivalent of the primate HSP27 and often the terms are used interchangeably. HSP27 confers protection at different levels as it can interact with several proteins implicated in cell death based upon its phosphorylation and oligomerization condition and not upon ATP. The main mechanisms for how HSP27 confers cytoprotection appear to be: molecular chaperoning, interference with cell death pathways, signaling of antiapoptotic pathways, stabilization of the cytoskeleton, and antioxidant activities. Serving as a chaperone, HSP27 can bind folded intermediate non-native proteins, inhibiting their aggregation, and in the presence of HSP70 these HSP27-bound proteins can be reactivated (Ehrnsperger, et al., 1997). Within the cytosol, HSP27 can sequester cytochrome C;

interfering with the formation of the apoptotic protease activating factor-1 (APAF-1)-cytochrome c multimeric apoptosome and the activation of procaspase 9 (Bruey, et al., 2000; Concannon, et al., 2001; Garrido, et al., 1999). HSP27 also directly interacts with procaspase-3, decreasing the activity of activated caspase-3 (Concannon, et al., 2001). HSP27 serves as a signaling messenger by causing the activation of serine/threonine kinase Akt thereby inhibiting Bcl-2 and caspase-9 (Cardone, et al., 1998). HSP25/27 has other actions. Phosphorylated HSP27 can stabilize F-actin and increase the number of cells retaining microfilament organization thus stabilizing membrane structure (Lavoie, et al., 1995). Additionally, HSP27 is able to increase glutathione levels, thereby reducing levels of ROS (Kretz-Remy, et al., 1996).

3.4.2 Heat Shock Protein 70

Over the last three decades, HSP70 has become the most thoroughly investigated protein of the HSP family of proteins. Like HSP25, HSP70 can inhibit cell death at various sites within the cell. However, unlike HSP25, HSP70 function is "ATP-dependent." HSP70 is typically found *in vivo* bound by ATP and HSP70 function is typically based upon the hydrolysis of the attached ATP molecule. HSP70 serves as a chaperone protein, inhibits stress signaling, prevents mitochondrial membrane permeabilization, and inhibits apoptotic pathways. HSP70 may chaperone kinases by binding to an unfolded carboxyl terminus, preventing aggregation, and allowing re-autophosphorylation of the kinase enzyme; thus stabilizing the enzyme and restoring function (Gao & Newton, 2002). HSP70 also binds the death receptors, DR4 and DR5, inhibiting Apo-2L/TRAIL-induced cell death (Guo, et al., (2005), and HSP70 blocks Bax translocation into the mitochondrial outer membrane. The latter effect prevents the permeabilization of the mitochondrial membrane and subsequent release of apoptosis-inducing factor (AIF) and cytochrome C (Stankiewicz , et al., 2005). HSP70 binds AIF within the cytosol; inhibiting its nuclear translocation and limiting nuclear condensation (Ruchalski, et al., 2006). Similar to HSP25, HSP70 prevents cell death by binding to Apaf-1 and interfering in the formation of the apoptosome complex and subsequent recruitment of procaspase-9 (Beere, et al., 2000). Lastly, HSP70 suppresses apoptotic signaling by binding precursor forms of caspase-3 and caspase-7; preventing their cleavage and activation (Komarova, et al., 2004).

3.5 Cleaved caspase 3

Both HSP25 and HSP70 inhibit the cleavage of caspase-3 (Concannon, et al., 2001; Komarova, et al., 2004). Cleaved caspase-3 (CC3) is a primary executioner of apoptosis as it is responsible for the total or partial proteolytic cleavage of numerous key cellular survival proteins (Fernandes-Alnemri , et al., 1994). One of those proteins being the abundant nuclear enzyme polymerase, which functions in DNA repair and protein modification during oxidative stress (Smith, 2001). Thus, induction of HSP25 and HSP70 may alleviate cerebral ischemic injury and resuscitation injury that results from the mitochondrial release of cytochrome C with subsequent cleavage of caspase-3.

4. Evidence of preconditioning and postconditioning in the brain

Wu and colleagues (Wu, et al., 2006) directly examined the roles of mPTP and the mK_{ATP} channel in preconditioning and postconditioning in a rat model of cerebral stroke. These investigators activated the mK_{ATP} channel with diazoxide 20 minutes before middle cerebral artery occlusion followed by reperfusion, or inhibited the mPTP by infusion of cyclosporin A 15 minutes before reperfusion. It was discovered that both measures significantly increased functional performance scores and reduced infarction volumes. Importantly, both of these effects were abolished by blocking the adenine nucleotide port located on the mPTP. Their results strongly suggested that the mK_{ATP} channel and mPTP activity during reperfusion share a common protective pathway; the Reperfusion Survival Kinase Pathway (RISK). More recently, Feng, Rhodes, and Bhatt (2010) discovered that hypoxic preconditioning could invoke neuroprotection through the activation of AKT, a kinase that is part of the aforementioned RISK pathway. These investigators subjected newborn rats to 3 hours of 8% oxygen followed by 24 hours of reoxygenation. Following reoxygenation, the right carotid artery was permanently ligated and again the rats were subjected to 8% oxygen but for 140 minutes instead of 3 hours. Compared to rats subjected to normoxia prior to carotid ligation, preconditioned rats had a significant reduction in cerebral injury. It was found that preconditioning preserved RISK pathway signaling and attenuated caspase-3 activity.

Acute models of postconditioning have emphasized the benefit of cerebral reperfusion under controlled conditions. For example, several groups have shown that carefully controlled periods of reperfusion, before the full return of cerebral circulation, results in reduced injury. Zhao and colleagues (2006) employed permanent middle cerebral artery occlusion in combination with transient common carotid artery occlusions. Shorter periods of repeated common carotid occlusion resulted in a reduction in infarct size. Pignataro, et al. (2008) also employed middle cerebral artery occlusion for 100 minutes. Reperfusion of the artery that included a 10-minute period of occlusion was found to be the most effective, although intermittent occlusions were also beneficial. Gao, Ren and Zhao (2008) found that three cycles of reperfusion of the common carotid artery, in conjunction with permanent middle artery occlusion, reduced infarct size, while ten cycles was not effective. These publications, as well as numerous reports with cardiac models, emphasis the criticality of the duration of cerebral ischemia (longer periods of ischemia result in more cerebral damage, including irreversibility), as well as the essential specifics of the timing, duration, number of cycles, and inter-reperfusion intervals for effective postconditioning.

As well, recent work has shown the benefit of pharmacological postconditioning in cerebral ischemia. O'Sullivan and colleagues (2007) employed a rat model of combined hemorrhagic shock and permanent unilateral common carotid artery occlusion. The administration of diazoxide at the time of hemorrhagic resuscitation significantly increased the expression of heat shock proteins in the cerebral cortex and hippocampus. Robin and colleagues (2011), using a middle cerebral artery occlusion model, found that in Wistar strain rats ischemic postconditioning decreased infarct size by 40% and improved neurological outcomes. Specifically, pharmacological postconditioning by diazoxide administration decreased cerebral infarct by 60%. In addition, these beneficial effects in both ischemic postconditioning and diazoxide postconditioning were blocked through the use of the K_{ATP} blocker, 5-hydroxydecanoate (5-HD), which blocked the inhibition of the mPTP opening caused by ischemic postconditioning and diazoxide.

In 2011, Wang and colleagues discovered that selective delta opioid peptide [D-Ala2, D-Leu5] enkephalin (DADLE) provided a postconditioning effect by protecting hippocampal CA1 neurons in a model of forebrain ischemia. In this investigation, DADLE triggered postconditioning neuroprotection for hippocampal CA1 neurons and improved spatial learning and memory in rats. This protection was dependent upon DADLE-induced activation of the PI3K/Akt signaling.

5. Conclusion

As reviewed, the majority of research related to pre- and post-conditioning has not been performed in studies related to cerebral ischemia. As recently stated by Keep and colleagues (2010), the question remains—"Is there a place for cerebral preconditioning in the clinic?" The clinical utility of cerebral conditioning is potentially limited by issues of safety, the relatively narrow therapeutic window, and the need to present the stimulus before the injury.

Brief periods of ischemia can enact classical and delayed conditioning. These momentary periods of ischemia have been shown to protect neuronal cells *in vitro* and to reduce injury *in vivo* in several experiment models and species (Koch, 2010). Since safety issues prevent deliberately inducing conditioning by cerebrovascular occlusion, research has focused on pharmacological agents, including volatile anesthetics, inhibitors of cellular metabolism, K_{ATP} channel activators, and inflammatory mediators (Keep, et al., 2010). Other agents that have been effective in producing conditioning are hyperbaric oxygen, cooling and hyperthermia, and acupuncture (Keep, et al., 2010). Recent research has also given credence to remote conditioning where ischemia to a hindlimb (e.g., by application of a tourniquet) protects the brain from later middle cerebral artery occlusion. Remote preconditioning or ischemia probably has the most practical use for clinical utilization. However, currently there are no clinical data to strongly support the use of any type of conditioning for brain protection.

From a clinical standpoint, a major problem with the application of conditioning is timing. With the exception of a planned neurosurgical intervention, classically employed technique such as vascular clamping is impractible as a pretreatment. Pharmacological agents, then. Given at the time of reperfusion may hold promise. Agents such as $MgSO_4$, erythropoietin, anti-hypertension drugs, anticoagulants, and statins all given to patients at risk for stroke have shown limited damage from a stroke should it occur (Keep, et al., 2010).

In addition, there is still little *clinical* evidence from basic research regarding the use of preconditioning for neuroprotection. Research models currently in use have at least four important limitations. First, experiments are routinely conducted on young, disease-free animals (Koch, 2010). The majority of patients who suffer cerebral ischemic events are older, and may have artherosclerosis, cardiac or kidney disease, or other co-morbidities, such as obesity, hypertension, diabetes, as well as additional risk factors such as sedentary lifestyle, and tobacco, alcohol, or illicit drug abuse. The 'chronic' ischemic state of these patients, with a chronic conditioning compensatory state, may not allow further conditioning protection with interventions. Secondly, both Keep, et al. (2010) and Koch (2010) noted that the effect of medications used by patients has a potential to interfere with preconditioning effects. Do certain prescribed medications or self-administered substances such as herbal products interfere with the conditioning signaling pathways? Third, the neuroprotective cascade might be very specific to gender, diet, genetic background, and age (Dirnagl, et al., 2009). Lastly, major issues to be resolved include determination of doses of preconditioning drugs that are safe and whether premorbid conditions, for example intermittent transient ischemic events, act as a conditioning stimulus event (Dirnagl, et al., 2009; Keep, et al., 2010; Koch, 2010).

Finally, optimal neuroprotection may be a combination of physiological manipulations (e.g., body temperature regulation) and pharmacological treatment(s). Gidday (2010) provides an excellent overview of the current state of pharmacological approaches for neuroprotection. Related to the present review, the translational possibilities require continued bench science to characterize the signal transduction pathways mediating neuroprotection, and whether or not they have potential clinical applicability. There are many "gaps" in understanding the mechanisms of action of the >20 drugs presently known to be beneficial (Gidday, 2010), and we must determine how best to employ these agents.

The landmark study by Murry and colleagues on cardiac tissue heralded new and exciting research regarding classic and delayed and remote preconditioning as well as the more clinically important postconditioning effect. Research continues with pharmacological or physical manipulations that can mimic pre- or post- conditioning and this could eventually have significant clinical ramifications. Further work is needed that considers the aforementioned limitations. Reducing the long-term effect of stroke or traumatic brain injury by preserving ischemic tissue can vastly improve the quality of life for patients. Likewise, billions of dollars saved from long-term care requirements, lost wages, family care-giver issues, and the reduced burden on our health care system will all stand to benefit from progress in this critical field of study.

6. Acknowledgments

The views expressed in this work are those of the authors and do not reflect those of the United States Army, Department of Defense, or the United States Governmental Institution.

7. References

Addison, P. D., Neligan, P. C., Ashrafpour, H., Khan, A., Zhong, A., Moses, M., Forrest, C. R. & Pang, C. Y. (2003). Noninvasive remote ischemic preconditioning for global protection of skeletal muscle against infarction. *Am J Physiol Heart Circ Physiol*, Vol. 285, No. 4, pp. H1435-H1443

Aguilar-Bryan, L. & Bryan, J. (1999). Molecular biology of adenosine triphosphate-sensitive potassium channels. *Endocr Rev*, Vol. 20, No. 2, pp. 101-135

Argaud, L., Gateau-Roesch, O., Muntean, D., Chalabreysse, L., Loufouat, J., Robert, D. & Ovize, M. (2005). Specific inhibition of the mitochondrial permeability transition prevents lethal reperfusion injury. *J Mol Cell Cardiol*, Vol. 38, No. 2, pp. 367-374

Armstrong, S. C. (2004). Protein kinase activation and myocardial ischemia/reperfusion injury. *Cardiovasc Res*, Vol. 61, No. 3, pp. 427-436

Beere, H. M., Wolf, B. B., Cain, K., Mosser, D. D., Mahboubi, A., Kuwana, T., Tailor, P., Morimoto, R. I., Cohen, G. M. & Green, D. R. (2000). Heat-shock protein 70 inhibits apoptosis by preventing recruitment of procaspase-9 to the Apaf-1 apoptosome. *Nat Cell Biol*, Vol. 2, No. 8, pp. 469-475

Bell, R. M. & Yellon, D. M. (2003a). Atorvastatin, administered at the onset of reperfusion, and independent of lipid lowering, protects the myocardium by up-regulating a pro-survival pathway. *J Am Coll Cardiol*, Vol. 41, No. 3, pp. 508-515

Bell, R. M. & Yellon, D. M. (2003b). Bradykinin limits infarction when administered as an adjunct to reperfusion in mouse heart: the role of PI3K, Akt and eNOS. *J Mol Cell Cardiol*, Vol. 35, No. 2, pp. 185-193

Bolli, R. (2000). The late phase of preconditioning. *Circ Res*, Vol. 87, No. 11, pp. 972-983

Bopassa, J.-C., Ferrera, R., Gateau-Roesch, O., Couture-Lepetit, E. & Ovize, M. (2006). PI 3-kinase regulates the mitochondrial transition pore in controlled reperfusion and postconditioning. *Cardiovasc Res*, Vol. 69, No. 1, pp. 178-185

Bruey, J. M., Ducasse, C., Bonniaud, P., Ravagnan, L., Susin, S. A., Diaz-Latoud, C., Gurbuxani, S., Arrigo, A. P., Kroemer, G., Solary, E. & Garrido, C. (2000). Hsp27 negatively regulates cell death by interacting with cytochrome c. *Nat Cell Biol*, Vol. 2, No. 9, pp. 645-652

Cardone, M. H., Roy, N., Stennicke, H. R., Salvesen, G. S., Franke, T. F., Stanbridge, E., Frisch, S. & Reed, J. C. (1998). Regulation of cell death protease caspase-9 by phosphorylation. *Science*, Vol. 282, No. 5392, pp. 1318-1321

Carini, R. & Albano, E. (2003). Recent insights on the mechanisms of liver preconditioning. *Gastroenterology*, Vol. 125, No. 5, pp. 1480-1491

Chiari, P. C., Bienengraeber, M. W., Pagel, P. S., Krolikowski, J. G., Kersten, J. R. & Warltier, D. C. (2005). Isoflurane protects against myocardial infarction during early reperfusion by activation of phosphatidylinositol-3-kinase signal transduction: evidence for anesthetic-induced postconditioning in rabbits. *Anesthesiology*, Vol. 102, No. 1, pp. 102-109

Cohen, M. V., Yang, X.-M. & Downey, J. M. (2007). The pH hypothesis of postconditioning: staccato reperfusion reintroduces oxygen and perpetuates myocardial acidosis. *Circulation*, Vol. 115, No. 14, pp. 1895-1903

Concannon, C. G., Orrenius, S. & Samali, A. (2001). Hsp27 inhibits cytochrome c-mediated caspase activation by sequestering both pro-caspase-3 and cytochrome c. *Gene Expr*, Vol. 9, No. 4-5, pp. 195-201

Darling, C. E., Jiang, R., Maynard, M., Whittaker, P., Vinten-Johansen, J. & Przyklenk, K. (2005). Postconditioning via stuttering reperfusion limits myocardial infarct size in rabbit hearts: role of ERK1/2. *Am J Physiol Heart Circ Physiol*, Vol. 289, No. 4, pp. H1618-H1626

Dickson, E. W., Blehar, D. J., Carraway, R. E., Heard, S. O., Steinberg, G. & Przyklenk, K. (2001). Naloxone blocks transferred preconditioning in isolated rabbit hearts. *J Mol Cell Cardiol*, Vol. 33, No. 9, pp. 1751-1756

Dickson, E. W., Lorbar, M., Porcaro, W. A., Fenton, R. A., Reinhardt, C. P., Gysembergh, A. & Przyklenk, K. (1999a). Rabbit heart can be "preconditioned" via transfer of coronary effluent. *Am J Physiol*, Vol. 277, No. 6 Pt 2, pp. H2451-H2457

Dickson, E. W., Reinhardt, C. P., Renzi, F. P., Becker, R. C., Porcaro, W. A. & Heard, S. O. (1999b). Ischemic preconditioning may be transferable via whole blood transfusion: preliminary evidence. *J Thromb Thrombolysis*, Vol. 8, No. 2, pp. 123-129

Dirnagl, U., K. Becker, &A. Meisel (2009). Preconditioning and tolerance against cerebral ischaemia: from experimental strategies to clinical use. *Lancet Neurol*, Vol. 8, No. 4, pp. 398-412

Ehrnsperger, M., Gräber, S., Gaestel, M. & Buchner, J. (1997). Binding of non-native protein to Hsp25 during heat shock creates a reservoir of folding intermediates for reactivation. *EMBO J*, Vol. 16, No. 2, pp. 221-229

Emerson, M. R., Nelson, S. R., Samson, F. E. & Pazdernik, T. L. (1999). Hypoxia preconditioning attenuates brain edema associated with kainic acid-induced status epilepticus in rats. *Brain Res*, Vol. 825, No. 1-2, pp. 189-193

Feng, J., Lucchinetti, E., Ahuja, P., Pasch, T., Perriard, J.-C. & Zaugg, M. (2005). Isoflurane postconditioning prevents opening of the mitochondrial permeability transition pore through inhibition of glycogen synthase kinase 3beta. *Anesthesiology*, Vol. 103, No. 5, pp. 987-995

Feng, Y., Rhodes, P. G. & Bhatt, A. J. (2010). Hypoxic preconditioning provides neuroprotection and increases vascular endothelial growth factor A, preserves the phosphorylation of Akt-Ser-473 and diminishes the increase in caspase-3 activity in neonatal rat hypoxic-ischemic model. *Brain Res*, Vol. 1325, 1-9

Fernandes-Alnemri, T., Litwack, G. & Alnemri, E. S. (1994). CPP32, a novel human apoptotic protein with homology to *Caenorhabditis elegans* cell death protein Ced-3 and mammalian interleukin-1 beta-converting enzyme. *J Biol Chem*, Vol. 269, No. 49, pp. 30761-30764

Ferranti, R., da Silva, M. M. & Kowaltowski, A. J. (2003). Mitochondrial ATP-sensitive K^+ channel opening decreases reactive oxygen species generation. *FEBS Lett*, Vol. 536, No. 1-3, pp. 51-55

Fujita, M., Asanuma, H., Hirata, A., Wakeno, M., Takahama, H., Sasaki, H., Kim, J., Takashima, S., Tsukamoto, O., Minamino, T., Shinozaki, Y., Tomoike, H., Hori, M. & Kitakaze, M. (2007). Prolonged transient acidosis during early reperfusion contributes to the cardioprotective effects of postconditioning. *Am J Physiol Heart Circ Physiol*, Vol. 292, No. 4, pp. H2004-H2008

Gao, T. & Newton, A. C. (2002). The turn motif is a phosphorylation switch that egulates the binding of Hsp70 to protein kinase C. *J Biol Chem*, Vol. 277, No. 35, pp. 31585-31592

Gao, X., Ren, C. & Zhao, H. (2008). Protective effects of ischemic postconditioning compared with gradual reperfusion or preconditioning. *J Neurosci Res*, Vol. 86, No. 11, pp. 2505-2511

Garlid, K. D., Paucek, P., Yarov-Yarovoy, V., Murray, H. N., Darbenzio, R. B., D'Alonzo, A. J., Lodge, N. J., Smith, M. A. & Grover, G. J. (1997). Cardioprotective effect of diazoxide and its interaction with mitochondrial ATP-sensitive K^+ channels. Possible mechanism of cardioprotection. *Circ Res*, Vol. 81, No. 6, pp. 1072-1082

Garrido, C., Bruey, J. M., Fromentin, A., Hammann, A., Arrigo, A. P. & Solary, E. (1999). HSP27 inhibits cytochrome c-dependent activation of procaspase-9. *FASEB J*, Vol. 13, No. 14, pp. 2061-2070

Garrido, C., Brunet, M., Didelot, C., Zermati, Y., Schmitt, E. & Kroemer, G. (2006). Heat shock proteins 27 and 70: anti-apoptotic proteins with tumorigenic properties. *Cell Cycle*, Vol. 5, No. 22, pp. 2592-2601

Gateau-Roesch, O., Argaud, L. & Ovize, M. (2006). Mitochondrial permeability transition pore and postconditioning. *Cardiovasc Res*, Vol. 70, No. 2, pp. 264-273

Gho, B. C., Schoemaker, R. G., van den Doel, M. A., Duncker, D. J. & Verdouw, P. D. (1996). Myocardial protection by brief ischemia in noncardiac tissue. *Circulation*, Vol. 94, No. 9, pp. 2193-2200

Gidday, J.M. (2010). Pharmacologic preconditioning: Translating the promise. *Transl Stroke Res*, Vol. 1, No. 1, pp. 19-30

Glazier, S. S., O'Rourke, D. M., Graham, D. I. & Welsh, F. A. (1994). Induction of ischemic tolerance following brief focal ischemia in rat brain. *J Cereb Blood Flow Metab*, Vol. 14, No. 4, pp. 545--553

Goto, M., Liu, Y., Yang, X. M., Ardell, J. L., Cohen, M. V. & Downey, J. M. (1995). Role of bradykinin in protection of ischemic preconditioning in rabbit hearts. *Circ Res*, Vol. 77, No. 3, pp. 611-621

Gross, E. R., Hsu, A. K. & Gross, G. J. (2004). Opioid-induced cardioprotection occurs via glycogen synthase kinase beta inhibition during reperfusion in intact rat hearts. *Circ Res*, Vol. 94, No. 7, pp. 960-966

Gross, G. J. (2005). Pharmacological preconditioning: Potential new treatment modalities for the ischemic myocardium. *Vascul Pharmacol*, Vol. 42, No. 5-6, pp. 199

Guo, F., Sigua, C., Bali, P., George, P., Fiskus, W., Scuto, A., Annavarapu, S., Mouttaki, A., Sondarva, G., Wei, S., Wu, J., Djeu, J., & Bhalla, K. (2005). Mechanistic role of heat shock protein 70 in Bcr-Abl-mediated resistance to apoptosis in human acute leukemia cells. *Blood*, Vol. 105, No. 3, pp. 1246-55

Halestrap, A. P. (2004). Does the mitochondrial permeability transition have a role in preconditioning?. *Circulation*, Vol. 110, No. 11, pp. e303

Honda, H. M., Korge, P. & Weiss, J. N. (2005). Mitochondria and ischemia/reperfusion injury. *Ann N Y Acad Sci*, Vol. 1047, 248-258

Hoshida, S., Yamashita, N., Otsu, K. & Hori, M. (2002). The importance of manganese superoxide dismutase in delayed preconditioning: involvement of reactive oxygen species and cytokines. *Cardiovasc Res*, Vol. 55, No. 3, pp. 495-505

Hu, K. & Nattel, S. (1995). Mechanisms of ischemic preconditioning in rat hearts. Involvement of alpha 1B-adrenoceptors, pertussis toxin-sensitive G proteins, and protein kinase C. *Circulation*, Vol. 92, No. 8, pp. 2259-2265

Ishida, T., Yarimizu, K., Gute, D. C. & Korthuis, R. J. (1997). Mechanisms of ischemic preconditioning. *Shock*, Vol. 8, No. 2, pp. 86-94

Jonassen, A. K., Sack, M. N., Mjøs, O. D. & Yellon, D. M. (2001). Myocardial protection by insulin at reperfusion requires early administration and is mediated via Akt and p70s6 kinase cell-survival signaling. *Circ Res*, Vol. 89, No. 12, pp. 1191-1198

Kadenbach, B., Ramzan, R., Moosdorf, R. & Vogt, S. (2011) The role of mitochondrial membrane potential in ischemic heart failure. *Mitochondrion*, Vol. 11, No. 5, pp. 700-706

Keep, R. F., Wang, M. M. Xiang, J. Hua, Y. & Xi, G. (2010). Is there a place for cerebral preconditioning in the clinic? *Transl Stroke Res*, Vol. 1, No. 1, pp. 4-18

Kilts, J. D., Grocott, H. P. & Kwatra, M. M., (2005). G alpha(q)-coupled receptors in human atrium function through protein kinase C epsilon and delta. *J Mol Cell Cardiol*, Vol. 38, No. 2, pp. 267-276

Kin, H., Zhao, Z.-Q., Sun, H.-Y., Wang, N.-P., Corvera, J. S., Halkos, M. E., Kerendi, F., Guyton, R. A. & Vinten-Johansen, J. (2004). Postconditioning attenuates myocardial ischemia-reperfusion injury by inhibiting events in the early minutes of reperfusion. *Cardiovasc Res*, Vol. 62, No. 1, pp. 74-85

Kirino, T. (2002). Ischemic tolerance. *J Cereb Blood Flow Metab* 22, Vol., No. 11, pp. 1283-1296

Koch, S. (2010). Preconditioning the human brain: Practical considerations for proving cerebral protection. *Transl Stroke Res*, Vol. 1, No. 3, pp. 161-169

Komarova, E. Y., Afanasyeva, E. A., Bulatova, M. M., Cheetham, M. E., Margulis, B. A. & Guzhova, I. V. (2004). Downstream caspases are novel targets for the antiapoptotic activity of the molecular chaperone hsp70. *Cell Stress Chaperones*, Vol. 9, No. 3, pp. 265-275

Kretz-Remy, C., Mehlen, P., Mirault, M. E. & Arrigo, A. P. (1996). Inhibition of I kappa B-alpha phosphorylation and degradation and subsequent NF-kappa B activation by glutathione peroxidase overexpression. *J Cell Biol*, Vol. 133, No. 5, pp. 1083-1093

Krolikowski, J. G., Weihrauch, D., Bienengraeber, M., Kersten, J. R., Warltier, D. C. & Pagel, P. S. (2006). Role of Erk1/2, p70s6K, and eNOS in isoflurane-induced cardioprotection during early reperfusion in vivo. *Can J Anaesth*, Vol. 53, No. 2, pp. 174-182

Lacza, Z., Snipes, J. A., Kis, B., Szabó, C., Grover, G. & Busija, D. W. (2003). Investigation of the subunit composition and the pharmacology of the mitochondrial ATP-dependent K^+ channel in the brain. *Brain Res*, Vol. 994, No. 1, pp. 27-36

Lavoie, J. N., Lambert, H., Hickey, E., Weber, L. A. & Landry, J. (1995). Modulation of cellular thermoresistance and actin filament stability accompanies phosphorylation-induced changes in the oligomeric structure of heat shock protein 27. *Mol Cell Biol*, Vol. 15, No. 1, pp. 505-516

Legtenberg, R. J., Rongen, G. A., Houston, R. J. E., Oeseburg, B. & Smits, P. (2002). The role of myocardial K_{ATP}-channel blockade in the protective effects of glibenclamide against ischaemia in the rat heart. *Pharmacol Toxicol*, Vol. 91, No. 2, pp. 51-56

Liem, D. A., te Lintel Hekkert, M., Manintveld, O. C., Boomsma, F., Verdouw, P. D. & Duncker, D. J. (2005). Myocardium tolerant to an adenosine-dependent ischemic preconditioning stimulus can still be protected by stimuli that employ alternative signaling pathways. *Am J Physiol Heart Circ Physiol*, Vol. 288, No. 3, pp. H1165-H1172

Lin, D.-T. & Lechleiter, J. D. (2002). Mitochondrial targeted cyclophilin D protects cells from cell death by peptidyl prolyl isomerization. *J Biol Chem*, Vol. 277, No. 34, pp. 31134-31141

Liu, G. S., Thornton, J., Winkle, D. M. V., Stanley, A. W., Olsson, R. A. & Downey, J. M. (1991). Protection against infarction afforded by preconditioning is mediated by A1 adenosine receptors in rabbit heart. *Circulation*, Vol. 84, No. 1, pp. 350-356

Livak, K. J., Freund, R., Schweber, M., Wensink, P. C. & Meselson, M. (1978). Sequence organization and transcription at two heat shock loci in *Drosophila*. *Proc Natl Acad Sci USA*, Vol. 75, No. 11, pp. 5613-5617

Madamanchi, N. R., Li, S., Patterson, C. & Runge, M. S. (2001). Reactive oxygen species regulate heat-shock protein 70 via the JAK/STAT pathway. *Arterioscler Thromb Vasc Biol*, Vol. 21, No. 3, pp. 321-326

Marber, M. S., Latchman, D. S., Walker, J. M. & Yellon, D. M. (1993). Cardiac stress protein elevation 24 hours after brief ischemia or heat stress is associated with resistance to myocardial infarction. *Circulation*, Vol. 88, No. 3, pp. 1264-1272

Maulik, N., Engelman, R. M., Rousou, J. A., Flack, J. E., Deaton, D. & Das, D. K. (1999). Ischemic preconditioning reduces apoptosis by upregulating anti-death gene Bcl-2. *Circulation*, Vol. 100, No. 19 Suppl, pp. II369-II375

Mitchell, M. B., Meng, X., Ao, L., Brown, J. M., Harken, A. H. & Banerjee, A. (1995). Preconditioning of isolated rat heart is mediated by protein kinase C. *Circ Res*, Vol. 76, No. 1, pp. 73-81

Mizumura, T., Nithipatikom, K. & Gross, G. J. (1995). Bimakalim, an ATP-sensitive potassium channel opener, mimics the effects of ischemic preconditioning to reduce infarct size, adenosine release, and neutrophil function in dogs. *Circulation*, Vol. 92, No. 5, pp. 1236-1245

Murry, C. E., Jennings, R. B. & Reimer, K. A. (1986). Preconditioning with ischemia: a delay of lethal cell injury in ischemic myocardium. *Circulation*, Vol. 74, No. 5, pp. 1124--1136

Noma, A. (1983). ATP-regulated K^+ channels in cardiac muscle. *Nature*, Vol. 305, No. 5930, pp. 147-148

Obal, D., Dettwiler, S., Favoccia, C., Scharbatke, H., Preckel, B. & Schlack, W. (2005). The influence of mitochondrial K_{ATP}-channels in the cardioprotection of preconditioning and postconditioning by sevoflurane in the rat *in vivo*. *Anesth Analg*, Vol. 101, No. 5, pp. 1252-1260

Ockaili, R. A., Bhargava, P. & Kukreja, R. C. (2001). Chemical preconditioning with 3-nitropropionic acid in hearts: role of mitochondrial K_{ATP} channel. *Am J Physiol Heart Circ Physiol*, Vol. 280, No. 5, pp. H2406-H2411

Okamoto, F., Allen, B. S., Buckberg, G. D., Bugyi, H. & Leaf, J. (1986). Reperfusion conditions: importance of ensuring gentle versus sudden reperfusion during relief of coronary occlusion. *J Thorac Cardiovasc Surg*, Vol. 92, No. 3 Pt 2, pp. 613-620

O'Sullivan J., Fu D., Alam H.B., & McCabe J.T. (2008). Diazoxide increases liver and kidney HSP25 and HSP70 after shock and stroke. *J Surg Res*, Vol. 49, No. 1, pp. 120-130

O'Sullivan, J. C., Yao, X.-L., Alam, H. & McCabe, J. T. (2007). Diazoxide, as a postconditioning and delayed preconditioning trigger, increases HSP25 and HSP70 in the central nervous system following combined cerebral stroke and hemorrhagic shock. *J Neurotrauma*, Vol. 24, No. 3, pp. 532-546

Pang, C. Y., Yang, R. Z., Zhong, A., Xu, N., Boyd, B. & Forrest, C. R. (1995). Acute ischaemic preconditioning protects against skeletal muscle infarction in the pig.. *Cardiovasc Res*, Vol. 29, No. 6, pp. 782-788

Patel, H. H., Moore, J., Hsu, A. K. & Gross, G. J. (2002). Cardioprotection at a distance: mesenteric artery occlusion protects the myocardium via an opioid sensitive mechanism. *J Mol Cell Cardiol*, Vol. 34, No. 10, pp. 1317-1323

Penna, C., Mancardi, D., Rastaldo, R., Losano, G. & Pagliaro, P. (2007). Intermittent activation of bradykinin B2 receptors and mitochondrial K_{ATP} channels trigger cardiac postconditioning through redox signaling. *Cardiovasc Res*, Vol. 75, No. 1, pp. 168-177

Penninger, J. M. & Kroemer, G. (2003). Mitochondria, AIF and caspases–rivaling for cell death execution. *Nat Cell Biol*, Vol. 5, No. 2, pp. 97-99

Peralta, C., Closa, D., Hotter, G., Gelpí, E., Prats, N. & Roselló-Catafau, J. (1996). Liver ischemic preconditioning is mediated by the inhibitory action of nitric oxide on endothelin. *Biochem Biophys Res Commun*, Vol. 229, No. 1, pp. 264--270

Philipp, S., Yang, X.-M., Cui, L., Davis, A. M., Downey, J. M. & Cohen, M. V. (2006). Postconditioning protects rabbit hearts through a protein kinase C-adenosine A2b receptor cascade. *Cardiovasc Res*, Vol. 70, No. 2, pp. 308-314

Pignataro, G., Meller, R., Inoue, K., Ordonez, A.N., Ashley, M.D., Xiong, Z. & Simon, R.P. (2008). *In vivo* and *in vitro* characterization of a novel neuroprotective strategy for stroke: ischemic postconditioning. J Cereb Blood Flow Metab, Vol. 28, No. 2, pp. 232-241

Przyklenk, K., Bauer, B., Ovize, M., Kloner, R. A. & Whittaker, P. (1993). Regional ischemic 'preconditioning' protects remote virgin myocardium from subsequent sustained coronary occlusion. *Circulation*, Vol. 87, No. 3, pp. 893-899

Ritossa, F. (1962). A new puffing pattern induced by heat shock and DNP in *Drosophilia*. *Experentia*, Vol. 18, No. 86, pp. 571-573

Rizvi, A., Tang, X. L., Qiu, Y., Xuan, Y. T., Takano, H., Jadoon, A. K. & Bolli, R. (1999). Increased protein synthesis is necessary for the development of late preconditioning against myocardial stunning. *Am J Physiol*, Vol. 277, No. 3 Pt 2, pp. H874-H884

Robin, E., Simerabet, M., Hassoun, S. M., Adamczyk, S., Tavernier, B., Vallet, B., Bordet, R. & Lebuffe, G. (2011). Postconditioning in focal cerebral ischemia: role of the mitochondrial ATP-dependent potassium channel. *Brain Res*, Vol. 1375, 137-146

Ruchalski, K., Mao, H., Li, Z., Wang, Z., Gillers, S., Wang, Y., Mosser, D. D., Gabai, V., Schwartz, J. H. & Borkan, S. C. (2006). Distinct hsp70 domains mediate apoptosis-inducing factor release and nuclear accumulation. *J Biol Chem*, Vol. 281, No. 12, pp. 7873-7880

Saitoh, S., Zhang, C., Tune, J. D., Potter, B., Kiyooka, T., Rogers, P. A., Knudson, J. D., Dick, G. M., Swafford, A. & Chilian, W. M. (2006). Hydrogen peroxide: a feed-forward dilator that couples myocardial metabolism to coronary blood flow. *Arterioscler Thromb Vasc Biol*, Vol. 26, No. 12, pp. 2614-2621

Schulman, D., Latchman, D. S. & Yellon, D. M. (2002). Urocortin protects the heart from reperfusion injury via upregulation of p42/p44 MAPK signaling pathway. *Am J Physiol Heart Circ Physiol*, Vol. 283, No. 4, pp. H1481-H1488

Schultz, J. E., Hsu, A. K. & Gross, G. J. (1998). Ischemic preconditioning in the intact rat heart is mediated by delta1- but not mu- or kappa-opioid receptors. *Circulation*, Vol. 97, No. 13, pp. 1282-1289

Shinmura, K., Tang, X. L., Wang, Y., Xuan, Y. T., Liu, S. Q., Takano, H., Bhatnagar, A. & Bolli, R. (2000). Cyclooxygenase-2 mediates the cardioprotective effects of the late phase of ischemic preconditioning in conscious rabbits. *Proc Natl Acad Sci U S A*, Vol. 97, No. 18, pp. 10197-10202

Smith, S. (2001). The world according to PARP. *Trends Biochem Sci*, Vol. 26, No. 3, pp. 174-179

Stankiewicz, A. R., Lachapelle, G., Foo, C. P. Z., Radicioni, S. M. & Mosser, D. D. (2005). Hsp70 inhibits heat-induced apoptosis upstream of mitochondria by preventing Bax translocation. *J Biol Chem*, Vol. 280, No. 46, pp. 38729-38739

Szabó, I. & Zoratti, M. (1992). The mitochondrial megachannel is the permeability transition pore. *J Bioenerg Biomembr*, Vol. 24, No. 1, pp. 111-117

Szewczyk, A. & Marbán, E. (1999). Mitochondria: a new target for K channel openers? *Trends Pharmacol Sci*, Vol. 20, No. 4, pp. 157-161

Takano, H., Manchikalapudi, S., Tang, X. L., Qiu, Y., Rizvi, A., Jadoon, A. K., Zhang, Q. & Bolli, R. (1998). Nitric oxide synthase is the mediator of late preconditioning against myocardial infarction in conscious rabbits. *Circulation*, Vol. 98, No. 5, pp. 441-449

Takano, H., Tang, X. L. & Bolli, R. (2000). Differential role of K_{ATP} channels in late preconditioning against myocardial stunning and infarction in rabbits. *Am J Physiol Heart Circ Physiol*, Vol. 279, No. 5, pp. H2350-H2359

Takayama, S., Reed, J. C. & Homma, S. (2003). Heat-shock proteins as regulators of apoptosis. *Oncogene*, Vol. 22, No. 56, pp. 9041-9047

Tong, H., Chen, W., Steenbergen, C. & Murphy, E. (2000). Ischemic preconditioning activates phosphatidylinositol-3-kinase upstream of protein kinase C. *Circ Res*, Vol. 87, No. 4, pp. 309-315

Tong, H., Imahashi, K., Steenbergen, C. & Murphy, E. (2002). Phosphorylation of glycogen synthase kinase-3beta during preconditioning through a phosphatidylinositol-3-kinase–dependent pathway is cardioprotective. *Circ Res*, Vol. 90, No. 4, pp. 377-379

Tsang, A., Hausenloy, D. J., Mocanu, M. M. & Yellon, D. M. (2004). Postconditioning: a form of "modified reperfusion" protects the myocardium by activating the phosphatidylinositol 3-kinase-Akt pathway. *Circ Res*, Vol. 95, No. 3, pp. 230-232

Vinten-Johansen, J., Jiang, R., Reeves, J. G., Mykytenko, J., Deneve, J. & Jobe, L. J. (2007). Inflammation, proinflammatory mediators and myocardial ischemia-reperfusion Injury. *Hematol Oncol Clin North Am*, Vol. 21, No. 1, pp. 123-145

Voellmy, R. & Boellmann, F. (2007). Chaperone regulation of the heat shock protein response. *Adv Exp Med Biol*, Vol. 594, 89-99

Wang, S., Duan, Y., Su, D., Li, W., Tan, J., Yang, D., Wang, W., Zhao, Z. & Wang, X., No. 2011). Delta opioid peptide [D-Ala2, D-Leu5] enkephalin (DADLE) triggers postconditioning against transient forebrain ischemia. *Eur J Pharmacol*, Vol. 658, No. 2-3, pp. 140-144

Wang, Y., Ahmad, N., Kudo, M. & Ashraf, M. (2004). Contribution of Akt and endothelial nitric oxide synthase to diazoxide-induced late preconditioning. *Am J Physiol Heart Circ Physiol*, Vol. 287, No. 3, pp. H1125-H1131

Wang, Y., Xu, H., Mizoguchi, K., Oe, M. & Maeta, H. (2001). Intestinal ischemia induces late preconditioning against myocardial infarction: a role for inducible nitric oxide synthase. *Cardiovasc Res*, Vol. 49, No. 2, pp. 391-398

Wu, L., Shen, F., Lin, L., Zhang, X., Bruce, I. C. & Xia, Q. (2006). The neuroprotection conferred by activating the mitochondrial ATP-sensitive K^+ channel is mediated by inhibiting the mitochondrial permeability transition pore. *Neurosci Lett*, Vol. 402, No. 1-2, pp. 184-189

Xiao, L., Lu, R., Hu, C. P., Deng, H. W. & Li, Y. J. (2001). Delayed cardioprotection by intestinal preconditioning is mediated by calcitonin gene-related peptide. *Eur J Pharmacol*, Vol. 427, No. 2, pp. 131-135

Yang, X.-M., Proctor, J. B., Cui, L., Krieg, T., Downey, J. M. & Cohen, M. V. (2004). Multiple, brief coronary occlusions during early reperfusion protect rabbit hearts by targeting cell signaling pathways. *J Am Coll Cardiol*, Vol. 44, No. 5, pp. 1103-1110

Yellon, D. M. & Downey, J. M. (2003). Preconditioning the myocardium: from cellular physiology to clinical cardiology. *Physiol Rev*, Vol. 83, No. 4, pp. 1113-1151

Zaugg, M., Lucchinetti, E., Spahn, D. R., Pasch, T. & Schaub, M. C. (2002). Volatile anesthetics mimic cardiac preconditioning by priming the activation of mitochondrial K_{ATP} channels via multiple signaling pathways. *Anesthesiology*, Vol. 97, No. 1, pp. 4-14

Zhao, H., Sapolsky, R.M. & Steinberg, G.K. (2006). Interrupting reperfusion as a stroke therapy: ischemic postconditioning reduces infarct size after focal ischemia in rats. *J Cereb Blood Flow Metab*, Vol. 26, No. 9, pp. 1114-1121

Zhao, Z.-Q., Corvera, J. S., Halkos, M. E., Kerendi, F., Wang, N.-P., Guyton, R. A. & Vinten-Johansen, J. (2003). Inhibition of myocardial injury by ischemic postconditioning during reperfusion: comparison with ischemic preconditioning. *Am J Physiol Heart Circ Physiol*, Vol. 285, No. 2, pp. H579-H588

Zhu, M., Feng, J., Lucchinetti, E., Fischer, G., Xu, L., Pedrazzini, T., Schaub, M. C. & Zaugg, M. (2006). Ischemic postconditioning protects remodeled myocardium via the PI3K-PKB/Akt reperfusion injury salvage kinase pathway. *Cardiovasc Res*, Vol. 72, No. 1, pp. 152-162

3

Fasudil (a Rho Kinase Inhibitor) Specifically Increases Cerebral Blood Flow in Area of Vasospasm After Subarachnoid Hemorrhage

Masato Shibuya, Kenko Meda and Akira Ikeda
Department of Neurosurgery, Chukyo Hospital, Nagoya,
Japan

1. Introduction

Subarachnoid hemorrhage due to a rupture of cerebral aneurysm is a severe disease with morbidity and mortality. Although, if patients' conditions are fair before surgery, they are rather safely operated by either clipping or coiling, vasospasm remains as a major complication of this disease. There are still many patients who suffer from vasospasm causing neurological deficits. Both strong vasoconstriction and inflammation are involved in the pathphysiological mechanism of vasospasm. In 1992 we had reported specific effects of a vasodilating drug "fasudil" in the treatment of vasospasm, but mechanisms how fasudil ameliorated vasospasm had not been clearly understood as it is today.

RhoA/Rho kinase had been found in 1996 and was revealed to act as molecular on-off switches that control multiple signaling pathways. Upregulated Rho kinase is known to be involved in various diseases from vascular disease to cancer. In cerebral vasospasm, upregulated Rho kinase was found to be involved in many aspects, such as increased calcium sensitivity, reduced production of nitric oxide, migration of inflammatory cells and their production of superoxide anions and increased blood viscosity. Interestingly, fasudil was found to specifically increase cerebral blood flow in the area with vasospasm. In the present paper pathophysiological mechanism of vasospasm and effects of fasudil are reviewed and mechanisms why fasudil increases cerebral blood flow in the area with vasospasm without so much changing that of normal flow area will be discussed.

2. Cerebral vasospasm following subarachnoid hemorrhage

Cerebral infarction due to delayed vasospasm is still the leading cause of a poor postoperative outcome of patients with a ruptured cerebral aneurysm especially if we consider deficits in higher neurological functions such as cognitive functions. Several days after a subarachnoid hemorrhage (SAH), blood vessels begin to be contracted by substances eluted from the blood clot such as oxyhemoglobin, endothelin, amines and many other chemical substances. Most of the patients show contraction of the blood vessels (angiographic spasm). In about one third of the patients, signs of neurological deficits appear (symptomatic spasm) on an average of day 7 after the hemorrhage (Bederson et al., 2009, Shibuya et al., 1992). Patients may even die of severe spasm, especially due to vasospasm of arteries supplying basal part of the brain: hypothalamus and brainstem. A representative case of a patient with severe vasospasm is shown in Fig. 1.

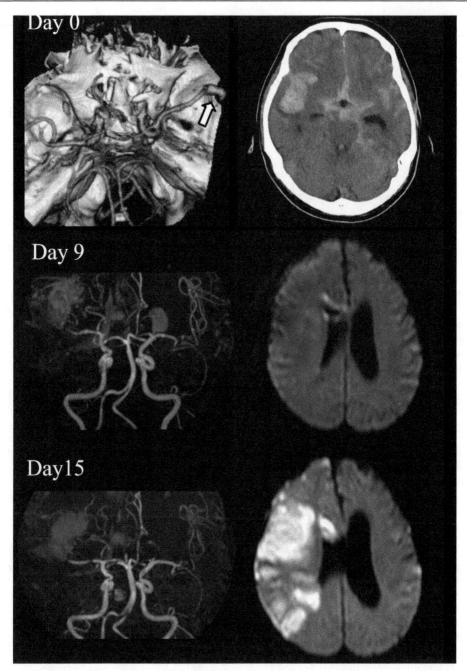

Fig. 1. Representative case of a patient with severe vasospasm.
Patient is a 70y/o male with a past history of prostatic cancer, hypertension and diabetes mellitus. He had a sudden onset of severe headache and lost consciousness two times at

home. He was slightly drowsy and disoriented (Hunt & Hess grade III) with mild weakness
in the left arm and leg. A head computed tomography (CT) (upper right) showed a diffuse
subarachnoid hemorrhage and a large hematoma in the right Sylvian fissure. A 3-D CT
angiogram (upper left) showed a 10mm long aneurysm at the bifurcation of the right middle
cerebral artery (MCA) (arrow). The aneurysm was clipped and subarachnoid space was
washed with urokinase on the same day. He smoothly recovered from surgery and he was
treated routinely postoperatively to prevent vasospasm with careful management of blood
pressure, water and electrolytes balance. Fasudil 30mg (i.v./30min, t.i.d.) was started on day
1. His postoperative course was smooth with clear consciousness and a mild left
hemiparesis.

A routine checkup, on day 9, by a magnetic resonance angiography (MRA, middle left)
showed a moderately severe vasospasm in the right MCA, a segmental vasospasm in the left
MCA and proximal portion of the right anterior cerebral artery (ACA). Diffusion weighted
magnetic resonance image (DWI) showed no abnormality (middle right). His blood pressure
was elevated with dopamine and daily dose of fasudil was increased to 60mg (i.v., t.i.d.) to
prevent development of further neurological deficits.

However, the next day (day 10), his left hemiparesis deteriorated and he became drowsy.
MRA on day 15 showed that vasospasm in bilateral MCAs progressed. Especially, distal
branches of the right MCA were hardly seen. Segmental vasospasm appeared in the
proximal portion of the right MCA, left ACA and distal portion of the vertebral arteries
(lower left). However, vasospasm in the proximal portion of the right ACA improved. DWI
on the same day showed an infarction in the right MCA territory (lower right). In spite of
deterioration of vasospasm on MRI and MRA on day 15, he began to recover his
consciousness the same day. Although he was communicable and could eat by himself, his
left hemiplegia did not improve and he was discharged to a rehabilitation hospital. Now,
two years after the onset, he is bed ridden and taken care at his home.

Vasospasm is not a simple contraction of blood vessels but it is complex pathological
phenomena consisting of abnormal contraction of blood vessels which is not easily relaxed
by usual calcium antagonists and inflammation. Tissue damage is seen in vascular
endothelium and smooth muscle cells in the medial wall caused by free radicals released
from inflammatory cells. Decreased production of nitric oxide (NO) is also contributing to
both contraction and tissue damage. Rho kinase has been found to be deeply implicated in
the pathophysiology of vasospasm (Miyagi et al., 2000; Sato et al., 2000) and use of a Rho
kinase inhibitor: fasudil dramatically improved patients' outcome (Shibuya et al., 1992)

3. Effects of Fasudil, a Rho kinase inhibitor on cerebral vasospasm

Fasudil HCl: (hexahydro-1-5-isoquinolinesulfonyl)-1H-1.4-diazepine HCl, (also called
HA1077, AT877, or Eril@) is originally considered to be an intracellular calcium antagonist.
By experimental studies in dogs we had found that fasudil dilated spastic arteries without
causing systemic hypotension, which could not been shown by any of the previously
presented drugs (Takayasu et al., 1986). The effectiveness was also confirmed in patients by
a double blind trial (Shibuya et al., 1992). Fasudil showed stronger brain protection from
ischemic damage than dilatation of the spastic artery itself, suggesting its possible effects in
patients with cerebral infarction as well. Fasudil is now routinely used in Japan for patients
with SAH. Zhao et al. (2007) in China showed by a randomized trial that fasudil was

significantly better for vasospasm than nimodipine which was most commonly used in the western countries.

After Rho kinase was found (Kimura et al., 1996), it became clear that upregulated Rho kinase worked unfavorably to the host in many vascular diseases and effects of fasudil on vasospasm mainly depended on its inhibition of Rho kinase. Fasudil was found to inhibit Rho kinase most strongly than any other protein kinases such as protein kinases C, A, and G (Hidaka et al., 2005). Fasudil is metabolized in human to hydroxyfasudil. Both fasudil and hydroxyfasudil are strong inhibitors of Rho kinase, however biological half-life of fasudil and hydroxyfasudil after an intravenous infusion of fasudil in human are 18 min and 6 hours, respectively. Thus major effect is considered to depend on hydroxyfasudil rather than fasudil itself.

Upregulated Rho kinase inhibits relaxation of the contracted blood vessels by inhibiting dephosphorylation of phosphorylated myosin light chain (MLC) either directly or through inhibition of endothelial NO synthase (eNOS). In an experimental model of vasospasm induced by $PGF_2\alpha$, double phosphorylation of MLC, at Thr18 in addition to Ser19, was found. This is considered to be the underlying mechanism of the strong contraction or increased sensitivity to Ca^{++}. Furthermore, fasudil was found to inhibit the second (pathological) phosphorylation at Thr18 of MLC more strongly (IC50: 0.3uM) than the first phosphorylation at Ser19 (IC50: 3uM) (Seto et al., 1991).

4. Fasudil specifically increases rCBF in area with vasospasm

Specific effect of fasudil on cerebral vasospasm has been suggested to depend on its inhibition of the abnormal phosphorylation of MLC. On the other hand, under normal situation, increased intracellular calcium phosphorylates MLC by activating calmodulin and myosin light chain kinase (MLCK) which is relaxed by dephosphorylation of MLC by phosphatase.

In a two hemorrhage canine model of SAH, basilar artery diameter is decreased to about 60% on day 7. Intravenous administration of a calcium antagonist nicardipine (0.1mg/kg, i.v./30min) did not dilate the spastic basilar artery but caused systemic hypotension. While fasudil (HA1077) (0.5~3mg/kg, i.v. /30min) significantly dilated the spastic artery without causing hypotension (Takayasu et al., 1986). It can be explained by specific inhibition of Rho kinase by fasudil. In other words, fasudil dilated spastic artery more specifically than normal or non-spastic arteries.

Specific vasodilating effect of fasudil has been shown by measuring regional cerebral blood flow (rCBF). In patients who had been operated on their ruptured aneurysms, Ueda (2000) compared the effects of fasudil on rCBF using 99mTc-HMPAO with that of nicardipine. Nicardipine (2mg, i.v.) decreased BP and increased pulse rate. It decreased rCBF in the low flow (spastic) area (to -10%, P<0.05) without changing rCBF of the normal flow area, suggesting a loss of autoregulation in the spastic area. On the other hand, fasudil (15 mg, i.v.) increased rCBF in the low flow area by 16% (P<0.05) without changing that of normal flow area.

Using CT perfusion method in patients with SAH, Ono et al. (2005) have examined changes in the cerebral blood perfusion (CBP) by fasudil (30mg, i.v./30min) in both normal (>40ml/100g/min) and low flow (<40ml) regions due to vasospasm. The mean CBP in the low flow area (34.4±4.7ml) was significantly increased (to 41.0±8.2 ml, P<0.05, n=43), whereas the mean CBP of the normal flow region (51.8±7.6ml) did not change after fasudil

(50.4±8.4ml, n=125). We also have shown by using 99mTc-HMPAO that fasudil (30-60mg/i.v./30 min) significantly increased rCBF in the operated side of the brain in patients showing ischemic signs of vasospasm. Such difference was not found in patients without vasospasm (Shibuya et al., 2008).

These data suggest that upregulated Rho kinase is involved in the decrease of rCBF in patients with vasospasm which was specifically improved by a Rho kinase inhibitor fasudil. On the other hand calcium antagonist dilated normal arteries more than spastic arteries leading to a systemic hypotension and a steal phenomenon, a steal of blood from a spastic region to a normal region.

5. Effects of fasudil on cerebral infarction

Rho kinase is also up-regulated in patients with cerebral infarction, both in ischemic brain and in migrated WBCs. It is involved in many aspects of ischemic brain damage caused by migration of inflammatory cells to the ischemic site and their production of free radicals by activated NADPH oxidase. Rho kinase elevates blood viscosity by producing the tissue factor (also called factor III, thrombokinase, or CD142) which triggers the coagulation cascade. Blood viscosity is also elevated by reduced plasticity of RBCs due to polymerization of actin fibers which is induced by activated Rho kinase and protein kinase C (Arai et al., 1993; Brabeck et al., 2003; Feske et al., 2009; Satoh et al., 2010). Effectiveness of fasudil on cerebral infarction has been shown both by experimental (Tsuchiya et al., 1993) and clinical studies (Shibuya et al., 2005). After specific effects of fasudil on cerebral vasospasm and infarction had been shown, it has been tried and showed effectiveness in various kinds of vascular diseases such as coronary ischemia, glaucoma, pulmonary hypertension, chronic kidney disease and so on (Dong et al., 2010, Schmandke et al., 2007).

6. Discussion

6.1 Rho kinase

Rho kinase is the immediate downstream target of RhoA, a small GTP binding protein belonging to Ras, Rho, Rab and Ran subfamilies and acts as molecular on-off switches that control multiple signaling pathways. Inactive form of Rho-GDP is activated by guanine nucleotide exchange factors (GEFs) and Guanine dissociation inhibitors (GDIs) through stimulation by lysophosphatidic acid (LPA) and sphyngosine-1-phosphate (S1P). Active form (GTP and membrane-bound) RhoA is inactivated by GTPase activating proteins (GAPs) to GDP bound form in cytosole. Rho kinase is a serine-threonine protein kinase that are involved in diverse cellular functions including vascular smooth muscle cell (SMC) contraction such as cerebral and coronary vasospasm, atherosclerosis, actin cytoskelton arrangement, cell adhesion, motility and gene expression (Noma et al., 2006).

6.2 Upregulated Rho kinase and increased sensitivity to calcium in vasospasm

Miyagi et al. (2000) showed that RhoA and mRNA of Rho kinase was increased in the basilar artery of SAH rats. Sato et al. (2000) clearly showed, in a two hemorrhage dog model, that Rho kinase was up-regulated with the decrease in basilar artery diameter and with the increase of phosphorylation of myosin binding subunit (MBS) of myosin phosphatase of the basilar artery, all of which were inhibited by a Rho kinase inhibitor Y27632. Activated Rho kinase inhibits MLC phosphatase by phosphorylating its component MBS at Thr697 (Feng et al., 1999) either directly or through activation of protein kinase C (PKC). PKC activated protein kinase C-potentiated inhibitory protein-17 (CPI-17) by phosphorylating at Thr38 (Koyama et al., 2000). In vasospastic condition, contraction force is increased without changes in intracellular concentration of Ca^{++}. Thus double (sometimes triple) phosphorylation of MLC by upregulated Rho kinase is considered to be the mechanism of so called increased sensitivity to Ca^{++}.

6.3 Involvement of inflammation in vasospasm

Inflammatory cells migrate to vasospasm or infarction sites and cause tissue injury by producing free radicals. When human WBCs were incubated in a Boyden chamber, WBCs migrated through a millipore filter by adding a chemoattractant such as formyl-methionyl-leucyl-phenylalanine (fMLP) to one side of the chamber. This migration was dose dependently inhibited by fasudil (Satoh et al., 1999). When WBCs were incubated with phorbol myristate acetate (PMA), a protein kinase C activator, they produced superoxide anion (O_2^{-}) by NADPH oxidase, which also was dose dependently inhibited by fasudil (Arai et al., 1993). Free radicals such as O_2^- are known to cause structural damage in endothelial cells and SMCs, leading to a decreased production of nitric oxide (NO) by endothelial NO synthase (eNOS).

6.4 Inhibition of NO synthase (eNOS) by Rho kinase

Nitric oxide (NO) plays an important role in the regulation of vascular tone, inhibition of platelet aggregation, suppression of SMC proliferation and prevention of leukocyte recruitment to the vessel wall. Activity of eNOS is controlled by a variety of signals surrounding blood vessels. Laminar shear stress, O_2 tension and transforming growth factor (TGF)β1 can regulate eNOS expression at the transcriptional level. Chronic hypoxia, tissue necrosis factor (TNF)α, thrombin, oxidized low density lipoprotein (LDL) and cellular proliferation are known to regulate eNOS expression at postscriptional level. Shear stress and vascular endothelial growth factor (VEGF) rapidly activated eNOS by phosphorylating at Ser1177. Hypoxia is known to upregulate Rho kinase which inhibits eNOS by phosphorylating at Thr495 (Flemming et al., 2001; Noma et al., 2006; Sugimoto et al., 2007). On the other hand, inhibition of Rho kinase by hydroxyfasudil increased phosphorylation of protein kinase Akt Ser473 and production of NO (Wolfrum et al., 2004). NO relaxes blood vessels by activating guanylate cyclase (which produced cyclic GMP) and protein kinase G, which activated MLC phosphatase by phosphorylating its component MBS at Ser695 (Nakamura & Ikebe, 2007, see also Fig. 2).

Pulmonary hypertension is a fatal disease in which eNOS activity is decreased. When human vascular endothelium was incuvated under hypoxic state of 3% O_2, both expression of mRNA of eNOS and eNOS activity were suppressed. The suppression was ameliorated by Rho kinase inhibitors, botulinus C3 transferase and fasudil (Takemoto et al., 2002). Actually, fasudil showed good results in patients with pulmonary hypertension (Fukumoto et al., 2005).

6.5 Increased blood viscosity in cerebral vasospasm and infarction

Blood viscosity is elevated in patients with acute cerebral infarction (Coull et al., 1991). However, it is not clear if this reflects a pre-existing risk factor or an acute phase response to the stroke itself or both. In rats model of temporary ischemia, by passing a nylon thread through the carotid artery for one hour and then removed, blood viscosity measured 24 hours later by a cone-plated discometer (at 37.5 rpm), was elevated from a control of 5.31 centipoise (cP) to 6.05 cP. Fasudil (1~10mg/kg) dose dependently inhibited the elevation of blood viscosity (Hitomi et al., 2000). Both production of the tissue factor (Zhang et al., 2007) and Rho kinase-activated polymerization of f-actin are considered to be involved in the increase of blood viscosity which were ameliorated by fasudil (Feske et al., 2009, Nagata et al., 20022Satoh et al., 2010).

RhoA/Rho kinase pathway has been shown to be involved in many other vascular diseases such as angiogenesis, atherosclerosis, cerebral and coronary spasm and infarction, glomerulosclerosis, hypertension, ischemia-reperfusion injury, neointimal proliferation, bronchial asthma, glaucoma and so on. Our current concepts about the Rho-kinase related mechanisms and effects of a Rho kinase inhibitor fasudil in cerebral vasospasm and infarction are shown in Fig. 2.

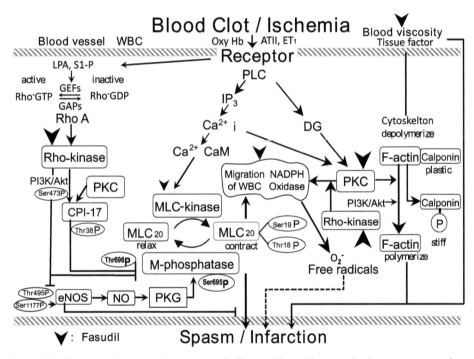

Fig. 2. Rho kinase related mechanisms and effects of fasudil in cerebral vasospasm and infarction

Chemical ligands eluted from subarachnoid blood clot or from ischemic brain such as oxyhemoglobin, angiotensin II and endothelin increase intracellular lysophosphatidic acid (LPA) and sphyngosine-1-phosphate (S1-P) which activate RhoA through activation of guanine nucleotide exchange factors (GEFs) from an inactive GDP-Rho in the cytosole to an active and membrane bound GTP-Rho. Activated Rho kinase contracts blood vessels by inhibiting myosin light chain (MLC) phosphatase by phosphorylating its component myosin binding subunit (MBS) at Thr696 through activation of protein kinase C-potentiated inhibitory protein-17 (CPI-17). Rho kinase also inhibits relaxation of contracted blood vessels by inhibiting endothelial nitric oxide synthase (eNOS) through inhibition of phosphatidylinositol-3kinase (PI3K)/protein kinase Akt. On the other hand, eNOS is activated by dephosphorylation at Thr495 or phosphorylation at Ser1177 when Rho kinase is inhibited. NO relaxes blood vessels by activating guanylate cyclase and protein kinase G (PKG). PKG activates MLC phosphatase by phosphorylating its component myosin binding subunit (MBS) at Ser695.

On the other hand, migration of inflammatory cells like WBCs and their production of free radicals by NADPH oxidase are stimulated by upregulated Rho kinase and protein kinase C. Rho kinase also increases blood viscosity by producing the tissue factor which triggers the coagulation cascade and also by decreasing plasticity of RBCs. Plasticity of RBCs is decreased when f-actin, consisting cytoskeleton, is polymerized by Rho kinase and protein kinase C.

These adverse phenomena: abnormal contraction of blood vessels, migration of inflammatory cells and their production of free radicals, increase of blood viscosity had all been ameliorated by a Rho kinase inhibitor fasudil which showed in turn that upregulated Rho kinase is involved in each of these sites (see text for references). Arrow head indicates acting points of fasudil.

7. Conclusion

Upregulated Rho kinase is deeply implicated in the complex mechanisms of delayed cerebral vasospasm after a subarachnoid hemorrhage, in both vasoconstriction and inflammation. Double phosphorylation of myosin light chain leading to pathological contraction, suppression of eNOS, production of free radicals are all induced by upregulated Rho kinase. Fasudil improved these situations by mainly inhibiting upregulated Rho kinase, which can explain why fasudil specifically increased cerebral blood flow in the area with vasospasm.

8. References

Arai, M., Sasaki, Y. & Nozawa, R. (1993) Inhibition by the protein kinase inhibitor HA1077 of the activation of NADPH oxidase in human neutrophils. *Biochem Pharmacol* 46:1487-1490

Bederson, J.B., Connolly, E.S.Jr, Batjer, H.H. et al. (2009) American Heart Association. Guidelines for the management of aneurysmal subarachnoid hemorrhage. Stroke 40:994-1025

Brabeck, C., Mittelbronn, M., Bekure, K. et al. (2003) Effect of cerebral infarctions on regional RhoA and RhoB expression. *Arch Neurol* 60:1245-1249

Coull, B.M., Beamer, N., de Garmo, P. et al. (1991) Chronic blood hyperviscosity in subjects with acute stroke, transient ischemic attack, and risk factors for stroke. *Stroke* 22:162-168

Dong, M., Yan, B.P., Liao J.K. et al. (2010) Rho-kinase inhibition: a novel therapeutic target for the treatment of cardiovascular diseases. Drug Discovery Today 15:622-629.

Feng, J., Ito, M., Ichikawa, K. et al. (1999) Inhibitory phosphorylation site for rho-associated kinase on smooth muscle myosin phosphatase. *J Biol Chem* 274:3744-3752

Feske, S.K., Sorond, F.A., Henderson, G.V. et al. (2009) Increased leukocyte ROCK activity in patients after ischemic attack. *Brain Res* 1257:89-93

Flemming, I., Fisslthaler, B., Dimmeler, S. et al. (2001) Phosphorylation of Thr 495 regulates Ca2+/calmodulin-dependent endothelial nitric oxide synthase activity. *Circ Res* 88:E68-E75.

Fukumoto, Y., Matoba, T., Ito, A. et al. (2005) Acute vasodilator effects of a Rho-kinase inhibitor fasudil in patients with severe pulmonary hypertension. *Heart* 91:391-392

Hidaka, H., Shibuya, M., Suzuki, Y. et al. (2005) Isoquinolinesulfonamide: A specific inhibitor of Rho-kinase and the clinical aspect of anti-Rho-kinase therapy. *HEP* 167:411-432

Hitomi, A., Satoh, S., Ikegaki, I. et al. (2000) Hemorrheological abnormalities in experimental cerebral ischemia and effects of protein kinase inhibitor on blood fluidity. *Life Sci* 67:1929-1939

Kimura, K., Ito, M., Amano, M. et al. (1996) Regulation of myosin phosphatase by Rho and Rho-associated kinase (Rho-kinase). *Science* 273:245-258

Koyama, M., Ito, M., Feng, J. et al. (2000) Phosphorylation of CPI-17, an inhibitory phosphoprotein of smooth muscle myosin phosphatase, by rho-kinse. *FEBS Let* 475:197-200

Miyagi, Y., Carpenter, R.C., Meguro, T. et al. (2000) Upregulation of RhoA and Rho kinase RNAs in the basilar artery of a rat model of subarachnoid hemorrhage. *J Neurosurg* 93:471-476

Nagata, K., Ishibashi, T., Sakamoto, T. et al. (2002) Rho/Rho-kinase is involved in the synthesis of tissue factor in human monocytes. *Atherosclerosis* 163:39-47

Nakamura, K. & Ikebe, M. (2007) cGMP-dependent relaxation of smooth muscle is coupled with the change in the phosphorylation of myosin phosphatase. *Circ Res* 101: 712-722

Noma, K., Oyama, N. & Liao, J.K. (2006) Physiological role of ROCKs in the cardiovascular system. *Am J physiol* 290:C661-C668

Ono, K., Shirotani, T., Yuba, K. et al. (2005) Cerebral circulation dynamics following fasudil intravenous infusion: a CT perfusion study. *Brain Nerve (Tokyo)* 57:779-783.

Sato, M., Tani, E., Fujikawa, H. et al. (2000) Involvement of Rho kinase mediated phosphorylation of myosin light chain in enhancement of cerebral vasospasm. *Circ Res* 87:195-200

Satoh, S., Hitomi, A., Ikegaki, I. et al. (2010) Amelioration of endothelial damage /dysfunction is a possible mechanism for neuroprotecive effects of Rho-kinase inhibitors against ischemic brain damage. *Brain Res Bull* 81:191-195

Satoh, S., Kobayashi, T., Hitomi, A. et al. (1999) Inhibition of neutrophil migration by a protein kinase inhibitor for the treatment of ischemic brain infarction. *Jpn J Pharmacol* 80:41-48

Schmandke, A., Schmandke, A. & Strittmatter, S.M. (2007) ROCK and Rho: Biochemistry and neuronal functions of Rho-associated protein kinases. Neuroscientist 13:454-469.

Seto, M., Sasaki, Y., Sasaki, Y. et al. (1991) Effect of HA1077, a protein kinase inhibitor, on myosin phosphorylation and a tension in smooth muscle. *Eur J Pharmacol* 195:267-272

Shibuya, M., Suzuki, Y., Sugita, K. et al. (1992) Effect of AT877 on cerebral vasospasm after aneurysmal subarachnoid hemorrhage. *J Neurosurg* 76: 571-577

Shibuya, M., Hirai, S, Seto, M. et al. (2005) Effects of fasudil in ischemic stroke: results of a prospective placebo-controlled double blind trial. *J Neurol Sci* 238:31-39

Shibuya, M, Ikeda, A., Ohsuka, K. et al. (2008) Fasudil (a rho kinase inhibitor) may specifically increase rCBF in spastic area. *Acta Neurochir Suppl* 104:275-278

Sugimoto, M., Nakayama, M., Gotoh, T.M. et al. (2007) Rho-kinase phosphorylates eNOS at threonine 495 in endothelial cells. *BBRC* 361:462-467

Takayasu, M., Suzuki, Y., Shibuya, M. et al. (1986) The effects of HA compound calcium antagonists on delayed cerebral vasospasm in dogs. *J Neurosurg* 65:80-85

Takemoto, M., Sun, J., Hiroki, J. et al. (2002) Rho-kinase mediates hypoxia-induced downregulation of endothelial nitric oxide synthase. *Circulation* 106:57-62

Tsuchiya, T., Sako, K., Yonemasu, Y. et al. (1993) The effects of HA1077, a novel protein kinase inhibitor, on reductions of cerebral blood flow and glucose metabolism following acute and/or chronic bilateral carotid ligation in Wistar rats. *Exp Brain Res* 97:233-238

Ueda, T. (2000) Effect on increase of cerebral blood flow with cerebral vasospasm by fasudil hydrochloride. *Med Pharmacy (Tokyo)* 42:753-759.

Wolfrum, S., Dendorfer, A., Rikitake, Y. et al (2004) Inhibition of Rho-kinase leads to rapid activation of phosphatidylinositol 3 kinase/protein kinase Akt and cardiovascular protection. *Atheroscler thromb Vasc Biol* 24:1842-1847

Zhao, J., Zhou, D., Guo, J. et al. (2006) Effect of fasudil hydrochloride, a protein kinase inhibitor, on cerebral vasospasm after aneurysmal subarachnoid hemorrhage. Results of a randomized trial of fasudil hydrochloride versus nimodipine. *Neurol Med Chir (Tokyo)* 46:421-428

Zhang, X.P., Hu, Y., Hong, M., et al., (2007) Plasma thrombomodulin, fibrinogen, and activity of tissue factor as risk factors for acute cerebral infarction. *Am J Clin Pathol* 128:287-292

4

Could Mannitol-Induced Delay of Anoxic Depolarization be Relevant in Stroke Patients?

Maurizio Balestrino*, Enrico Adriano and Patrizia Garbati
Department of Neuroscience, Ophtalmology and Genetics, University of Genova,
Italy

1. Introduction

The use of hyperosmotic agents in stroke is still a matter of debate, since their usefulness has repeatedely been suggested but not conclusively demonstrated (Righetti E et al., 2002). Better understanding of the possible mechanism of protection by hyperosmotic agents may help identifying clinical situations where they may be more useful. It is generally assumed that their effect in stroke is due to their capacity to reduce brain edema. However, increasing extracellular osmolarity has direct effects on neuronal electrical function (Osehobo and Andrew, 1993; Rudehill et al., 1993), and one of us has previously reported that adding mannitol to the perfusing medium of brain slices delays anoxic depolarization (AD) (Balestrino, 1995a; Balestrino, 1995b). Since the latter is a factor in causing neuronal damage in anoxia and ischemia (Balestrino and Somjen, 1986; Jarvis et al., 2001; Kaminogo et al., 1998; Somjen et al., 1990), this may be another mechanism of brain protection by hyperosmotic agents in stroke. This study investigates whether or not this delay occurs at values of hyperosmolarity that may be obtained in clinical practice. We first carried out a survey of the literature on osmolarity changes after administration of hyperosmotic agents in vivo, under both clinical and experimental conditions. Then, we did a dose-response study of mannitol-induced delay of AD. Finally we compared the two sets of data to gauge whether or not mannitol-induced delay of AD occurs in the range of hyperosmolarity that might be obtained in clinical practice.

2. Materials and methods

Sprague-Dawley female rats (155-190g.) were anaesthetised with ether and decapitated. The left hippocampus was dissected free and cut in 600 μm thick transversal slices. Slices were immediately transferred into an "interface" recording chamber (Fine Science Tools, Vancouver B. C. Canada) and incubated at $35\pm1°C$. They were bathed by Artificial CerebroSpinal Fluid (ACSF) flowing at 2 ml/min and having the following composition: NaCl 130 mM, KCl 3.5 mM, NaH_2PO_4 1.25 mM, $NaHCO_3$ 24 mM, $CaCl_2$ 2.4 mM, $MgSO_4$ 1.2 mM, glucose 10 mM. This medium was continuously bubbled with 95% O_2 / 5% CO_2, resulting in a pH of 7.35-7.40. The same warmed, humidified 95% O_2 / 5% CO_2 mixture aerated the slices representing the gas phase. Anoxia was induced by replacing oxygen with

---

* Corresponding Author

nitrogen in the gas phase. The DC-coupled, ground-referenced extracellular potential of the tissue was constantly monitored in the cell body layer of CA1. As soon as the sudden fall in this potential that is the hallmark of AD was observed, oxygen flow was restored. A cross-over study design was observed, with the same slice being subjected to anoxia, at 30′ intervals, both in the presence and in the absence of mannitol. Each slice was subjected to two anoxic episodes. The sequence of treatments (mannitol first, or control ACSF first) was alternated in consecutive experiments, to minimize the bias due to possible effects of repeated anoxia *per se* on AD latency. In two experiments, the same slice was subjected to three anoxic episodes the first one in mannitol, the second in control ACSF, the third one in mannitol again. For statistical analysis, in each experiment the difference in latency between AD in mannitol and AD in control ACSF was computed, and used as a gauge of mannitol efficacy in that experiment.

3. Results

3.1 Literature search on serum osmolarity changes in vivo
Results are summarized in figure 1 and in Table 1.

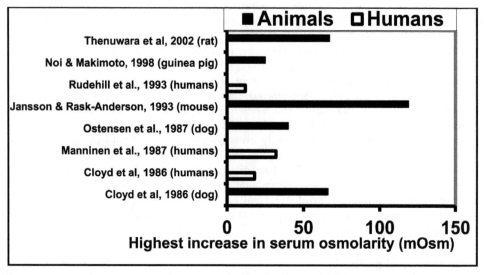

Fig. 1. **Increases in serum osmolarity reported in the literature:** This figure depicts the highest increase in serum osmolarity reported in each of the papers listed in Table 1. It refers to papers quoted in the Reference List. This figure is meant to graphically visualize the highest reported increases. Refer to Table I and to text for further information.

In human patients, use of mannitol at the dose of 0.5-2 g/Kg body weight is reported (Cloyd et al., 1986; Newman, 1979; Rudehill et al., 1993). Such a dose leads, still in human patients, to a maximum increase in serum osmolarity of about 10-32 mOsm (Cloyd et al., 1986; Manninen et al., 1987; Rudehill et al., 1993). When experimental animals are considered, administration of 1 g/Kg body weight to rats yelded a serum osmolarity increase of 4 mOsm (Thenuwara et al., 2002). In dogs, mannitol administration of 0.5, 1 or 1.5 g/Kg lead to a peak increase (mean±SD) of 43±18, 66±18 and 52±23 mOsm, respectively, during the brief time of the infusion, and to the

Paper	Animal species	Osmotic agent infused	Dose	Serum osmolarity increase
(Cloyd et al., 1986)	Humans	Mannitol	0.5, 0.7 g/Kg	10 - 18 mOsm
(Cloyd et al., 1986)	Dog	Mannitol	0.5, 1, 1.5 g/Kg	43-66 mOsm
(Jansson and Rask-Anderson, 1993)	Mice	Glycerol	1.3, 2.6 and 5.2 g /kg	12-119 mOsm
(Manninen et al., 1987)	Humans	Mannitol	1, 2 g/Kg	32 mOsm
(Newman, 1979)	Humans	Mannitol	2 g/Kg	Not reported
(Noi and Makimoto, 1998)	Guinea pig	Glycerol	30-min infusion of 50% glycerol	6 mOsm
(Noi and Makimoto, 1998)	Guinea pig	Urographin®	30-min infusion of 76% Urographin®	25 mOsm
(Ostensen et al., 1987)	Dog	Mannitol		40 mOsm
(Rudehill et al., 1993)	Humans	Mannitol	1 g/Kg	12 mOsm.
(Thenuwara et al., 2002)	Rat	Mannitol	1, 4, 8 g/Kg, with or without furosemide	4-67 mOsm

Table 1. **Literature data on changes in serum osmolarity after i.v. infusion of osmotic agents.** The table summarizes available literature data on changes in serum osmolarity after i.v. infusion of osmotic agents. When different changes in osmolarity are reported following different doses of osmotic agent, in the table the range of increases is given. The values given in the table are either the numbers provided by the Authors or those obtained by measuring graphs in their papers. In the latter case, the value is obviously less precise. When the Authors reported mean±SD for pre- and post-infusion osmolarity, in the table the corresponding difference between means is given.

lower increase of 10 mOsm or less afterwards (Rudehill et al., 1993). Higher doses of mannitol (4 g/Kg and 8 g/Kg, with or without the addition of furosemide) lead, in rats, to a rather high serum osmolarity increase, reaching an average as high as 67 mOsm (Thenuwara et al., 2002). Under experimental conditions in vivo, glycerol infusion leads to average increases in serum osmolarity of 6 mOsm in guinea pigs (Noi and Makimoto, 1998) and of up to 119 mOsm in dogs (Jansson and Rask-Anderson, 1993). Using Urografin® infusion, a 25 mOsm increase in serum osmolarity was obtained in guinea pigs (Noi and Makimoto, 1998).

3.2 Effects of increasing mannitol in vitro
The previously shown robust effect of mannitol in delaying AD was first confirmed in double wash-out experiments, where the same slice was subjected to transient anoxia in the presence of mannitol, then in control ACSF, then again in the presence of mannitol. These experiments are illustrated in figure 2. Mannitol concentrations of 100 and 500 mM were used in these experiments, as they were those that had been previously shown to most reliably delay AD (Balestrino, 1995).

The effects of mannitol where then investigated at different concentrations. Fig. 3 summarizes these results. As it can be seen, 1 and 10 mM were not effective in delaying AD. Twenty-five mM significantly delayed AD, while 50 mM did not show a statistically significant effect. The quite high concentrations of 100 and 500 mM significantly increased the latency of AD.

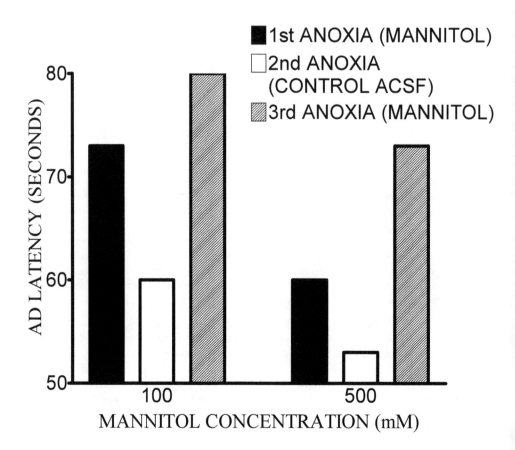

Fig. 2. **Double wash-out experiments showing mannitol effectiveness in delaying anoxic depolarization.** In two different slices, anoxia was induced in mannitol-fortified Artificial CerebroSpinal Fluid (ACSF), then in control ACSF, then again in ACSF with added mannitol. In one experiment (set of bars at left) 100 mM mannitol were used, in the other (set of bars at right) 500 mM mannitol were used. Bars represent latency of AD in each anoxia episode. Control ACSF reversibly decreased AD latency, thus confirming the previously published efficacy of mannitol in increasing AD latency.

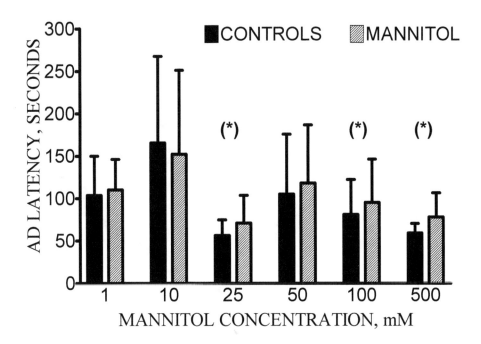

Fig. 3. **Effects of different mannitol concentrations in delaying anoxic depolarization.** The bars show latency of AD (mean± SD)in both control and mannitol-fortified ACSF for different mannitol concentrations. Asterisks mark the groups in which the difference is statistically significant (p<0.03, t-test for paired data). N=3 for 1mM, N=4 for 10 mM, N=8 for 25 mM, N=7 for 50 mM, N=6 for 100 mM, N=6 for 500 mM. See text for experiment design.

Figure 4 shows an example of AD delay by mannitol.

In a further analysis, we calculated for each slice the difference between the latency of AD in mannitol and the latency of AD in control ACSF. Such a difference was used as a gauge of mannitol effectiveness in that particular slice. If the difference had been positive, it would have indicated that latency in mannitol was longer that in control (i.e., AD occurred later), thus showing protection by mannitol and quantifying its degree. The opposite would have been true for a negative difference. Results are shown in Figure 5. As it can be seen, above 10 mM all concentrations of mannitol delay AD to a comparable extent. Such a finding has already been reported, from our laboratory, for AD delay by creatine (Balestrino, 1995).

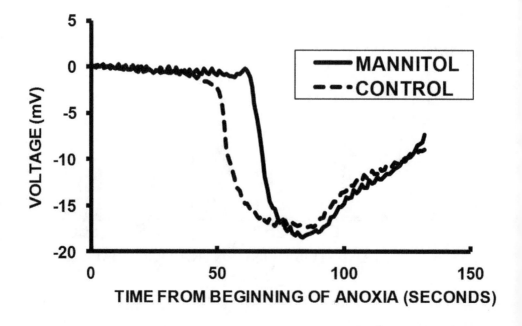

Fig. 4. **Sample anoxic depolarization in control and mannitol-treated ACSF.** Two different anoxic episodes in the same slice. The dotted line represents DC tracing (showing anoxic depolarization) during anoxia in control ACSF, the solid line represents the same tracing during anoxia in ACSF with added mannitol. AD occurs later in mannitol-fortified ACSF.

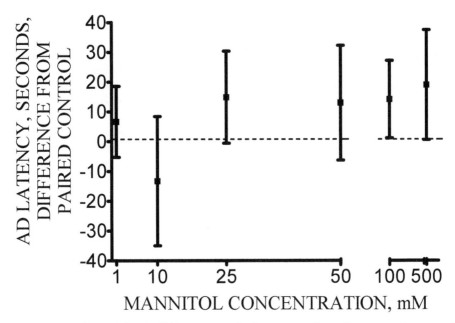

Fig. 5. **Measure of AD delay in different mannitol concentrations.** Same experiments as in figure 3. This figure depicts more precisely the increase in AD latency determined by mannitol at each concentration. For each slice, the difference (AD latency in ACSF with mannitol) – (AD latency in control ACSF) was computed. A positive difference means that AD latency was longer in mannitol (i.e., AD occurred later), the opposite is true for a negative difference. Data were grouped for mannitol concentration. For each concentration, mean±SD is provided. Number of experiments as in figure 3. Concentrations of 25 mM mannitol and higher all delay AD to the same extent.

4. Discussion

The effectiveness of hyperosmolarity in delaying AD was confirmed by these findings. Delay of AD may be relevant to neuroprotection in stroke, because AD is a factor in the generation of anoxic damage, and its delay has been associated with better outcome under experimental conditions (Balestrino and Somjen, 1986; Jarvis et al., 2001; Kaminogo et al., 1998; Somjen et al., 1990). The present study indicates that significant delay of AD is obtained at mannitol concentrations greater than 10 mM, 25 mM being the lowest effective dose among those tested. An overview of the literature showed that in human patients serum osmolarity increases, under common clinical settings, by 10-32 mOsm after administration of 1 g/Kg mannitol (Table 1 and fig. 1). This is equivalent to adding 10-32 mM mannitol to in vitro slices[1]. At the lower end of this range, such an

---

[1] Since the molecule of mannitol does not split in acqueous solutions, the molarity of mannitol in solution (here expressed in mM) corresponds to the consequent increase in osmolarity (1mM=1mOsm).

increase would be insufficient (10 mM (Cloyd et al., 1986; Rudehill et al., 1993)) or perhaps barely sufficient (18 mM (Cloyd et al., 1986)) to afford delay of AD. In the upper end, a 32 mM increase (Manninen et al., 1987) would probably be somehow effective in delaying AD. In fact, we showed that in vitro the addition of 25 mM mannitol (increasing osmolarity by 25 mOsm) significantly delays AD. The delay in AD was not significant after addition of 50 mM (increasing osmolarity by 50 mOsm), indicating that these osmolarity increases (25-50 mOsm) are of borderline efficacy. However, much higher increases, up to 100 mOsm and more, were reliably effective in vitro, and have been reported under experimental conditions in laboratory animals, apparently without severe adverse effects (Table 1 and figure 1). The latter increases would be in a range that does cause AD delay (compare figure 5 with figure 1). If further studies suggested that a comparable increase in serum osmolarity can be safely obtained in human patients, it might be useful not only by decreasing brain edema, but also by having a direct effect on tissue depolarization.

Two more considerations are in order.

First, in human stroke mannitol or other hyperosmotic agents would be adiminstered when AD has already occurred. In fact, AD is an event that occurs in the core of an infarction soon after ischemia. Nevertheless, under experimental conditions continuous or repeated depolarizations have been demonstrated in the hours following stroke (Chen et al., 1993; Ohta et al., 1997). Their reduction has been associated with better outcome (Chen et al., 1993). Given the striking similarity of these events with "classical" AD, it is very likely that hyperosmolarity can delay or suppress these waveforms as well, thus providing protection.

Second, the changes reported in the literature are in serum, not in the interstitial space of the brain. To the best of our knowledge, no study has yet measured increases in osmolarity in the interstitial space of the brain, probably due to the technical difficulty of this investigation. However, it is reasonable to assume that an increase in osmotic pressure in the serum draws water from the brain interstitial space, thus increasing its osmolarity to a comparable degree. Therefore, increase in serum osmolarity should be comparable, at least to an extent, to increase in osmolarity of the brain interstitial space.

Finally, it should be noted that future clinical studies on hyperosmotic agents in stroke should take into account the increase in serum osmolarity that was obtained in the single patients. In fact, our data indicate that the latter is a critical variable in determining whether the hyperosmotic therapy will be effective or not.

Summing up, we conclude that the increase in serum osmolarity that is commonly obtained in clinical practice is not sufficient to delay AD. Larger increases in serum osmolarity have been, however, reported in animal experiments. If further studies indicated that such increases were safe in humans as well as in animals, they might provide brain protection by decreasing AD and AD-like depolarizations. Future clinical studies on hyperosmotic agents in stroke should measure and take into account the degree of changes that were obtained in serum osmolarity.

5. Acknowledgment

We thank Prof. Aroldo Cupello for his useful comments on the manuscript.

6. References

Balestrino M. (1995) Studies on anoxic depolarization. In: Brain Slices in Basic and Clinical Research (A.Schurr, B.M.Rigor, eds), pp 273-293 Boca Raton, Florida: CRC Press.

Balestrino M (Pathophysiology of anoxic depolarization: new findings and a working hypothesis. J Neurosci Methods 59:99-103.1995).

Balestrino M, Somjen GG (Chlorpromazine protects brain tissue in hypoxia by delaying spreading depression-mediated calcium influx. Brain Res 385:219-226.1986).

Chen Q, Chopp M, Bodzin G, Chen H (Temperature modulation of cerebral depolarization during focal cerebral ischemia in rats: correlation with ischemic injury. J Cereb Blood Flow Metab 13:389-394.1993).

Cloyd JC, Snyder BD, Cleeremans B, Bundlie SR, Blomquist CH, Lakatua DJ (Mannitol pharmacokinetics and serum osmolality in dogs and humans. J Pharmacol Exp Ther 236:301-306.1986).

Jansson B, Rask-Anderson H (Correlations between serum osmolality and endolymphatic sac response using hypertonic glycerol. ORL J Otorhinolaryngol Relat Spec 55:185-192.1993).

Jarvis CR, Anderson TR, Andrew RD (Anoxic Depolarization Mediates Acute Damage Independent of Glutamate in Neocortical Brain Slices. Cerebral Cortex 11:249-259.2001).

Kaminogo M, Suyama K, Ichikura A, Onizuka M, Shibata S (Anoxic depolarization determines ischemic brain injury. Neurol Res 20:343-348.1998).

Manninen P, Lam A, Gelb A, Brown S (The effect of high-dose mannitol on serum and urine electrolytes and osmolality in neurosurgical patients. Canadian Journal of Anesthesia / Journal canadien d'anesthésie 34:442-446.1987).

Newman SL (Monitoring serum osmolality in mannitol treatment of Reye's syndrome. N Engl J Med 301:945-946.1979).

Noi O, Makimoto K (Comparative effects of glycerol and Urografin on cochlear blood flow and serum osmolarity. Hear Res 123:55-60.1998).

Ohta K, Graf R, Rosner G, Heiss WD (Profiles of cortical tissue depolarization in cat focal cerebral ischemia in relation to calcium ion homeostasis and nitric oxide production. J Cereb Blood Flow Metab 17:1170-1181.1997).

Osehobo EP, Andrew RD (Osmotic effects upon the theta rhythm, a natural brain oscillation in the hippocampal slice. Exp Neurol 124:192-199.1993).

Ostensen J, Bugge JF, Stokke ES, Langberg H, Kiil F (Mechanism of osmotic diuresis studied by infusion of NaHCO3 and mannitol in dogs. Acta Physiol Scand 131:397-409.1987).

Righetti E, Celani MG, Cantisani T, Sterzi R, Boysen G, Ricci S (2002) Glycerol for acute stroke (Cochrane Review). In: The Cochrane Library, Issue 2 2002 Oxford: Update Software.

Rudehill A, Gordon E, Ohman G, Lindqvist C, Andersson P (Pharmacokinetics and effects of mannitol on hemodynamics, blood and cerebrospinal fluid electrolytes, and osmolality during intracranial surgery. J Neurosurg Anesthesiol 5:12.1993).

Somjen GG, Aitken PG, Balestrino M, Herreras O, Kawasaki K (Spreading depression-like depolarization and selective vulnerability of neurons. A brief review. Stroke 21:III179-III183.1990).

Thenuwara K, Todd MM, Brian JE, Jr. (Effect of mannitol and furosemide on plasma osmolality and brain water. Anesthesiology 96:416-421.2002).

5

Nrf2 Activation, an Innovative Therapeutic Alternative in Cerebral Ischemia

Carlos Silva-Islas, Ricardo A. Santana,
Ana L. Colín-González and Perla D. Maldonado
*Patología Vascular Cerebral, Instituto Nacional de Neurología y Neurocirugía Manuel
Velasco Suárez
México*

1. Introduction

Cerebrovascular disease is the second cause of death and the most frequent cause of non-traumatic disability in adults worldwide, according to the World Health Organization (WHO, 2005). Noteworthy, acute ischemic stroke accounts for about 85% of all cases (Diez-Tejedor et al., 2001). The most common cause of stroke is a sudden occlusion of a blood vessel, resulting in activation of a series of biochemical events eventually leading to neuronal death (Dirgnal et al., 1999). Although return of blood flow (reperfusion) in ischemic brain tissue is essential for restoring normal function, paradoxically it can result in a secondary damage, where oxidative stress mediators play a critical role (Wong & Crack, 2008).

Antioxidant therapies have been used to determine whether oxidative stress may constitute a valuable therapeutic target in cerebral ischemia. Indeed, free radical scavengers (direct antioxidants) and agents that decrease free radicals production reduce damage in experimental models of cerebral ischemia. Despite experimental evidence supports the concept that free radicals production represents a valuable therapeutic target in stroke, negative results have been obtained in a number of clinical trials when some direct antioxidant agents have been evaluated (Aguilera et al., 2007). At present, this discrepancy is unclear; however, administration of treatment outside the temporal window of efficacy and difficulties in the establishment of the onset of ischemia and reperfusion in humans (Hsu et al., 2000) are factors that likely contributing to these differences. Clearly, development of preclinical testing must consider these factors in order to improve successful transition to clinical studies.

NF-E2-Related Factor-2 (Nrf2) is a transcription factor that play a crucial role in the cellular protection against oxidative stress. Nrf2 is referred to as the "master regulator" of the antioxidant response due to the fact that it modulates the expression of several genes including phase 2 and antioxidant enzymes playing an important role in detoxification of reactive oxygen species (ROS) and electrophilic species, including heme oxygenase-1, NAD(P)H:quinone oxidoreductase, glutathione-S-transferase, gamma-glutamyl cysteine ligase, glutathione reductase, etc. Recent studies demonstrate that dysfunction of Nrf2-driven pathways impairs cellular redox state thus oxidative stress.

Since ischemia and reperfusion insults generate an oxidative stress state, and considering that up to date there is no effective treatment to reverse morphological and behavioral alterations induced by stroke, it is conceivable that administration of antioxidants may limit oxidative damage and ameliorate progression of the disease. In this context, Nrf2 inducers are promising indirect antioxidant agents that are effective to attenuate oxidative stress and tissue/cell damage in different *in vivo* and *in vitro* experimental paradigms; therefore, here we review some compounds capable of inducing cellular antioxidant responses in order to understand their usefulness in prevention and treatment of cerebral ischemia-induced damage through activation of the Nrf2/ARE pathway.

2. Mechanism related to cerebral ischemic damage

Brain tissue requires high and constant supply of oxygen and glucose provided for the vascular system to maintain its viability and normal functions. Vascular obstruction – either transitory or permanent - of cerebral blood flow (ischemia) is accompanied by an immediate drop in neurological activity ultimately leading to cell death. The brain is not affected homogeneously and so, cerebral ischemia generates differentially damaged areas. Complete loss of blood flow produces an *infarct zone* where necrotic cell death is observed. The infarct area is surrounded by a *penumbra zone*, which is located between the *infarct zone* and the non-damaged area, or normally irrigated tissue. Cells belonging to the *penumbra zone* are still irrigated by collateral arteries, which maintain them viable for a variable period of time, although not functional (Figure 1). This is the area that shall be rescued, and the potential target for intervention with neuroprotective treatments (Dirgnal et al., 1999).

The return of blood flow (reperfusion) is associated with a decrease in the infarct size and clinical outcome. Although reperfusion is determinant for cell function recovery, after prolonged periods of ischemia, it also exerts negative side-effects. If blood flow is not restored within hours, the penumbra region will become part of the infarct zone. In some patients, reperfusion may exacerbate brain injury (*e.g.,* some patients show edema or intracranial hemorrhage) (Kuroda & Siesjo, 1997). In animal models, reperfusion can induce larger infarct areas that can be associated with permanent vessel occlusion (Aronowski et al., 1997).

The reduction and return of blood flow triggers a cascade of events further leading to neuronal death (Dirgnal et al., 1999; Durukan & Tatlisumak, 2007). Such sequence includes:

1. *Energy failure.* This is the first event of the ischemic cascade. Cells need oxygen and glucose to undergo oxidative phosphorylation for energy production, consequently during ischemia ATP production is decreased (Figure 2).
2. *Depolarization of membrane.* The impairment of ATP production disrupts Na^+/K^+-ATPase and Ca^{2+}/H^+-ATPase pumps and reverses the Na^+/Ca^{2+}-transporter. Upon these conditions, cells are unable to maintain membrane potential and Ca^{2+} voltage-dependent channels are activated, leading to depolarization of cellular membrane (Figure 3).
3. *Excitotoxicity and increase in intracellular Ca^{2+} levels.* After depolarization, excitotoxic amino acids - mostly glutamate - are released to the synaptic cleft. Glutamate activates N-methyl-D-aspartic acid (NMDA), α-amino-3-hydroxy-5-methylisoxazole-4-propionic acid (AMPA), and metabotropic glutamate receptors, thereby increasing intracellular

Ca²⁺ levels. In turn, voltage gated Ca^{2+} channels together with reverse operation of the Na^+/Ca^{2+} exchanger also increase intracellular Ca^{2+} levels (Figure 3). Once in the cytoplasmic domain, Ca^{2+} activates a variety of Ca^{2+} dependent enzymes, including protein kinase C, phospholipase A2, phospholipase C, cyclooxygenase-2, Ca^{2+}-dependent nitric oxide synthase, proteases and endonucleases, hence triggering protein phosphorylation, proteolysis, and mitochondrial damage.

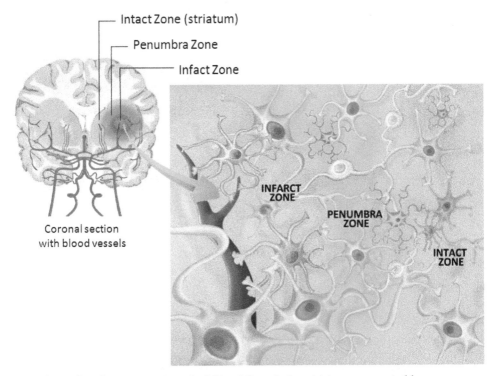

Fig. 1. Vascular obstruction of cerebral blood flow (ischemia) is accompanied by an immediate drop in neurological activity ultimately leading to cell death (*infarct zone*). Infarct core is surrounded by an area supplied with oxygen and glucose by collateral blood vessels (*penumbra zone*). Cells from the penumbra area are not functional; however, they remain viable for a variable period of time.

4. *Generation of free radicals and oxidative stress.* Reactive oxygen (ROS) and nitrogen (RNS) species generation is increased during ischemia, but particularly during reperfusion, and they eventually lead to oxidative stress. ROS and RNS cause lipid peroxidation, membrane injury, disruption of cellular processes, and DNA damage. Moreover, oxidative stress contributes to the disruption of the blood-brain barrier, hence allowing the infiltration of neutrophils and other cells (see below) (Chan, 2001).

5. *Inflammation and apoptosis.* Cerebral injury is a potent triggering of inflammatory cytokines and proteases secretion by microglia, leukocytes and resident cells of the neurovascular unit. Once the neurovascular barriers are breached, multiple neuroinflammatory cascades are activated, further leading to secondary brain injury

(Danton & Dietrich, 2003). Post-ischemic inflammation contributes to brain injury and has been linked to apoptosis. Cell death in cerebral ischemia is mainly dependent of the localization of the cells. For instance, in the core region, cell death is caused mainly by necrosis, while apoptosis predominates in the penumbra area.

ISCHEMIA

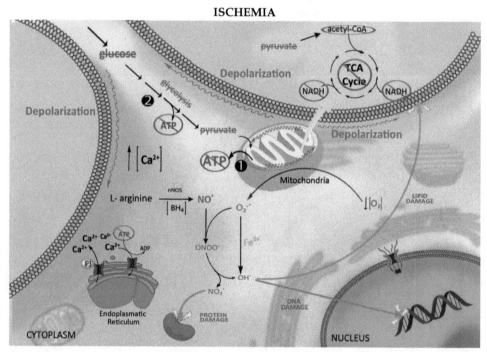

Fig. 2. The reduction of blood flow decreases oxygen and glucose levels; consequently, ATP production *(Energy failure)* (❶), glycolysis(❷) and ATP-dependent processes are blocked. Upon these conditions, oxidative damage is generated by residual oxygen in mitochondria. Pathways that are inhibited during ischemia are crossed out in the image. TCA cycle, tricarboxylic acid cycle; nNOS, neuronal nitric oxide synthase.

3. Oxidative stress is one of the most important events in ischemia/reperfusion-induced cerebral damage

In cells, the predominant ROS and RNS produced are superoxide anion ($O_2^{-\bullet}$), hydrogen peroxide (H_2O_2), hydroxyl radical ($^{\bullet}OH$), nitric oxide ($^{\bullet}NO$), peroxynitrite anion ($ONOO^-$), and nitrogen dioxide ($^{\bullet}NO_2$). In normal conditions, natural defense against ROS and RNS is provided by antioxidant molecules such as glutathione (GSH), ascorbic acid, α-tocopherol, and a number of antioxidant enzymes, including superoxide dismutase (SOD), glutathione peroxidase (GPx), and catalase (CAT). SOD converts $O_2^{-\bullet}$ to H_2O_2, whereas GPx and CAT convert H2O2 to H2O. However, an imbalance in the formation and clearance of ROS and RNS can lead to oxidative stress and subsequent changes affecting the cell dynamics (Aguilera et al., 2007; Margaill et al., 2005).

ISCHEMIA

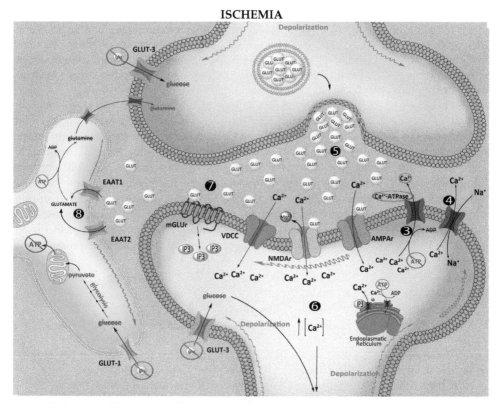

Fig. 3. Reduction of blood flow decreases ATP production, disrupts ATP-dependent pumps (❸) and reverses the Na$^+$/Ca^{2+} transporter (❹). Upon these conditions, cells are unable to maintain membrane potential (*Depolarization of membrane*). After depolarization, glutamate (GLUT) is released and activates N-methyl-D-aspartic acid (NMDAr) and α-amino-3-hydroxy-5-methylisoxazole-4-propionic acid (AMPAr) receptors(❺, *Excitotoxicity*), hence directly increasing intracellular Ca^{2+} levels (❻). On one hand, GLUT activates metabotropic glutamate receptors (mGLUr) (❼), which releases inositol 1,4,5-triphosphate (IP3), a molecule that binds to its receptor at the endoplasmatic reticulum to release more Ca^{2+} (❻, *Increase of intracellular Ca^{2+} level*). On the other hand, voltage gated Ca^{2+} channels (VDCC) and the reverse operation of the Na+/Ca^{2+}-exchanger increase intracellular Ca^{2+} levels. Energy disruption also affects astrocytes, causing a deficient activity of glutamate transporters (EAAT1 and EAAT2) (❽).

ROS and RNS produce cellular damage through lipid peroxidation, nucleic acid alteration and inactivation of enzymes (Figure 4); they also modify cellular signaling and gene regulation, contributing to breakdown of the blood-brain barrier and edema generation (Moro et al., 2005). Oxidative stress can ultimately induce neuronal damage, leading to neuronal death by apoptosis or necrosis (Loh et al., 2006).

The brain is particularly sensitive to oxidative stress since 20% of the total oxygen consumed by the body is used by this organ, which constitutes only 2% of the total body weight. This feature makes the brain the major generator of ROS and RNS when compared with other organs (Dringen, 2000). Moreover, in brain there are numerous conditions favoring ROS and RNS production, including: 1) a high unsaturated lipid content, 2) chemical reactions involving dopamine oxidation (Heiss, 2002; Hou & MacManus, 2002), 3) high concentrations of iron in various regions, and 4) lower antioxidant systems than other organs such as kidney or liver (Dringen, 2000).

As previously described, physiopathological mechanisms leading to neuronal injury in cerebral stroke are complex and multifactorial. However, several studies suggest that oxidative stress, secondary to ROS and RNS production, actively participates during post-ischemic brain damage (Peters et al., 1998; Rodrigo et al., 2005). During ischemia, free radical production in the infarct zone decreases or remains without change, while it increases during reperfusion. However, free radical production in the penumbral zone increases during both events (Liu et al., 2003). Despite the low oxygen tension produced during ischemia, exist an increase in ROS formation after 1.6 h of ischemia, the highest ROS production ($489 \pm 330\%$ of control) occurs after 20 min of reperfusion, and remains increased at least for 3 h (Peters et al., 1998). Christensen et al. (1994) reported that ROS production is maximal during the first hour of reperfusion.

Main sources of ROS, RNS, and free radicals during reperfusion are summarized as follows (Aguilera et al., 2007; Margaill et al., 2005):

1. Mitochondrial respiratory chain generates $O_2^{-\bullet}$.
2. Xanthine oxidase produces $O_2^{-\bullet}$ when it catalyzes oxidation of hypoxhantine to uric acid.
3. Cyclooxygenase 2 (COX-2) produces $O_2^{-\bullet}$ during oxidative metabolism of arachidonic acid, a delayed process in ischemia reperfusion.
4. NADPH oxidase (NOX) produces $O_2^{-\bullet}$ during NADPH oxidation.
5. Nitric oxide synthases (NOS) produce $^\bullet NO$ in normal conditions. $^\bullet NO$ produced can react with $O_2^{-\bullet}$ and generate the strong oxidant ONOO-. Tetrahydrobiopterin (BH4) is an important regulator of NOS function because it is required to maintain enzymatic coupling. Loss or oxidation of BH4 to 7,8-dihydrobiopterin (BH2) is associated with NOS uncoupling, resulting in the production of $O_2^{-\bullet}$ rather than $^\bullet NO$ (Crabtree & Channon, 2011) (Figure 4).

4. Direct and indirect antioxidants

Living systems have developed multiple lines of defense against oxidative stress. Cellular protection against oxidative stress is a process more complex than cellular protection against electrophiles. In this process two types of molecules participate (Dinkova-Kostova et al., 2007):

1. *Direct antioxidants*. Compounds of low molecular weight (ascorbate, glutathione, tocopherols, lipoid acid, ubiquinones, carotenes) that can undergo redox reactions and scavenge reactive oxidation products (peroxides), as well as ROS and RNS ($^\bullet OH$, ONOO-). Direct antioxidants are consumed or modified in the process of their antioxidant action (ROS scavenger). Thus, it is necessary to replenish or regenerate them.
2. *Indirect antioxidants*. These agents may or may not have redox activity, and exert many of their effects through upregulation of phase 2 and antioxidant enzymes. In turn, theses enzymes act catalytically, exhibit long half-lives, and display a wide variety of antioxidant activities, in addition to their capacities to detoxify electrophiles.

REPERFUSION

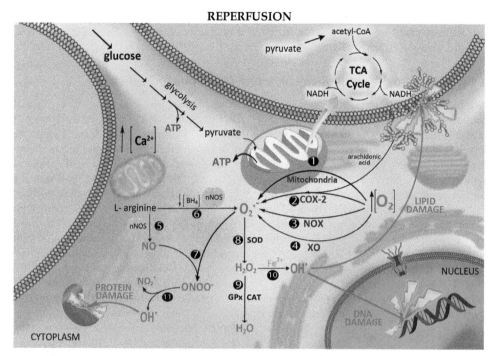

Fig. 4. Main sources of superoxide anion ($O_2^{-\bullet}$) during reperfusion are summarized as follows: mitochondrial respiratory chain ❶; cyclooxygenase-2 (COX-2) ❷; NADPH oxidase (NOX) ❸; xanthine oxidase (XO) ❹; and nitric oxide synthase (NOS), responsible for nitric oxide ($^\bullet NO$) formation ❺, or $O_2^{-\bullet}$ if tetrahydrobiopterin (BH4) is deficient ❻. $O_2^{-\bullet}$ can react with $^\bullet NO$ to generate peroxynitrite anion (ONOO-) ❼, or be degraded by superoxide dismutase (SOD) to hydrogen peroxide (H_2O_2) ❽. Then, H_2O_2 can be catabolized by glutathione peroxidase (GPx) or catalase (CAT) to H_2O ❾, or react with Fe^{2+} to form hydroxyl radicals ($^\bullet OH$) via the Fenton reaction ❿. ONOO- can be degraded to nitrogen dioxide radical ($NO_2^\bullet$) and $^\bullet OH$ (11), responsible for damaging lipids, proteins and DNA.

However, the distinction between direct and indirect antioxidants is complicated by a close reciprocal relation between these two types of agents, as is showed in the following examples (Dinkova-Kostova et al., 2007):

1. Whilst glutathione is the main protective direct antioxidant present in high concentrations (mM) in tissues, its rate of synthesis is controlled by γ-glutamate cysteine ligase (GCL), a typical phase 2 enzyme that is upregulated by phase 2 inducers which are, by definition, indirect antioxidants. The complexity of this reciprocal relation is further enhanced by the mandatory participation of glutathione in activities of several antioxidant enzymes (glutathione peroxidase, glutathione-S-transferases, glutathione reductase).

2. At least one phase 2 enzyme, heme oxygenase-1 (HO-1) generates carbon monoxide and biliverdin/biliruvin, which are small direct antioxidant molecules.

3. Some direct antioxidants are inducers of the phase 2 response; e.g., the vicinal dithiol lipoic acid and reduced Michale reaction acceptors such as hydroquinones.

4. Phase 2 enzymes NADPH:quinone oxidoreductase-1 (NQO1) and glutathione reductase
    are responsible for regeneration of reduced and active forms of oxidized tocopherols,
    and ubiquinone and glutathione, respectively.

5. Indirect antioxidants induce a cytoprotective phase 2 response

Aerobic cells have developed an elaborated mechanism for their protection against
oxidative stress, known as "phase 2 response" (Dinkova-Kostova & Talaly, 2008; Kensler et
al., 2007; Kobayashi & Yamamoto, 2006; Motohashi & Yamamoto, 2004). Phase 2 response
involves a group of genes that are regulated by a common molecular signaling pathway
depending of the transcription factor Nrf2, and can be coordinately induced by a variety of
synthetic and natural agents (Dinkova-Kostova et al., 2005a; Talalay, 2000). Extensive
studies on chemistry of inducers have disclosed that all are chemically reactive without
having common structural features (Dinkova-Kostova et al., 2004), and all react with
sulfhydryl groups (Dinkova-Kostova et al., 2001) of highly reactive cysteine residues of
Keap1, the cellular sensor that is integrally involved in the mechanism of induction (Itoh et
al., 2003; Wakabayashi et al., 2004). The known inducers belong to at least nine chemical
classes (Dinkova-Kostova et al., 2004): (i) diphenols, phenylenediamines and quinones; (ii)
Michael reaction acceptors; (iii) isothiocyanates/dithiocarbamates; (iv) 1,2-dithiole-3-
thiones/oxathiolene oxides; (v) hydroperoxides; (vi) trivalent arsenicals; (vii) heavy metals;
(viii) vicinal dimercaptans; and (ix) carotenoids.

It is now widely recognized that the up-regulation of the phase 2 response is a powerful,
highly efficient and promising strategy for protection against several diseases including
ischemic stroke (Alfieri et al., 2011; Talalay, 2000). Experimental evidence shows the
powerful protective effects of phase 2 response: (*i*) its up-regulation protects cells, animals,
and humans against a wide variety of damaging agents including ROS, RNS, carcinogens,
electrophiles, and radiation (Kensler et al., 2007; Kobayashi & Yamamoto, 2006; Motohashi
& Yamamoto, 2004; Talalay et al., 2007); (*ii*) when the phase 2 response is disrupted, cells are
much more susceptible to oxidative damage; and (*iii*) numerous anticarcinogens have been
identified and isolated from natural sources by bioassays that monitor induction of Nrf2-
dependent enzymes such as NAD(P)H:quinone oxidoreductase (NQO1) (Kang & Pezzuto,
2004; Zhang et al., 1992).

5.1 Phase 2 proteins and enzymes

In the past, enzymatic protection against oxidants focused largely on classical enzymes such
as SOD, CAT, and various types of peroxidases (Halliwell & Gutteridge, 1999), now this is
changing. Phase 2 proteins were originally perceived as only promoters of xenobiotic
conjugation with endogenous ligands (e.g., glutathione, glucuronic acid) to generate more
water-soluble and easily excretable products. This restricted view of the nature and
functions of phase 2 proteins and enzymes has gradually been expanded. Nowadays,
several genes are considered part of the phase 2 response. Enzymes encoded by these genes
have chemically versatile antioxidant properties, share common regulatory mechanisms,
and are highly inducible by a variety of agents including dietary components (Ramos-
Gomez et al., 2001; Talalay, 2000).

Phase 2 proteins catalyze diverse reactions that collectively result in broad protection
against the continuous damaging effects of ROS, RNS and electrophiles. They are expressed

at low basal levels, but can be markedly elevated by various small molecules (indirect antioxidants).

Using an oligonucleotide microarray analysis, Lee et al. (2003a) reported that *tert*-butylhydroquinone (t-BHQ), a well know Nrf2 inducer, stimulated a group of genes responsible for conferring protection against oxidative stress or inflammation in primary cortical astrocytes. The major functional categories are detoxification enzymes, antioxidant proteins, NADPH-producing proteins, growth factors, defense/immune/inflammation-related proteins, and signaling proteins (Table 1). It has been proposed that proteins within these functional categories are vital to cell's defense system, suggesting that an orchestrated change in the modulation of Nrf2/ARE pathway would stimulate a synergistic protective effect.

Proteins and enzymes directly related with an antioxidant protective effect can be divided into 3 major groups (Lee et al., 2003a):

Group 1. Genes involved in glutathione (GSH) homeostasis. GSTs catalyze the nucleophilic addition of GSH to an electrophilic group of a broad spectrum of xenobiotic compounds. GPx and PRx metabolize H_2O_2 to H_2O and oxidized GSH (GSSG), and GR regenerates GSH. Ideally, in association with an increased utilization of GSH, there would also be an increased production of GSH. The rate-limiting step in the GSH biosynthesis is mediated by GCLM/GCLC. The coordinate regulation of these genes can evoke a synergistic effect in the maintenance of GSH levels, as well as in detoxification of reactive intermediates (Figure 5).

Group 2. Genes involved in H_2O_2 detoxification and iron homeostasis. SOD and HO-1 are very important for cellular defense against oxidative stress. SOD detoxifies $O_2^{-\bullet}$ resulting H_2O_2, and HO-1 generates a potent radical scavenger, bilirubin. However, SOD and HO-1 can induce more oxidative stress because they increase the cellular concentrations of H_2O_2 and free iron, respectively; which together can generate •OH through the Fenton reaction. For complete detoxification of superoxide, H_2O_2 should be further metabolized to H_2O by GPx, CAT, or PRx. CAT directly detoxifies H_2O_2, whereas PRx uses GSH (Figure 6) and/or thioredoxin (Trx) as an electron donor for peroxidation of H_2O_2, resulting in generation of GSSG or oxidized thioredoxin, respectively (Figure 6). GSSG and oxidized thioredoxin are converted to their reduced forms by GR and TXNRD1, respectively. In addition, proper management of free iron is also important for minimizing oxidative stress, and this can be best achieved by ferritin. Ferritin converts Fe^{2+} to Fe^{3+} (ferroxidase activity) and sequesters it, thereby avoiding the participation of Fe^{2+} in the Fenton reaction (Orino et al., 2001). Thus, up-regulation of HO-1 together with ferritin constitutes a physiological strategy to increase the antioxidant potential while •OH formation is minimized.

Group 3. Genes involved in NADPH homeostasis. NQO1, GR, and TXNRD1 are important in detoxifying quinones and maintaining the cellular redox balance. One common feature of these proteins is the fact that they use NADPH as an electron donor. So, for efficient detoxification and maintenance of cellular redox status, it would be beneficial to up-regulate these proteins together with the appropriate reducing potential (NADPH) to support enzymatic reactions. G6PD/malic enzyme can directly generate NADPH, and transketolase/transaldolase can increase NADPH production by regenerating substrates for G6PD (Figure 7). These Nrf2-dependent genes would also contribute to cell's detoxification potential and cellular redox balance.

GENE	GENE	GENE
Detoxification	*Antioxidant/reducing potential*	*Transcription*
✓ NAD(P)H:quinone oxidoreductase-1 (NQO1)[a]	✓ γ-glutamate cysteine ligase modifier subunit (GCLM)[a]	✓ CCAAT/enhancer-binding protein-β
✓ Glutathione-S-transferase (GST) A4[a]	✓ γ-glutamate cysteine ligase catalytic subunit (GCLC)[a]	✓ Zinc finger protein of cerebellum-2
✓ GST Pi2[a]		✓ TG-interacting factor
✓ GST Mu1[a]	✓ Hemo oxygenase-1 (HO-1) (decycling)[a]	✓ MafG
✓ GST Mu3[a]		✓ Activating transcription factor-4
✓ GST Omega1[a]	✓ Thioredoxin reductase-1 (TXNRD-1)	*Growth*
✓ GST microsomal-1[a]	✓ Thioredoxin (Trx)[a]	✓ Proliferin
✓ UDP glycosyltransferase 1A6[a]	✓ Ferritin light chain-1[a]	✓ Proliferin-2
✓ Epoxide hydrolase-1[a]	✓ Ferritin H subunit[a]	✓ Nerve growth factor- β
✓ Aldehyde dehydrogenase-2	✓ Type I peroxiredoxin (PRx)	✓ Platelet-derived growth factor-α
✓ Aldehyde dehydrogenase-9	✓ 1-Cys PRx protein-2	*Defense/immune/inflammation*
✓ Aldehyde oxidase-1	✓ Transferrin receptor	✓ Macrophage C-type lectin
✓ Cytochrome P450 1B1	✓ Cu, Zn superoxide dismutase (CuZnSOD)[a]	✓ EST, similar to dithiolethione-inducible-1
Signaling	✓ Catalase-1 (CAT)	✓ PAF acetylhydrolase
✓ Protein kinase, cAMP-dependent regulatory, type Iβ	✓ Glutathione peroxidase-4 (GPx)	✓ P lysozyme structural
✓ AW125016 4 1.9 0.07 NR	✓ Glutathione reductase-1 (GR)	✓ Lysozyme M
✓ Mitogen-activated protein kinase-10	✓ Glucose-6-phosphate dehydrogenase (G-6PD), X-linked	✓ Prostaglandin-endoperoxide synthase-2
	✓ G-6PDH-2	✓ Matrix metalloproteinase-12
	✓ Transaldolase-1	
	✓ Transketolase	
	✓ Solute carrier family-1/4	
	✓ Glycine transporter-	
	✓ Malic enzyme, supernatant[a]	

[a]Known to contain or to potentially have an ARE sequence.
Modified of Lee et al., 2003a.

Table 1. Nrf2-dependent genes induced by *tert*-butylhydroquinone in primary cortical astrocytes

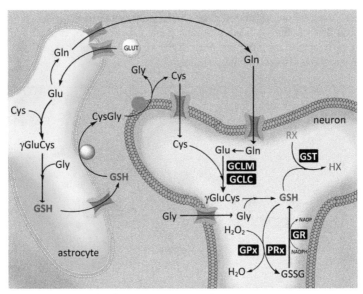

Fig. 5. Genes involved in glutathione (GSH) homeostasis are indicated in black boxes. GST, glutathione-S-transferase; GCLM, γ-glutamate cysteine ligase modifier subunit; GCLC, γ-glutamate cysteine ligase catalytic subunit; GPx, glutathione peroxidase; PRx, peroxiredoxin; GR, glutathione reductase.

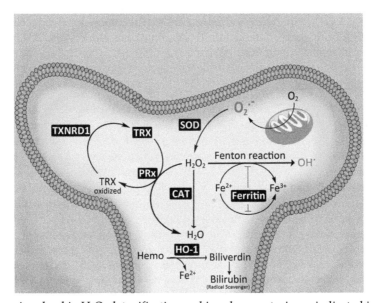

Fig. 6. Genes involved in H_2O_2 detoxification and iron homeostasis are indicated in black boxes. SOD, superoxide dismutase; CAT, catalase; PRx, peroxiredoxin; Trx, thioredoxin; HO-1, hemo oxygenase-1; TXNRD1, thioredoxin reductase-1.

Together, these coordinately regulated gene clusters presented in Figures 5, 6 and 7 strongly support the hypothesis that Nrf2-dependent gene expression is crucial for an efficient detoxification of reactive metabolites and ROS, as well as for the cellular capacity to counteract stressing events such as inflammation.

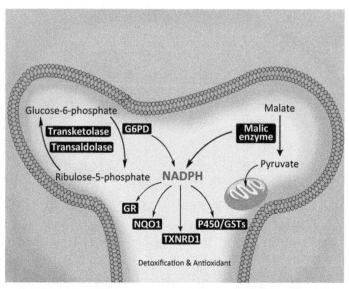

Fig. 7. Genes involved in NADPH homeostasis are indicated in black boxes. P450, cytochrome P450; GST, glutathione-S-transferase; TXNRD1, thioredoxin reductase-1; NQO1, NAD(P)H:quinone oxidoreductase-1; GR, glutathione reductase; G6PD, glucose-6-phosphate dehydrogenase.

6. Nrf2 characteristics

The transcription factor Nrf2 (Nuclear factor-E2-related factor 2) is the guardian of redox homeostasis because it regulates basal and inducible expression of array ride of antioxidant and cytoprotective genes, providing a level of protection required for normal cellular activities and against various oxidative stress-related pathologies, including ischemic stroke (Cho & Kleeberger, 2009; Nguyen et al., 2004; Van Muiswinkel & Kuiperij, 2005). Nrf2 is highly expressed in detoxification organs - such as liver and kidney - and organs exposed to the external environment - such as skin, lung and digestive tract - (Motohashi et al., 2002), whereas in the brain its levels are low (Moi et al., 1994).

Nrf2 is a member of the cap 'n' collar (CNC) family basic region-leucine zipper transcription factor (Katsuoka et al., 2005; Sykiotis & Bohmann, 2010). Nrf2 protein has six highly conserved regions, called Nrf2-ECH homology (Neh) domains. Neh1 is located in the half C-terminal of the molecule and constitutes the basic DNA binding domain and the leucine zipper for dimerization. Neh2 domain is located in the proximal N-terminus of Nrf2 and represents the region through which Nrf2 associates with the cytoplasmic protein Keap1 (kelch-like ECH-associated protein 1) (Itoh et al., 1999). Neh6 is a redox-insensitive degron, which is essential for maximal turnover of Nrf2 in stressed cells, as well as for its degradation (McMahon et al., 2004). Neh3 domain is required for transcriptional activation of the protein (Nioi et al., 2005). Neh4 and Neh5 domains are required for its binding to ARE (Figure 8, *upper panel*).

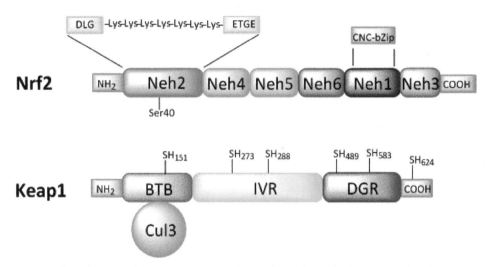

Fig. 8. Nrf2 and Keap1 domains. *Upper panel*: in Nrf2, Neh1 is the basic DNA binding domain and the leucine zipper for dimerization. Neh2 is the Keap1 (kelch-like ECH-associated protein 1) binding domain. Neh3 is required for transcriptional activation of the protein. Neh4 and Neh5 domains are required for the binding to ARE. Neh6 is essential for both Nrf2 turnover in stressed cells and for its degradation. *Lower panel*: in Keap1, BTB domain functions as a substrate adaptor protein for a Cul3-dependent ubiquitin ligase complex. IVR domain is a domain of intervention which is distinguished for its high number of cysteine residues. DGR domain is associated with actin filaments, giving stability to Keap1.

Under oxidant conditions, Nrf2 binds with high affinity to the *cis*-acting enhancer sequence called Antioxidant Response Element (ARE, 5´-GTGACnnnGC-3´), located in the 5´-flanking regions of a broad range of antioxidant and cytoprotective genes that act against oxidative/electrophilic damage (Nguyen et al., 2004; Rushmore et al., 1991). The binding of Nrf2 to ARE requires its heterodimerization with small Maf proteins (Katsuoka et al., 2005), which stimulates transcription of downstream genes, with participation of transcriptional co-activators - mainly CREB-binding protein (CBP) -, through the Neh4 and Neh5 domains (Figure 8, *upper panel*) in the transcription factor. These co-activators act synergistically to attain maximum its activity (Katoh et al., 2001).

7. Regulation of Nrf2: Keap1 (ARE elements)

Nrf2 activity is primarily regulated by suppressor protein Keap1 (Figure 8, *lower panel*), a member of the BTB (Broad complex/Tramtrack/Bric-a-brac)-Kelch protein family (Cullinan et al., 2004), that under normal conditions (unstressed) forms a complex with Nrf2 within the cytosol. This complex is associated with actin filaments through its double glycine repeat

(DGR) domain (Figure 10, *left panel*), which plays an important role in retention of Nrf2 (Kang et al., 2004).

BTB domain of Keap1 functions as an adaptor for Cul3-dependent E3 ubiquitin ligase complex that interacts with the seven lysine residues located in the Neh2 domain of Nrf2, promoting its ubiquitination (Kobayashi et al., 2004; Zhang et al., 2004) and its continuous degradation by 26S proteasome (Nguyen et al., 2003). This is supported by the relatively short half-life of Nrf2 (10-30 min) in absence of cellular stress (McMahon et al., 2003). Upon oxidative stress conditions, the interaction between Nrf2 and Keap1 is disrupted through changes in certain domains of Keap1, hence promoting the release of Nrf2 (Eggler et al., 2005).

The human Keap1 protein contains 27 cysteine residues, some of which are highly reactive to a wide variety of chemical stimuli. Furthermore, a large amount of evidence has emerged suggesting that certain cysteines of Keap1 may be targets of Nrf2 inducers such as sulforaphane, which reacts with thiol groups of Keap1 to form resistant thionoacyl adducts by hydrolysis and transacylation reactions (Hong et al., 2005) (Figure 9).

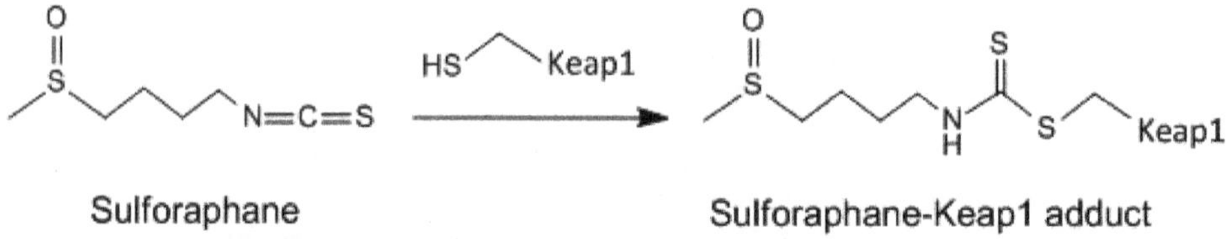

Sulforaphane   Sulforaphane-Keap1 adduct

Fig. 9. Formation of adducts between sulforaphane and Keap1.

It has been reported that Cys151 in BTB domain of Keap1 is required for inhibition of Keap1-dependent Nrf2 degradation stimulated by sulforaphane and oxidative stress (Zhang & Hannink, 2003). Cys273 and Cys288, located in the IVR domain of Keap1, are essential for its repressive activity under basal conditions. It has been suggested that this effect also responds to sulforaphane (Kobayashi et al., 2006). On the other hand, it has been reported that Cys489, Cys583, and Cys624 were most reactive toward sulforaphane (Hong et al., 2005). Therefore, the responsiveness of Nrf2 to inducers, such as sulforaphane, involves redox-dependent alterations of thiol groups in several domains of Keap1, which acts like a sensor responding to oxidative and environment stress through dynamic changes in cystein reducing status (Jung & Kwak, 2010). In turn, Keap1 is considered as a zinc metalloprotein because the chemical modification of critical cysteine residues is modulated by thiol-bound zinc (approximately 1 mol per subunit), which is displaced by the reaction with inducers or other classical sulfhydryl reagents, such as sulforaphane (Dinkova-Kostova et al., 2005b).

Another important event in the activation of Nrf2 may be its phosphorylation. The protein kinase-dependent signal transduction pathways have been implicated in the release of Nrf2 from Keap1-mediated repression, mainly by protein kinase C, whose target is a single serine residue, Ser40 (Bloom & Jaiswal, 2003; Huang et al., 2002). To explain how Keap1/Nrf2 complex respond to basal or inducible stimuli, it has been proposed the "hinge and latch" model (Tong et al., 2006a), which suggests that a single Nrf2 molecule makes contacts with two domains of Keap1 homodimer (McMahon et al., 2006; Tong et al., 2006a). Neh2 domain of Nrf2 contains two sites for Keap1 binding, termed motifs DLG and ETGE. These motifs exhibit different affinity for Keap1; the affinity of ETGE is greater than DLG (Tong et al., 2006b). The term "hinge" indicates that the interaction of high affinity is not affected by inducers; in contrast, inducers abolish the low-affinity interaction mediated by the "latch", thereby disrupting the presentation of Nrf2 to the ubiquitination machinery of Keap1 (Li & Kong, 2009) (Figure 10, *right panel*). Other models that describe the interaction between Nrf2 and Keap1 have provided conflicting information when contrasted with the "hinge and latch" model (Lo & Hannink, 2006; 2008).

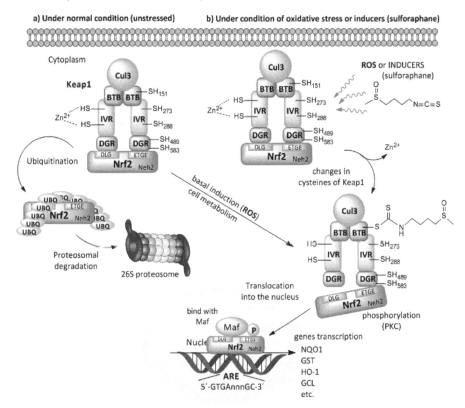

Fig. 10. Effect of sulforaphane on Nrf2/Keap1 complex. *Left panel*: Upon unstressed conditions, this complex is dissociated and Nrf2 can either suffer proteosomal degradation or respond to stimuli typical of basal cell metabolism. In the later, Nrf2 is phosphorylated and translocated to the nucleus forming heterodimers with Maf and acting on ARE. *Right panel*: Under stress oxidative conditions, or in the presence of inducers, several cysteine residues suffer changes inducing its Nrf2 dissociation and further translocation of this factor to nucleus, where it will induce phase 2 genes transcription.

Sulforaphane induces a phase 2 response as a result of gene expression modulation through Nrf2/ARE pathway. ARE-driven targets include NAD(P)H:quinone oxidereductase (NQO1), heme oxygenase-1 (HO-1) and γ-glutamylcysteine ligase (γGCL). The induction of these enzymes has been observed both in *in vivo* and *in vitro* experiments after sulforaphane treatment.

8. Nrf2 in cerebral ischemia

Nrf2 has been detected in neuronal and glial cells (Chen et al., 2011; Li et al., 2011; Shah et al., 2010; Yang et al., 2009). Previous studies using gel-shift assay found that ischemic brains selectively upregulates ARE-mediated gene expression, whereas binding activities of other stress response elements were unchanged, including metal response element, interleukin-6, and STAT (signal transducer and activator of transcription) response elements (Campage et al., 2000).

Middle cerebral artery occlusion (permanent or transient) is a classical and well-characterized model inducing cerebral ischemia in rats that involves a cytotoxic response occurring within few minutes from the onset of cerebral ischemia, and encompasses oxidative stress, pro-inflammatory responses and cell death (Ikeda et al., 2003; Longa et al., 1989; Simonyi et al., 2005). Yang et al. (2009) used permanent focal ischemia to detect the expression of Nrf2. They found that Nrf2 protein and mRNA were upregulated when is compared with normal control, showing a peak at 24 h and localizing with nuclei and cytoplasm of neurons and astrocytes. Alternatively, Nrf2 was presented in the injured regions of cortices with cerebral ischemic/reperfusion, and markedly increased in both cytoplasm and nuclei (Li et al., 2011). Meanwhile, Keap1 immunoreactivity was significantly reduced. Besides, an altered expression of thioredoxin, glutathione, and heme oxigenase was detected (Tanaka et al., 2011).

Oligemia is another model that was used to determine Nrf2 localization. It consists in a reduction in the mean arterial pressure to 30-40 mm Hg, resulting in a 50% reduction in cerebral blood flow after reperfusion. This blood flow reduction presents an increase in oxidative stress through lipid peroxidation (Heim et al., 1995; Läer et al., 1993) and an augmented $^\bullet OH$ production during the reperfusion phase (Heim et al., 2000). In this model, Nrf2 was specifically upregulated 1 h after the surgery. Nrf2-positive neurons were found in the Purkinje cells of the cerebellar cortex and in the pyramidal neurons of the cingulate cortex (Liverman et al., 2004).

Additionally, Nrf2 knockout (Nrf2$^{-/-}$) mice have been used to understand the role of Nrf2 during ischemia-mediated oxidative brain insult.

In vitro studies showed that neurons and astrocytes from Nrf2 knockout (Nrf2$^{-/-}$) mice were more sensitive to oxidative stress, Ca^{2+} influx and mitochondrial toxicity than neurons and astrocytes from wild type animals; however, when the cells were transfected with a functional Nrf2 construct, they became less prone to oxidative stress (Kraft et al., 2004; Lee et al., 2003a; Lee and Johnson, 2004). Consistent with these results, dominant negative-Nrf2 stable cells and Nrf2-sensitized neuroblastoma cells silenced with siRNA were more amenable to apoptosis induced by nitric oxide (Dhakshinamoorthy & Porter, 2004). Also, increasing Nrf2 activity in mixed neuronal/glial cultures was highly neuroprotective in *in vitro* models that simulated components of stroke damage, such as oxidative glutamate toxicity, H$_2$O$_2$ exposure, metabolic inhibition by rotenone, and Ca^{2+} overload (Duffy et al., 1998; Kraft et al., 2004; Lee et al., 2003b; Murphy et al., 1991; Shih et al., 2003).

In vivo, using permanent middle cerebral artery occlussion by cauterization, Shih et al. (2005) did not observe significant difference in infarct size between Nrf2$^{-/-}$ and Nrf2$^{+/+}$ mice 24 h after stroke. However, 7 days after permanent focal ischemia, they observed a two-fold increase in infarct volume with Nrf2$^{-/-}$ mice, while the infarct size of Nrf2$^{+/+}$ mice did not increase in size between 24 h and 7 days. On the other hand, Nrf2 knockout (Nrf2$^{-/-}$) mice subjected to 90 min middle cerebral artery occlusion followed by 24 h reperfusion, showed an infarct volume and neurological deficit significantly larger than in wild type mice (Shah et al., 2007).

Taking together, these data suggest that Nrf2 is upregulated in permanent ischemia and ischemic/reperfusion, an augment that is related with a decreased expression of Keap1 and an altered expression of antioxidant proteins. Thus, this upregulation may be due to an alteration in the redox state, a mechanism through which cells active an antioxidant response to protect themselves from future oxidant damage. Moreover, it has been demonstrated that Nrf2 activation induces the expression of the Nrf2 gene itself (Lee et al., 2005), indicating that the administration of Nrf2 inducers may be an important neuroprotective antioxidant mechanism that can limit stroke damage.

9. Effect of Nrf2 inducers in cerebral ischemia

A wide range of dietary phytochemicals or supplements with medicinal properties have been reported to activate adaptive stress responses related with the induction of cytoprotective genes through Nrf2 induction (Surh et al., 2008). The mechanism of action of such phytochemicals can therefore be considered as a form of hormesis where a stressor triggers an adaptive response which increases resistance to more severe stress and disease (Calabrese et al., 2007). Unfortunately, few of these compounds have been tested in brain ischemic models; some of them are sulforaphane, curcumin and ter-butilhydroquinone, among others.

Sulforaphane

Sulforaphane is a natural dietary isothiocyanate present in cruciferous vegetables of the genus *Brassica* such as broccoli, brussel sprouts, cauliflower, cabbage, etc. Several studies have shown the neuroprotective properties of sulforaphane against ischemia/reperfusion damage. It has been found that sulforaphane (5 mg/kg) reduced the cerebral infarct volume in a carotid/middle cerebral artery occlusion common model in rodents when it was administered 15 min after injury (Zhao et al., 2006). Other groups reported that an injection of sulforaphane (5 mg/kg) 30 min before the onset of ischemia reduced the infarct size in a neonatal hypoxia-ischemia model (Ping et al., 2010). In both studies, the protective effects of sulforaphane were associated with its well-known capacity to induce the expression of HO-1 mRNA and protein through Nrf2/ARE pathway.

Other *in vivo* studies support the ability of sulforaphane as inducer of phase II enzymes in brain increasing HO-1, NQO1 and GST mRNA levels (Chen et al., 2011). It has also shown in *in vitro* studies that pretreatment and post-treatment with sulforaphane reduced hippocampal death of astrocytes and neurons induced by transient exposure to O_2 and glucose deprivation. This protective effect was associated with nuclear accumulation of Nrf2 accompanied by an increase in NQO1, HO-1 and GCL mRNA levels, and a decrease in DNA oxidation (Danilov et al., 2009; Soane et al., 2010). Altogether, these studies indicate that sulforaphane could be considered as a useful tool for pre- and post-treatment of brain injury due its well-know capacity as inducer of Nrf2.

Curcumin

Curcumin is a diferuloylmethane derived from the rhizomes of turmeric (*Curcuma longa* Linn, Zingiberaceae) widely used in Indian curry with a favorable safe profile. Its chemopreventive effects have been related with its antioxidant and anti-inflammatory properties (Surh & Chun, 2007; Thangapazham et al., 2006). However, its mechanism of action is still poorly understood.

Curcumin has a protective effect against neurodegeneration in cerebral ischemia through the preservation of the blood-brain barrier integrity, and a decrease of the ischemia-induced lipid peroxidation, mitochondrial dysfunction and anti-apoptotic effects (Sun et al., 2008).

Yang et al., (2009) observed that the systematic administration of curcumin (100 mg/kg) 15 min after middle cerebral artery permanent occlusion increased Nrf2 nuclear translocation and Nrf2 and HO-1 gene and protein levels at 24 h onset of reperfusion. Curcumin reduced neurologic deficit, brain edema and infarct volume at 24 h after stroke. These results show that curcumin maybe an effective therapeutic drug for the treatment of brain injury toward a potential mechanism of upregulation Nrf2/ARE pathway at gene and protein levels.

However, the bioavailability of curcumin is very limited due to poor absorption, rapid metabolism and quick systemic elimination. Moreover, it has a poor blood-brain barrier penetration following acute administration. To improve its bioavailability, pharmacokinetics and interaction with multiple viable targets, new curcumin derivatives are being synthesized (Lapchak, 2001).

tert-Butylhydroquinone (t-BHQ)

tert-butylhydroquinone (t-BHQ), a metabolite of the widely used food antioxidant butylated hydroxyanisole, has already been approved for human use (Food and Agriculture Organization of the United Nations/World Health Organization, 1999; National Toxicology Program, 1997). t-BHQ possesses an oxidizable 1,4 diphenolic structure that confers its potent ability to dissociate Keap1/Nrf2 complex (Van Ommen et al., 1992). T-BHQ can protect neuronal cells against the oxidative insult initiated by dopamine, H_2O_2, *tert*-butyl hydroperoxide, NMDA and glutamate (Duffy et al., 1998; Kraft et al., 2004; Li et al., 2002; Murphy et al., 1991; Shah et al., 2007).

Shih et al., (2005) determined the neuroprotective effect of tBHQ in ischemic injury in two different ischemia/reperfusion models - middle cerebral artery occlusion and endothelin-1 vasoconstriction - in rats and mice, using different routes of administration: intacerebroventricular, intraperitoneal, and dietary. Intracerebroventricular administration of t-BHQ (1 μL/h) during 3 days before rats were subjected to 1.5 h of ischemia and 24 h reperfusion showed a significant reduction of infarction in the cortex and a significant reduction in the neuronal scores. Intraperitoneal administration of t-BHQ (16.7 mg/Kg; 3 times/8h) 24 h before middle cerebral artery occlusion improved functional recovery up to 1 month after MCAO, showing a long-term benefit in ischemic damage and sensimotor deficit. Nrf2$^{+/+}$ and Nrf2$^{+/-}$ mice fed with 1% t-BHQ during one week before permanent focal ischemia did not show changes in infarct area after 7 days, while Nrf2$^{-/-}$ mice were less tolerant to the diet, losing 20% body weight and showing a continuous growth of infarct area, thus suggesting that loss of Nrf2 function promotes peri-infact zone. Finally, Nrf2$^{+/+}$ and Nrf2$^{-/-}$ mice were fed with t-BHQ after endothelin-1 administration into cortical parenchyma. Nrf2$^{+/+}$ mice showed a decrease in endothelin-1-induced infarction while Nrf2$^{-/-}$ mice showed an exacerbated injury (Shih et al., 2003; 2005).

Collectively, these data suggest that t-BHQ may have a therapeutic potential for ischemic injury by increasing brain antioxidant capacity though the up-regulation of Nrf2 expression.

10. Presumable protective effect of garlic compounds in cerebral ischemia

Numerous studies have shown that garlic and its compounds exhibit a diverse biological activity, including anti-tumorigenic, anti-atherosclerosis, detoxification, anti-inflammatory, and antioxidant (Aguilera et al., 2010; Ali et al., 2000; Fisher et al., 2007; Fukushima et al., 1997; Mathew & Biju, 2008). The effect of different garlic preparations (aged garlic extract, aqueous garlic extract, garlic oil) and isolated compounds (S-allylcysteine) in cerebral ischemia, has been associated to its ability to scavenge ROS, acting as direct antioxidants (Kim et al., 2006a).

Gupta et al. (2003) found that garlic oil administration 90 min before the ischemia/reperfusion diminished the infarct area and associated this effect to its antioxidant properties. Saleem et al. (2006) showed that aqueous garlic extract treatment increased neurobehavioral score, decreased malondialdehyde levels, increased GSH content, and prevented the depletion in GPx, GR, GST and Na^+/K^+-ATPasa activities. Moreover, CAT and SOD activities were increased by aqueous garlic extract. Aguilera et al. (2010) reported that the major protective effect exerted by aged garlic extract was observed when it was administered at the onset of reperfusion. In this work, aged garlic extract prevented the ischemia/reperfusion-induced increase in nitrotyrosine levels and the decrease in GPx, SOD and CAT activities both in cortex and striatum.

Numagami et al. (1996) demonstrated that aged garlic extract compounds that present a thioallyl group (particularly S-allylcysteine) exhibited a strong antioxidant capacity in a model of cerebral ischemia in rats. Indeed, S-allylcysteine reduced the infarct volume and brain edema, while prevented $ONOO^-$ formation and lipid peroxidation (Numagami & Ohnishi, 2001). More recently, S-allylcysteine (300 mg/kg, i.p.) produced a protective effect on cerebral ischemic injury in rats due to the inhibition of extracellular signal-regulated kinase activity (Kim et al., 2006a). The fact that S-allylcysteine can cross the blood-brain barrier turned it soon of potential interest to be tested in neurotoxic models. In fact, the prophylactic impact and rescue properties of S-allylcysteine in ischemia/reperfusion injury are being recently discussed and reinforced (Sener et al., 2007). In addition, S-allylcysteine is a stable compound (Lawson, 1998) and is easily absorbed by gastrointestinal tract after oral administration (Kodera et al., 2002). One of its advantages in regard to other garlic compounds, such as allicin and dialyl sulfide, is its limited toxicity established by its higher lethal oral dose (Amagase et al., 2001). Pharmacokinetic studies demonstrate fast absorption and distribution phases followed by a slow elimination phase for oral administration, as well as fast distribution and slow elimination phases for i.v. administration (Nagae et al., 1994; Yan & Zeng, 2005). Pharmacokinetics of S-allylcysteine in humans by oral garlic administration revealed a half-life of 10 h and clearance time of 30 h (Kodera et al., 2002), suggesting a high bioavailability. After its oral administration, S-allylcysteine is absorbed by gastrointestinal tract, and its higher concentrations are detected in plasma and kidney up to 8 h post-intake (Nagae et al., 1994; Yan & Zeng, 2005).

On the other hand, garlic oil-derived organosulfur compounds such as diallyl trisulfide, dialyl disulfide, and dialyl sulfide provide significant protection against carcinogenesis, and this protection is likely related with their antioxidant properties (Maldonado et al., 2009). Moreover, the lipophilic characteristics of these compounds allow crossing the blood-brain barrier as follows: dialyl sulfide crosses the blood-brain barrier easier than dialyl disulfide > diallyl trisulfide > S-allylcysteine (Kim et al., 2006b).

Recently, it has been reported that some garlic compounds (diallyl trisulfide, dialyl disulfide, dialyl sulfide and S-ally-L-cysteine) are able to activate Nrf2 factor in liver, kidney, intestine and lung. (Chen et al., 2004; Fisher et al., 2007; Fukao et al., 2004; Gong et al., 2004; Guyonnet et al., 1999; Kalayarasan et al., 2008; 2009; Wu et al., 2002). However, there is no information on Nrf2 induction by these garlic compounds in the brain.

Altogether, these data indicate that S-ally-L-cysteine, diallyl trisulfide, dialyl disulfide, and dialyl sulfide may be alternative treatments for cerebral ischemia through Nrf2 upregulation.

11. Conclusion

Nowadays is widely recognized that up-regulation of phase 2 response is a powerful, highly efficient and promising antioxidant strategy for protection against several diseases, including ischemic stroke. A wide range of dietary phytochemicals with medicinal properties have been reported to activate adaptive stress responses related with the induction of cytoprotective genes through Nrf2/ARE pathway. Unfortunately, few of these compounds (sulforaphane, curcumin, ter-butilhydroquinone) have been tested in cerebral ischemia experimental models. Moreover, these compounds have characteristics that limit their use as therapeutic agents in ischemic stroke. For example, sulforaphane is expensive, while curcumin poorly crosses the blood-brain barrier. Due to this, new agents should be evaluated. In this context, some garlic compounds (diallyl sulfide, diallyl disulfide, diallyl trisulfide and S-allylcysteine) could be promising agents for treatment of ischemic stroke because their physicochemical properties are promising, their absorption is high and most of them can easily cross the blood-brain barrier. Moreover, they have the ability to active Nrf2 factor and induce a phase 2 response in several models of hepatic and renal damage.

12. Acknowledgements

This study was supported by CONACYT (Grant No. 103527 to PDM).

13. Abbreviation list

ARE	Antioxidant Response Element
BH2	Dihydrobiopterin
BH4	Tetrahydrobiopterin
CAT	Catalase
G6PD	Glucose-6phosphate dehydrogenase
GCLC	Glutamate cysteine ligase catalitic subunit
GCLM	Glutamate cysteine ligase modifier subunit
GPx	Glutathione Peroxidase
GSH	Reduced Glutathione
GSSG	Oxidized Glutathione
HO-1	Heme oxygenase-1
NQO1	NADPH:quinone oxidoreductase-1
Keap1	Kelch-like ECH-associated protein 1
Nrf2	Nuclear Factor-E2-related Factor 2
RNS	Reactive Nitrogen Species

ROS	Reactive Oxygen Species
SOD	Superoxide Dismutase
tBHQ	tert-butylhydroquinone
TXNRD1	Thioredoxine Reductase-1

14. References

Aguilera, P.; Chánez-Cárdenas, M.E. & Maldonado, P.D. (2007). Recent Advances in the Use of Antioxidant Treatments in Cerebral Ischemia, In: *New Perspectives on Brain Cell Damage, Neurodegeneration and Neuroprotective Strategies*, A. Santamaría & M.E. Jiménez-Capdeville, (Ed.), 145–159, Research Signpost, ISBN 81-308-0164-7, Kerala, India.

Aguilera, P.; Chánez-Cárdenas, M.E.; Ortiz-Plata, A.; León-Aparicio, D.; Barrera, D.; Ezpinoza-Rojo, M.; Villeda-Hernández, J.; Sánchez-García, A. & Maldonado P.D. (2010). Aged Garlic Extract Delays the Appearance of Infarct Area in Cerebral Ischemia Model, an Effect Likely Conditioned by the Celular Antioxidant System. *Phytomedicine*, Vol.17, No.4-3, (March), pp. 241-247, ISSN 0944-7113 (Print)

Alfieri, A.; Srivastava, S.; Siow, R.C.; Modo, M.; Fraser, P.A. & Mann, G.E. (2011). Targeting the Nrf2-Keap1 Antioxidant Defence Pathway for Neurovascular Protection in Stroke. *Journal of Physiologie*, Vol.589, No.Pt17, (September), pp. 4125-4136, ISSN 0022-3751 (Print)

Ali, M.; Al-Qattan, K.K.; Al-Enezi, F.; Khanafer, R.M. & Mustafa, T. (2000). Effect of Allicin From Garlic Powder on Serum Lipids and Blood Pressure in Rats Fed With a High Cholesterol Diet. *Prostaglandins, leukotrienes, and essential fatty acids*, Vol.62, No.4, (April), pp. 253-259, ISSN 0952-3278 (Print)

Amagase, H.; Petesch, B.L.; Matsuura, H.; Kasuga, S. & Itakura, Y. (2001). Intake of Garlic and Its Bioactive Components. *Journal of Nutrition*, Vol.131, No.3s, (March), pp. 955S-962S, ISSN 0022-3166 (Print)

Aronowski, J.; Strong, R. & Grotta, J.C. (1997). Reperfusion Injury: Demonstration of Brain Damage Produced by Reperfusion After Transient Focal Ischemia in Rats. *Journal of Cerebral Blood Flow and Metabolism*, Vol.17, No.10, (October), pp. 1048–1056, ISSN 0271-678X (Print)

Bloom, D.A. & Jaiswal, A.K. (2003). Phosphorylation of Nrf2 at Ser40 by Protein Kinase C in Response to Antioxidants Leads to the Release of Nrf2 From INrf2, but is not Required for Nrf2 Stabilization/Accumulation in the Nucleus and Transcriptional Activation of Antioxidant Response Element-Mediated NAD(P)H:Quinone Oxidoreductase-1 Gene Expression. *The Journal of Biological Chemistry*, Vol.278, No.45, (November), pp. 44675-44682, ISSN 0021-9258 (Print)

Calabrese, E.J.; Bachmann, K.A.; Bailer, A.J.; Bolger, P.M.; Borak, J.; Cai, L.; Cedergreen, N.; Cherian, M.G.; Chiueh, C.C.; Clarkson, T.W.; Cook, R.R.; Diamond, D.M.; Doolittle, D.J.; Dorato, M.A.; Duke, S.O.; Feinendegen, L.; Gardner, D.E.; Hart, R.W.; Hastings, K.L.; Hayes, A.W.; Hoffmann, G.R.; Ives, J.A.; Jaworowski, Z.; Johnson, T.E.; Jonas, W.B.; Kaminski, N.E.; Keller, J.G.; Klaunig, J.E.; Knudsen, T.B.; Kozumbo, W.J.; Lettieri, T.; Liu, S.Z.; Maisseu, A.; Maynard, K.I.; Masoro, E.J.; McClellan, R.O.; Mehendale, H.M.; Mothersill, C.; Newlin, D.B.; Nigg, H.N.; Oehme, F.W.; Phalen, R.F.; Philbert, M.A.; Rattan, S.I.; Riviere, J.E.; Rodricks, J.; Sapolsky, R.M.; Scott, B.R.; Seymour, C.; Sinclair, D.A.; Smith-Sonneborn, J.; Snow,

E.T.; Spear, L.; Stevenson, D.E.; Thomas, Y.; Tubiana, M.; Williams, G.M. & Mattson, M.P. (2007). Biological Stress Response Terminology: Integrating the Concepts of Adaptive Response and Preconditioning Stress Within a Hormetic Dose-Response Framework. *Toxicology and Applied Pharmacology*, Vol.222, No.1, (July), pp. 122-128, ISSN 0041-008X (Print)

Campagne, M.V.; Thibodeaux, H.; van Bruggen, N.; Cairns, B. & Lowe, D.G. (2000). Increased Binding Activity at an Antioxidant-Responsive Element in the Metallothionein-1 Promoter and Rapid Induction of Metallothionein-1 and -2 in Response to Cerebral Ischemia and Reperfusion. *The Journal of Neuroscience: the Official Journal of the Society for Neuroscience*, Vol.20, No.14, (July), pp. 5200-5207, ISSN 0270-6474 (Print)

Chan, P.H. (2001). Reactive oxygen radicals in signaling and damage in the ischemic brain. *Journal of Cerebral Blood Flow and Metabolism*, Vol. 21, No. 1, (January), pp. 2-14, ISSN 0271-678X (Print)

Chen, C.; Pung, D.; Leong, V.; Hebbar, V.; Shen, G.; Nair, S.; Li, W. & Kong, A.N. (2004). Induction of Detoxifying Enzymes by Garlic Organosulfur Compounds Through Transcription Factor Nrf2: Effect of Chemical Structure and Stress Signals. *Free Radical Biology & Medicine*, Vol.37, No.10, (November), pp. 1578-1590, ISSN 0891-5849 (Print)

Chen, G.; Fang, Q.; Zhang, J.; Zhou, D. & Wang, Z. (2011). Role of the Nrf2-ARE Pathway in Early Brain Injury After Experimental Subarachnoid Hemorrhage. *Journal of Neuroscience Research*, Vol.89, No.4, (April), pp. 515-523, ISSN 0360-4012 (Print)

Cho, H.Y. & Kleeberger, S.R. (2009). Nrf2 Protects Against Airway Disorders. *Toxicology and Applied Pharmacology*, Vol.244, No.1, (April), pp. 43-56, ISSN 0041-008X (Print)

Christensen, T.; Bruhn, T.; Balchen, T. & Diemer, N.H. (1994). Evidence for Formation of Hydroxyl Radicals During Reperfusion After Global Cerebral Ischaemia in Rats Using Salicylate Trapping and Microdialysis. *Neurobiology of Disease*, Vol.1, No.3, (December), pp. 131–138, ISSN 0969-9961 (Print)

Crabtree, M.J. & Channon, K.M. (2011). Synthesis and Recycling of Tetrahydrobiopterin in Endothelial Function and Vascular Disease. *Nitric Oxide*, Vol.25, No.2, (August), pp. 81-88, ISSN 1089-8603 (Print)

Cullinan, S.B.; Gordan, J.D.; Jin, J.; Harper, J.W. & Diehl, J.A. (2004). The Keap1-BTB Protein is an Adaptor That Bridges Nrf2 to a Cul3-Based E3 Ligase: Oxidative Stress Sensing by a Cul3-Keap1 Ligase. *Molecular and Cellular Biology*, Vol.24, No.19, (October), pp. 8477-8486, ISSN 0270-7306 (Print)

Danilov, C.A.; Chandrasekaran, K.; Racz, J.; Soane, L.; Zielke, C. & Fiskum, G. (2009). Sulforaphane Protects Astrocytes Against Oxidative Stress and Delayed Death Caused by Oxygen and Glucose Deprivation. *Glia*, Vol.57, No.6, (April), pp. 645-656, ISSN 0894-1491 (Print)

Danton, G.H. & Dietrich, W.D. (2003). Inflammatory Mechanism After Ischemia and Stroke. *Journal of Neuropathology and Experimental Neurology*, Vol.62, No.2, (February), pp. 127-136, ISSN 0022-3069 (Print)

Dhakshinamoorthy, S. & Porter, A.G. (2004). Nitric Oxide-Induced Transcriptional Up-Regulation of Protective Genes by Nrf2 Via the Antioxidant Response Element Counteracts Apoptosis of Neuroblastoma Cells. *The Journal of Biological Chemistry*, Vol.279, No.19, (May), pp. 20096–20107, ISSN 0021-9258 (Print)

Díez-Tejedor, E.; Del Brutto, O.; Álvarez-Sabín, J.; Muñoz, M. & Abiusi, G. (2001). Classification of the Cerebrovascular Diseases. *Revista de Neurologia*, Vol.33, No.5, (September), pp. 455-464, ISSN 0210-0010 (Print)

Dinkova-Kostova, A.T.; Massiah, M.A.; Bozak, R.E.; Hicks, R.J. & Talalay, P. (2001). Potency of Michael Reaction Acceptors as Inducers of Enzymes That Protect Against Carcinogenesis Depends on Their Reactivity With Sulfhydryl Groups. *Proceedings of the National Academy of Sciences of the United States of America*, Vol.98, No.6, (March), pp. 3404-3409, ISSN 0027-8424 (Print)

Dinkova-Kostova, A.T.; Fahey, J.W. & Talalay, P. (2004) Chemical Structures of Inducers of Nicotinamide Quinone Oxidoreductase 1 (NQO1). *Methods in Enzymology*, Vol.382, pp. 423-448, ISSN 0076-6879 (Print)

Dinkova-Kostova, A.T.; Holtzclaw, W.D. & Kensler, T.W. (2005a) The Role of Keap1 in Celular Protective Responses. *Chemical Research in Toxicology*, Vol.18, No.12, (December), pp. 1779-1791. ISSN 0893-228X (Print)

Dinkova-Kostova, A.T.; Holtzclaw, W.D. & Wakabayashi, N. (2005b). Keap1, the Sensor for Electrophiles and Oxidants That Regulates the Phase 2 Response, is a Zinc Metalloprotein. *Biochemistry*, Vol.44, No.18, (May), pp. 6889-6899, ISSN 0006-2960 (Print)

Dinkova-Kostova, A.T.; Cheah, J.; Samouilov, A.; Zweier, J.L.; Bozak, R.E.; Hicks, R.J. & Talalay, P. (2007). Phenolic Michael Reaction Acceptors: Combined Direct and Indirect Antioxidant Defenses Against Electrophiles and Oxidants. *Medicinal Chemistry*, Vol.3, No.3, (May), pp. 261-268, ISSN 1573-4064 (Print)

Dinkova-Kostova, A.T. & Talalay, P. (2008). Direct and Indirect Antioxidant Properties of Inducers of Cytoprotective Proteins. *Molecular Nutrition & Food Ressearch*, Vol.52, No.Suppl1, (June), pp. S128–S138, ISSN 1613-4125 (Print)

Dirnagl, U.; Iadecola, C. & Moskowitz, M.A. (1999). Pathobiology of Ischaemic Stroke: An Integrated View. *Trends in Neuroscience*, Vol.22, No.9, (September), pp. 391-397, ISSN 0166-2236 (Print)

Dringen, R. (2000). Metabolism and Functions of Glutathione in Brain. *Progress in Neurobiology*, Vol.62, No.6, (December), pp. 649-671, ISSN 0301-0082 (Print)

Duffy, S.; So, A. & Murphy, T.H. (1998). Activation of Endogenous Antioxidant Defenses in Neuronal Cells Prevents Free Radical-Mediated Damage. *Journal of Neurochemistry*, Vol.71, No.1, (July), pp. 69–77, ISSN 0022-3042 (Print)

Durukan, A. & Tatlisumak, T. (2007). Acute Ischemic Stroke: Overview of Major Experimental Rodent Models, Pathophysiology, and Therapy of Focal Cerebral Ischemia. *Pharmacology, Biochemistry, and Behavior*, Vol.87, No.1, (May), pp. 179-197, ISSN 0091-3057 (Print)

Eggler, A.L.; Liu, G.; Pezzuto, J.M.; van Breemen, R.B. & Mesecar, A.D. (2005). Modifying Specific Cysteines of the Electrophile-Sensing Human Keap1 Protein is Insufficient to Disrupt Binding to the Nrf2 Domain Neh2. *Proceedings of the National Academy of Sciences of the United States of America*, Vol.102, No.29, (July), pp. 10070-10075, ISSN 0027-8424 (Print)

Fisher, C.D., Augustine, L.M.; Maher, J.M.; Nelson, D.M.; Slitt, A.L.; Klaassen, C.D.; Lehman-McKeeman, L.D. & Cherrington, N.J. (2007). Induction of Drug Metabolizing Enzymes by Garlic and Allyl Sulfide Compounds Via Activation of Constitutive Androstane Receptor and Nuclear Factor E2-Related Factor 2. *Drug*

Metabolism and Disposition: The Biological Fate of Chemicals, Vol. 35, No. 6, (June), pp. 995-1000, ISSN 0090-9556 (Print)

Food and Agriculture Organization of the United Nations/World Health Organization. (1999). Evaluation of certain food additives and contaminants (forty-ninth report of the Joint FAO/WHO Expert Committee on Food Additives). World Health Organ Tech Rep Ser 884:i-viii, pp. 1–96.

Fukao, T.; Hosono, T.; Misawa, S.; Seki, T. & Ariga, T. (2004). The Effects of Allyl Sulfides on the Induction of Phase II Detoxification Enzymes and Liver Injury by Carbon Tetrachloride. *Food and Chemical Toxicology: An International Journal Publisher for the British Industrial Biological Research Association*, Vol42, No.5, (May), pp. 743-749, ISSN 0278-6915 (Print)

Fukushima, S.; Takada, N.; Hori, T. & Wanibuchi, H. (1997). Cancer Prevention by Organosulfur Compounds From Garlic and Onion. *Journal of Cellular Biochemistry. Supplement*, Vol.27, pp. 100-105, ISSN 0733-1959 (Print)

Gong, P.; Hu, B. & Cederbaum, A.I. (2004). Diallyl Sulfide Induces Heme Oxygenase-1 Through MAPK Pathway. *Archives of Biochemistry and Biophysics*, Vol.432, No.2, (December), pp. 252-260, ISSN 0003-9861 (Print)

Gupta, R.; Singh, M. & Sharma, A. (2003). Neuroprotective Effect of Antioxidants on Ischemia and Reperfusion-Induced Cerebral Injury. *Pharmacological Research: the Official Journal of the Italian Pharmacological Society*, Vol.48, No.2, (August), pp. 209-215, ISSN 1043-6618 (Print)

Guyonnet, D.; Siess, M.H.; Le Bon, A.M. & Suschetet, M. (1999). Modulation of Phase II Enzymes by Organosulfur Compounds From Allium Vegetables in Rat Tissues. *Toxicology and Applied Pharmacology*, Vol.154, No.1, (January), pp. 50-58, ISSN 0041-008X (Print)

Halliwell, B. & Gutteridge, J. (1999). *Free Radicals in Biology and Medicine*, Oxford Univ. Press, ISBN 13 9780198568698, New York

Heim, C.; Melzacka, M.; Kolasiewicz, W.; Jaros, T.; Sieklucka, M.; Wesemann, W. & Sontag, K.H. (1995). Cerebral Oligemic Hypoxia and Iron Toxicity in the Mesolimbic System of Rats. *Journal of Neural Transmission. Supplementum*, Vol.46, pp. 165-173, ISSN 0303-6995 (Print)

Heim, C.; Zhang, J.; Lan, J.; Sieklucka, M.; Kurz, T.; Riederer, P.; Gerlach, M. & Sontag K.H. (2000). Cerebral Oligaemia Episode Triggers Free Radical Formation and Late Cognitive Deficiencies. *The European Journal of Neuroscience*, Vol.12, No.4, (February), pp. 715-725, ISSN 0953-816X (Print)

Heiss, W.D. (2002). Stroke--Acute Interventions. *Journal of Neural Transmission. Supplementum*, Vol.63, pp. 37-57, ISSN 0303-6995 (Print)

Hong, F.; Freeman, M.L. & Liebler, D.C. (2005). Identification of Sensor Cysteines in Human Keap1 Modified by the Cancer Chemopreventive Agent Sulforaphane. *Chemical Research in Toxicolog*, Vol.18, No.12, (December), pp. 1917-1926, ISSN 0893-228X (Print)

Hou, ST. & MacManus, J.P. (2002). Molecular Mechanisms of Cerebral Ischemia-Induced Neuronal Death. *International Review of Cytology*, Vol.221, pp. 93-148, ISSN 0074-7696 (Print)

Huang, H.C.; Nguyen, T. & Pickett. C.B. (2002). Phosphorylation of Nrf2 at Ser-40 by Protein Kinase C Regulates Antioxidant Response Element-Mediated Transcription. *The*

Journal of Biological Chemistry, Vol.277, No.45, (November), pp. 42769-42774, ISSN 0021-9258 (Print)

Hsu, C.Y.; Ahmed, S.H. & Lees, K.R. (2000). The Therapeutic Time Window--Theoretical and Practical Considerations. *Journal of Stroke and Cerebrovascular Diseases: The Official Journal of National Stroke Association*, Vol.9, No.6 Pt2, (November), pp. 24–31, ISSN 1052-3057 (Print)

Ikeda, K.; Negishi, H. & Yamori, Y. (2003). Antioxidant Nutrients and Hypoxia/Ischemia Brain Injury in Rodents. *Toxicology*, Vol.189, No.1-2, (July), pp. 55–61, ISSN 0300-483X (Print)

Itoh, K.; Wakabayashi, N.; Katoh, Y.; Ishii, T.; Igarashi, K.; Engel, J.D. & Yamamoto, M. (1999). Keap1 Represses Nuclear Activation of Antioxidant Responsive Elements by Nrf2 Through Binding to the Amino-Terminal Neh2 Domain. *Genes & Development*, Vol.13, No.1, (January), pp. 76-86, ISSN 0890-9369 (Print)

Itoh,K.; Wakabayashi,N.; Katoh,Y.; Ishii,T.; O'Connor,T. & Yamamoto, M. (2003). Keap1 Regulates Both Cytoplasmic--Nuclear Shuttling and Degradation of Nrf2 in Response to Electrophiles. *Genes to Cells: Devoted to Molecular & Cellular Mechanisms*, Vol.8, No.4, (April), pp. 379–391, ISSN 1356-9597 (Print)

Jung, K.A. & Kwak, M.K. (2010). The Nrf2 System as a Potential Target for the Development of Indirect Antioxidants. *Molecules*, Vol.15, No.10, (Octuber), pp. 7266-7291, ISSN 1420-3049 (Electronic)

Kalayarasan, S.; Sriram, N.; Sureshkumar, A. & Sudhandiran, G. (2008). Chromium (VI)-Induced Oxidative Stress and Apoptosis is Reduced by Garlic and Its Derivative S-allylcysteine Through the Activation of Nrf2 in the Hepatocytes of Wistar Rats. *Journal of Applied Toxicology: JAT*, Vol.28, No.7, (Octuber), pp. 908-919, ISSN 0260-437X (Print)

Kalayarasan, S.; Prabhu, P.N.; Sriram, N.; Manikandan, R.; Arumugam, M.,& Sudhandiran, G. (2009). Diallyl Sulfide Enhances Antioxidants and Inhibits Inflammation Through the Activation of Nrf2 Against Gentamicin-Induced Nephrotoxicity in Wistar Rats. *European Journal of Pharmacology*, Vol.606, No.1-3, (March), pp. 162-171, ISSN 0014-2999 (Print)

Kang, M.I.; Kobayashi, A.; Wakabayashi, N.; Kim, S.G. & Yamamoto, M. (2004). Scaffolding of Keap1 to the Actin Cytoskeleton Controls the Function of Nrf2 as Key Regulator of Cytoprotective Phase 2 Genes. *Proceedings of the National Academy of Sciences of the United States of America*, Vol.101, No.7, (February), pp. 2046-2051, ISSN 0027-8424 (Print)

Kang, Y.H. & Pezzuto, J.M. (2004). Induction of Quinone Reductase as a Primary Screen for Natural Product Anticarcinogens. *Methods in Enzymology*, Vol.382, pp. 380–414, ISSN 0076-6879 (Print)

Katoh, Y.; Itoh, K.; Yoshida, E.; Miyagishi, M.; Fukamizu, A. & Yamamoto, M. (2001). Two Domains of Nrf2 Cooperatively Bind CBP, a CREB Binding Protein, and Synergistically Activate Transcription. *Genes to Cells: Devoted to Molecular & Cellular Mechanisms*, Vol.6, No.10, (October), pp. 857-868, ISSN 1356-9597 (Print)

Katsuoka, F.; Motohashi, H.; Ishii, T.; Aburatani, H.; Engel, J.D. & Yamamoto, M. (2005). Genetic Evidence That Small Maf Proteins are Essential for the Activation of Antioxidant Response Element-Dependent Genes. *Molecular and Cellular Biology*, Vol.25, No.18, (September), pp. 8044-8051, ISSN 0270-7306 (Print)

Kensler, T.W.; Wakabayashi, N. & Biswal, S. (2007). Cell Survival Responses to Environmental Stresses Via the Keap1-Nrf2-ARE Pathway. *Annual Review of Pharmacology and Toxicology*, Vol.47, pp. 89–116, ISSN 0362-1642 (Print)

Kim, J. M.; Chang, N.; Kim, W.K. & Chun, H.S. (2006a). Dietary S-allyl-L-Cysteine Reduces Mortality With Decreased Incidence of Stroke and Behavioral Changes in Stroke-Prone Spontaneously Hypertensive Rats. *Bioscience, Biotechnology, and Biochemistry*, Vol.70, No.8, (August), pp. 1969-1971, ISSN 0916-8451 (Print)

Kim, J.M., Chang, H.J.; Kim, W.K.; Chang, N. & Chun, H.S. (2006b). Structure-Activity Relationship of Neuroprotective and Reactive Oxygen Species Scavenging Activities for Allium Organosulfur Compounds. *Journal of Agricultural and Food Chemistry*, Vol.54, No.18, (September), pp. 6547-6553, ISSN 0021-8561 (Print)

Kobayashi, A.; Kang, M.I.; Okawa, H.; Ohtsuji, M.; Zenke, Y.; Chiba, T.; Igarashi, K. & Yamamoto, M. (2004). Oxidative Stress Sensor Keap1 Functions As an Adaptor for Cul3-based E3 Ligase to Regulate Proteasomal Degradation of Nrf2. *Molecular and Cellular Biology*, Vol.24, No.16, (August), pp. 7130-7139, ISSN 0270-7306 (Print)

Kobayashi, A.; Kang, M.I.; Watai, Y.; Tong, K.I.; Shibata, T.; Uchida, K. & Yamamoto, M. (2006). Oxidative and Electrophilic Stresses Activate Nrf2 Through Inhibition of Ubiquitination Activity of Keap1. *Molecular and Cellular Biology*, Vol.26, No.1, (January), pp. 221-229, ISSN 0270-7306 (Print)

Kobayashi, M. & Yamamoto, M. (2006). Nrf2-Keap1 Regulation of Cellular Defense Mechanisms Against Electrophiles and Reactive Oxygen Species. *Advances in Enzyme Regulation*, Vol.46, pp. 113–140, ISSN 0065-2571 (Print)

Kodera, Y.; Suzuki, A.; Imada, O.; Kasuga, S.; Sumioka, I.; Kanezawa, A.; Taru, N.; Fujikawa, M.; Nagae, S.; Masamoto, K.; Maeshige, K. & Ono, K. (2002). Physical, Chemical, and Biological Properties of S-Allylcysteine, an Amino Acid Derived From Garlic. *Journal of Agricultural and Food Chemistry*, Vol.50, No.3, (January), pp. 622-632, ISSN 0021-8561

Kraft, A.D.; Johnson, D.A. & Johnson, J.A. (2004). Nuclear Factor E2-Related Factor 2-Dependent Antioxidant Response Element Activation by Tert-butylhydroquinone and Sulforaphane Occurring Preferentially in Astrocytes Conditions Neurons Against Oxidative Insult. *Journal of Neuroscience*, Vol.24, No.5, (February), pp. 1101-1112, ISSN 0270-6474 (Print)

Kuroda, S. & Siesjo, B.K. (1997). Reperfusion Damage Following Focal Ischemia: Pathophysiology and Therapeutic Windows. *Clinical Neuroscience (New York, N.Y.)*, Vol.4, No.4, pp. 199–212, ISSN 1065-6766 (Print)

Läer, S.; Block, F.; Huether, G.; Heim, C. & Sontag, K.H. (1993). Effect of Transient Reduction of Cerebral Blood Flow in Normotensive Rats on Striatal Dopamine-Release. *Journal of Neural Transmission. General Section*, Vol.92, No.2-3, pp. 203-211, ISSN 0300-9564 (Print)

Lapchak, P.A. (2001). Neuroprotective and Neurotrophic Curcuminoids to Treat Stroke: a Translational Perspective. *Expert Opinion on Investigational Drugs*, Vol.20, No.1, (January), pp. 13-22, ISSN 1354-3784 (Print)

Lawson, L.D. (1998). Garlic: a Review of Its Medicinal Effects and Indicated Active Compounds, In: *Phytomedicines of Europe: Chemistry and Biological Activity*, L.D. Lawson, & R. Bauer, (Ed.), 176-209, ACS symposium series 691, American Chemical Society, ISBN13 9780841235595, Washington, United States

Lee, J.M.; Calkins, M.J.; Chan, K.; Kan, Y.W. & Johnson, J.A. (2003a). Identification of the NF-E2-Related Factor-2-Dependent Genes Conferring Protection Against Oxidative Stress in Primary Cortical Astrocytes Using Oligonucleotide Microarray Analysis. *The Journal of Biological Chemistry*, Vol.278, No.14, (April), pp. 12029-12038, ISSN 0021-9258 (Print)

Lee, J.M.; Shih, A.Y.; Murphy, T.H. & Johnson, J.A. (2003b). NF-E2-Related Factor-2 Mediates Neuroprotection Against Mitochondrial Complex I Inhibitors and Increased Concentrations of Intracellular Calcium in Primary Cortical Neurons. *The Journal of Biological Chemistry*, Vol.278, No.39, (September), pp. 37948–37956, ISSN 0021-9258 (Print)

Lee, J.M. & Johnson, J.A. (2004). An Important Role of Nrf2-ARE Pathway in the Cellular Defense Mechanism. *Journal of Biochemistry and Molecular Biology*, Vol.37, No.2, (March), pp. 139-143, ISSN 1225-8687 (Print)

Lee, J.M.; Li, J.; Johnson, D.A.; Stein, T.D.; Kraft, A.D.; Calkins, M.J.; Jakel, R.J. & Johnson, J.A. (2005). Nrf2, a Multi-Organ Protector? *The FASEB Journal: official Publication of the Federation of American Societies for Experimental Biology*, Vol.19, No.9, (July), pp. 1061-1066, ISSN 0892-6638 (Print)

Li, J.; Lee, J.M. & Johnson, J.A. (2002). Microarray Analysis Reveals an Antioxidant Responsive Element-Driven Gene Set Involved in Conferring Protection From an Oxidative Stress-Induced Apoptosis in IMR-32 Cells. *The Journal of Biological Chemistry*, Vol.277, No.1, (January), pp. 388-394, ISSN 0021-9258 (Print)

Li, W. & Kong, A.N. (2009). Molecular Mechanisms of Nrf2-Mediated Antioxidant Response. *Molecular Carcinogenesis*, Vol.48, No.2, (February), pp. 91-104, ISSN 0899-1987 (Print)

Li, M.; Zhang, X.; Cui, L.; Yang, R.; Wang, L.; Liu, L. & Du, W. (2011). The Neuroprotection of Oxymatrine in Cerebral Ischemia/Reperfusion is Related to Nuclear Factor Erythroid 2-Related Factor 2 (Nrf2)-Mediated Antioxidant Response: Role of Nrf2 and Hemeoxygenase-1 Expression. *Biological & Pharmaceutical Bulletin*, Vol.34, No.5, pp. 595-601, ISSN 0918-6158 (Print)

Liu, S.; Liu, M.; Peterson, S.; Miyake, M.; Vallyathan, V. & Liu, K.J. (2003). Hydroxyl Radical Formation is Greater in Striatal Core Than in Penumbra in a Rat Model of Ischemic Stroke. *Journal of Neuroscience Research*, Vol.71, No.6, (March), pp. 882-888, ISSN 0077-7846 (Print)

Liverman, C.S.; Cui, L.; Yong, C.; Choudhuri, R.; Klein, R.M.; Welch, K.M. & Berman, N.E. (2004). Response of the Brain to Oligemia: Gene Expression, c-Fos, and Nrf2 Localization. *Brain Research. Molecular Brain Research*, Vol.126, No.1, (July), pp. 57-66, ISSN 0169-328X (Print)

Lo, S.C. & Hannink; M. (2006). PGAM5, a Bcl-XL-Interacting Protein, is a Novel Substrate for the Redox-Regulated Keap1-Dependent Ubiquitin Ligase Complex. *The Journal of Biological Chemistry*, Vol.281, No.49, (December), pp. 37893-37903, ISSN 0021-9258 (Print)

Lo, S.C. & Hannink, M. (2008). PGAM5 Tethers a Ternary Complex Containing Keap1 and Nrf2 to Mitochondria. *Experimental Cell Research*, Vol.314, No.8, (May), pp. 1789-17803, ISSN 0014-4827 (Print)

Loh, K.P.; Huang, S.H.; De Silva, R.; Tan, B.K. & Zhu, Y.Z. (2006). Oxidative Stress: Apoptosis in Neuronal Injury. *Current Alzheimer Research*, Vol.3, No.4, (September), pp. 327–337, ISSN 1567-2050 (Print)

Longa, E.Z.; Weinstein, P.R.; Carlson, S. & Cummins, R. (1989). Reversible Middle Cerebral Artery Occlusion Without Craniectomy in Rats. *Stroke*, Vol.20, No.1, (January), pp. 84–91, ISSN 0039-2499 (Print)

Maldonado, P.D.; Limón, D.; Galván-Arzate, S.; Santamaria, A. & Pedraza-Chaverri, J. (2009). Medicinal Properties of Garlic: Importance of Its Antioxidant Activity, In: *Garlic Consumption and Health*, M. Pãcurar, & G. Krejci, (Ed.), 61-116, Nova Science Publisher, ISBN 978-1-60741-642-5, New York, United States

Mathew, B.C. & Biju, R.S. (2008). Neuroprotective Effects of Garlic a Review. *The Libyan Journal of Medicine*, Vol.3, No.1, (March), pp. 23-33, ISSN 1993-2820 (Print)

Margaill, I.; Plotkine, M. & Lerouet, D. (2005). Antioxidant Strategies in the Treatment of Stroke. *Free Radical Biology & Medicine*, Vol.39, No.4, (August), pp. 429-443, ISSN 0891-5849 (Print)

McMahon, M.; Itoh, K.; Yamamoto, M. & Hayes, J.D. (2003). Keap1-Dependent Proteasomal Degradation of Transcription Factor Nrf2 Contributes to the Negative Regulation of Antioxidant Response Element-Driven Gene Expression. *The Journal of Biological Chemistry*, Vol.278, No.24, (June), pp. 21592-21600, ISSN 0021-9258 (Print)

McMahon, M.; Thomas, N.; Itoh, K.; Yamamoto, M. & Hayes J.D. (2004). Redox-Regulated Turnover of Nrf2 is Determined by at Least Two Separate Protein Domains, the Redox-Sensitive Neh2 Degron and the Redox-Insensitive Neh6 Degron. *The Journal of Biological Chemistry*, Vol.279, No.30, (July), pp. 31556-31567, ISSN 0021-9258 (Print)

McMahon, M.; Thomas, N.; Itoh, K.; Yamamoto, M. & Hayes, J.D. (2006). Dimerization of Substrate Adaptors Can Facilitate Cullin-Mediated Ubiquitylation of Proteins by a "Tethering" Mechanism: a Two-Site Interaction Model for the Nrf2-Keap1 Complex. *The Journal of Biological Chemistry*, Vol.281, No.34, (August), pp. 24756-24768, ISSN 0021-9258 (Print)

Moi, P.; Chan, K.; Asunis, I.; Cao, A. & Kan, Y.W. (1994). Isolation of NF-E2-Related Factor 2 (Nrf2), a NF-E2-Like Basic Leucine Zipper Transcriptional Activator That Binds to the Tandem NF-E2/AP1 Repeat of the Beta-Globin Locus Control Region. *Proceedings of the National Academy of Sciences of the United States of America*, Vol.91, No.21, (October), pp. 9926-9930, ISSN 0027-8424 (Print)

Moro, M.A.; Almeida, A.; Bolaños, J.P. & Lizasoain, I. (2005). Mitochondrial Respiratory Chain and Free Radical Generation in Stroke. *Free Radical Biology & Medicine*, Vol.39, No.10, (November), pp. 1291-1304, ISSN 0891-5849 (Print)

Motohashi, H.; O'Connor, T.; Katsuoka, F.; Engel, J.D. & Yamamoto, M. (2002). Integration and Diversity of the Regulatory Network Composed of Maf and CNC Families of Transcription Factors. *Gene*, Vol.294, No.1-2, (July), pp. 1-12, ISSN 0378-1119 (Print)

Motohashi, H. & Yamamoto, M. (2004). Nrf2-Keap1 Defines a Physiologically Important Stress Response Mechanism. *Trends Molecular Medicine*, Vol.10, No.11, (November), pp. 549–557, ISSN 1471-4914 (Print)

Murphy, T.H.; De Long, M.J. & Coyle, J.T. (1991). Enhanced NAD(P)H:quinone Reductase Activity Prevents Glutamate Toxicity Produced by Oxidative Stress. *Journal of Neurochemistry*, Vol.56, No.3, (March), pp. 990–995, ISSN 0022-3042 (Print)

Nagae, S.; Ushijima, M.; Hatono, S.; Imai, J.; Fasuga, S.; Matsuura, H.; Iyakura, Y. & Higashi, Y. (1994). Pharmacokinetics of the Garlic Compound S-Allylcysteine. *Planta Medica*, Vol.60, No.3, (June), pp. 214-217, ISSN 0032-0943

National Toxicology Program. (1997). NTP toxicology and carcinogenesis studies of t-butylhydroquinone (CAS no. 1948 –33-0) in F344/N rats and B6C3F(1) mice (feed studies). Natl Toxicol Program Tech Rep Ser 459:1–326

Nguyen, T.; Sherratt, P.J.; Huang, H.C.; Yang, C.S. & Pickett, C.B. (2003). Increased Protein Stability as a Mechanism That Enhances Nrf2-Mediated Transcriptional Activation of the Antioxidant Response Element. Degradation of Nrf2 by the 26 S Proteasome. *The Journal of Biological Chemistry*. Vol.278, No.7, (February), pp. 4536-4541, ISSN 0021-9258 (Print)

Nguyen, T.; Yang, C.S. & Pickett, C.B. (2004). The Pathways and Molecular Mechanisms Regulating Nrf2 Activation in Response to Chemical Stress. *Free Radical Biology & Medicine*, Vol.37, No.4, (August), pp. 433-441, ISSN 0891-5849 (Print)

Nioi, P.; Nguyen, T.; Sherratt, P.J. & Pickett, C.B. (2005). The Carboxy-Terminal Neh3 Domain of Nrf2 is Required for Transcriptional Activation. *Molecular and Cellular Biology*, Vol.25, No.24, (December), pp. 10895-10906, ISSN 0270-7306 (Print)

Numagami, Y.; Sato, S. & Ohnishi, S.T. (1996). Attenuation of Rat Ischemic Brain Damage by Aged Garlic Extracts: a Possible Protecting Mechanism as Antioxidants. *Neurochemistry International*, Vol.29, No.2, (August), pp. 135-143, ISSN 0197-0186 (Print)

Numagami, Y. & Ohnishi, S.T. (2001). S-Allylcysteine Inhibits Free Radical Production, Lipid Peroxidation and Neuronal Damage in Rat Brain Ischemia *Journal of Nutrition*, Vol.131, No.3s, (March), pp. 1100S-1105S, ISSN 0022-3166 (Print)

Orino, K.; Lehman, L.; Tsuji, Y.; Ayaki, H.; Torti, S.V. & Torti, F.M. (2001). Ferritin and the Response to Oxidative Stress. *The Biochemical Journal*, Vol.357, No.Pt1, (July), pp. 241-247, ISSN 0264-6021 (Print)

Peters, O.; Back, T.; Lindauer, U.; Busch, C.; Megow, D.; Dreier, J. & Dirnagl, U. (1998). Increased Formation of Reactive Oxygen Species After Permanent and Reversible Middle Cerebral Artery Occlusion in the Rat. *Journal of Cerebral Blood Flow and Metabolism*, Vol.18, No.2, (February), pp. 196–205, ISSN 0271-678X (Print)

Ping, Z.; Liu, W.; Kang, Z.; Cai, J.; Wang, Q.; Cheng, N.; Wang, S.; Wang, S.; Zhang, J.H. & Sun, X. (2010). Sulforaphane Protects Brains Against Hypoxic-Ischemic Injury Through Induction of Nrf2-Dependent Phase 2 Enzyme. *Brain Research*, Vol.1343, (July), pp. 178-185, ISSN 0006-8993 (Print)

Ramos-Gomez, M.; Kwak, M.K.; Dolan, P.M.; Itoh, K.; Yamamoto, M.; Talalay, P. & Kensler, T.W. (2001). Sensitivity to Carcinogenesis is Increased and Chemoprotective Efficacy of Enzyme Inducers is Lost in Nrf2 Transcription Factor-Deficient Mice. *Proceedings of the National Academy of Sciences of the United States of America*, Vol.98, No.6, (March), pp. 3410-3415, ISSN 0027-8424 (Print)

Rodrigo, J.; Fernandez, A.P.; Serrano, J.; Peinado, M.A. & Martinez, A. (2005). The Role of Free Radicals in Cerebral Hypoxia and Ischemia. *Free Radical Biology & Medicine*, Vol.39, No.1, (July), pp. 26–50, ISSN 0891-5849 (Print)

Rushmore, T.H.; Morton, M.R. & Pickett, C.B. (1991). The Antioxidant Responsive Element. Activation by Oxidative Stress and Identification of the DNA Consensus Sequence

Required for Functional Activity. *The Journal of Biological Chemistry*, Vol.266, No.18, (June), pp. 11632-11639, ISSN 0021-9258 (Print)

Saleem, S.; Ahmad, M.; Ahmad, A.S.; Yousuf, S.; Ansari, M.A.; Khan, M.B.; Ishrat, T. & Islam, F. (2006). Behavioral and Histologic Neuroprotection of Aqueous Garlic Extract After Reversible Focal Cerebral Ischemia. *Journal of Medicinal Food*, Vol.9, No.4, (Winter), pp. 537-544, ISSN 1096-620X (Print)

Sener, G.; Sakarcan, A. & Yegen, B.C. (2007). Role of Garlic in the Prevention of Ischemia Reperfusion Injury. *Molecular Nutrition & Food Research*, Vol.51, No.11, (November), pp. 1345-1352, ISSN 1613-4125 (Print)

Shah, Z.A.; Li, R.C.; Thimmulappa, R.K.; Kensler, T.W.; Yamamoto, M.; Biswal, S. & Doré, S. (2007). Role of Reactive Oxygen Species in Modulation of Nrf2 Following Ischemic Reperfusion Injury. *Neuroscience*, Vol.147, No.1, (June), pp. 53-59, ISSN 0306-4522 (Print)

Shah, Z.A.; Li, R.C.; Ahmad, A.S.; Kensler, T.W.; Yamamoto, M.; Biswal, S. & Doré, S. (2010). The Flavanol (-)-Epicatechin Prevents Stroke Damage Through the Nrf2/HO1 Pathway. *Journal of Cerebral Blood Flow and Metabolism*, Vol.30, No.12, (December), pp. 1951-1961, ISSN 0271-678X (Print)

Shih, A.Y.; Johnson, D.A.; Wong, G.; Kraft, A.D.; Jiang, L.; Erb, H.; Johnson, J.A. & Murphy, T.H. (2003). Coordinate Regulation of Glutathione Biosynthesis and Release by Nrf2-Expressing Glia Potently Protects Neurons From Oxidative Stress. *Journal of Neuroscience*, Vol.23, No.8, (April), pp. 3394–3406, ISSN 0270-6474 (Print)

Shih, A.Y.; Li, P. & Murphy, T.H. (2005). A Small-Molecule-Inducible Nrf2-Mediated Antioxidant Response Provides Effective Prophylaxis Against Cerebral Ischemia in Vivo. *Journal of Neuroscience*, Vol.25, No.44, (November), pp. 10321-10335, ISSN 0270-6474 (Print)

Simonyi, A.; Wang, Q.; Miller, R.L.; Yusof, M.; Shelat, P.B.; Sun, A.Y. & Sun, G.Y. (2005). Polyphenols in Cerebral Ischemia: Novel Targets for Neuroprotection. *Molecular Neurobiology*, Vol.31, No.1-3, pp. 135–148, ISSN 0893-7648 (Print)

Soane, L.; Li Dai, W.; Fiskum, G. & Bambrick, L.L. (2010). Sulforaphane Protects Immature Hippocampal Neurons Against Death Caused by Exposure to Hemin or to Oxygen and Glucose Deprivation. *Journal of Neuroscience Research*, Vol.88, No.6, (May), pp. 1355-1363, ISSN 0360-4012 (Print)

Sun, A.Y.; Wang, Q.; Simonyi, A. & Sun, G.Y. (2008). Botanical Phenolics and Brain Health. *Neuromolecular Medicine*, Vol.10, No.4, pp. 259-274, ISSN 1535-1084 (Print)

Surh, Y.J. & Chun, K.S. (2007). Cancer Chemopreventive Effects of Curcumin. *Advances in Experimental Medicine and Biology*, Vol.595, pp. 149–172, ISSN 0065-2598 (Print)

Surh, Y.J.; Kundu, J.K. & Na, H.K. (2008). Nrf2 as a Master Redox Switch in Turning on the Cellular Signaling Involved in the Induction of Cytoprotective Genes by Some Chemopreventive Phytochemicals. *Planta Medica*, Vol.74, No.13, (Octuber), pp. 1526-1539, ISSN 0032-0943

Sykiotis, G.P. & Bohmann, D. (2010). Stress-Activated Cap'n'collar Transcription Factors in Aging and Human Disease. *Science Signaling*, Vol.3, No.112 (March), pp. re3, ISSN 1937-9145 (Electronic)

Talalay, P. (2000). Chemoprotection Against Cancer by Induction of Phase 2 Enzymes. *Biofactors*, Vol.12, No.1-4, pp. 5–11, ISSN 0951-6433 (Print)

Talalay, P.; Fahey, J.W.; Healy, Z.R.; Wehage, S.L.; Benedict, A.L.; Min, C. & Dinkova-Kostova, A.T. (2007). Sulforaphane Mobilizes Cellular Defenses that Protect Skin Against Damage by UV Radiation. *Proceedings of the National Academy of Sciences of the United States of America*, Vol.104, No.44, (Octuber), pp. 17500–17505, ISSN 0027-8424 (Print)

Tanaka, N.; Ikeda, Y.; Ohta, Y.; Deguchi, K.; Tian, F.; Shang, J.; Matsuura, T. & Abe, K. (2011). Expression of Keap1-Nrf2 System and Antioxidative Proteins in Mouse Brain After Transient Middle Cerebral Artery Occlusion. *Brain Research*, Vol.1370, (January), pp. 246-253, ISSN 0006-8993 (Print)

Thangapazham, R.L.; Sharma, A. & Maheshwari, R.K. (2006). Multiple Molecular Targets in Cancer Chemoprevention by Curcumin. *The AAPS Journal*, Vol.8, No.3, (July), pp. E443–E449, ISSN 1550-7416

Tong, K.I.; Kobayashi, A.; Katsuoka, F. & Yamamoto, M. (2006a). Two-Site Substrate Recognition Model for the Keap1-Nrf2 System: a Hinge and Latch Mechanism. *Biological Chemistry*, Vol.387, No.10-11, (October-November), pp. 1311-1320, ISSN 1431-6730 (Print)

Tong, K.I.; Katoh, Y.; Kusunoki, H.; Itoh, K.; Tanaka, T. & Yamamoto, M. (2006b). Keap1 Recruits Neh2 Through Binding to ETGE and DLG Motifs: Characterization of the Two-Site Molecular Recognition Model. *Molecular and Cellular Biology*, Vol.26, No.8, (April), pp. 2887-2900, ISSN 0270-7306 (Print)

Van Muiswinkel, F.L. & Kuiperij, H.B. (2005). The Nrf2-ARE Signalling Pathway: Promising Drug Target to Combat Oxidative Stress in Neurodegenerative Disorders. *Current Drug Targets. CNS Neurological Disorders*, Vol.4, No.3, (June), pp. 267-281, ISSN 1568-007X (Print)

Van Ommen, B.; Koster, A.; Verhagen, H. & vanBladeren, P.J. (1992). The Glutathione Conjugates of Tert-Butyl Hydroquinone as Potent Redox Cycling Agents and Possible Reactive Agents Underlying the Toxicity of Butylated Hydroxyanisole. *Biochemical and Biophysical Research Communications*, Vol.189, No.1, (November), pp. 309-314, ISSN 0006-291X (Print)

Wakabayashi, N.; Dinkova-Kostova, A.T.; Holtzclaw, W.D.; Kang, M.I.; Kobayashi, A.; Yamamoto, M.; Kensler, T.W. & Talalay, P. (2004). Protection Against Electrophile and Oxidant Stress by Induction of the Phase 2 Response: Fate of Cysteines of the Keap1 Sensor Modified by Inducers. *Proceedings of the National Academy of Sciences of the United States of America*, Vol.101, No.7, (February), pp. 2040−2045, ISSN 0027-8424 (Print)

WHO. (2005). Preventing chronic diseases: a vital investment. Geneva: World Health Organization.

Wong, C.H. & Crack, P.J. (2008). Modulation of Neuro-Inflammation and Vascular Response by Oxidative Stress Following Cerebral Ischemia-Reperfusion Injury. *Current Medicinal Chemistry*, Vol.15, No.1, pp. 1-14, ISSN 0929-8673 (Print)

Wu, C.C.; Sheen, L.Y.; Chen, H.W.; Kuo, W.W.; Tsai, S.J. & Lii, C.K. (2002). Differential Effects of Garlic Oil and its Three Major Organosulfur Components on the Hepatic Detoxification System in Rats. *Journal of Agricultural and Food Chemistry*, Vol.50, No.2, (January), pp. 378- 383, ISSN 0021-8561 (Print)

Yan, C.K. & Zeng, F.D. (2005). Pharmacokinetics and Tissue Distribution of S-Allylcysteine in Rats. *Asian Journal of Drug Metabolism and Pharmacokinetics*, 5, pp. 61-69

Yang, C.; Zhang, X.; Fan, H. & Liu, Y. (2009). Curcumin Upregulates Transcription Factor Nrf2, HO-1 Expression and Protects Rat Brains Against Focal Ischemia. *Brain Research*, Vol.1282, (July), pp. 133-141, ISSN 0006-8993 (Print)

Zhang, Y.; Talalay, P.; Cho, C-G. & Posner, G.H. (1992). A Major Inducer of Anticarcinogenic Protective Enzymes From Broccoli: Isolation and Elucidation of Structure. *Proceedings of the National Academy of Sciences of the United States of America*, Vol.89, No.6, (March), pp. 2399–2403, ISSN 0027-8424 (Print)

Zhang, D.D. & Hannink, M. (2003). Distinct Cysteine Residues in Keap1 are Required for Keap1-Dependent Ubiquitination of Nrf2 and for Stabilization of Nrf2 by Chemopreventive Agents and Oxidative Stress. *Molecular and Cellular Biology*, Vol.23, No.22, (November), pp. 8137-8151, ISSN 0270-7306 (Print)

Zhang, D.D.; Lo, S.C.; Cross, J.V.; Templeton, D.J. & Hannink M. (2004). Keap1 is a Redox-Regulated Substrate Adaptor Protein for a Cul3-Dependent Ubiquitin Ligase Complex. *Molecular and Cellular Biology*, Vol.24, No.24, (December), pp. 10941-10953, ISSN 0270-7306 (Print)

Zhao, J.; Kobori, N.; Aronowski, J. & Dash, P.K. (2006). Sulforaphane Reduces Infarct Volume Following Focal Cerebral Ischemia in Rodents. *Neuroscience Letters*, Vol.393, No.2-3, (January), pp. 108-112, ISSN 0304-3940 (Print)

6

Endogenous Agents That Contribute to Generate or Prevent Ischemic Damage

Ornella Piazza[1] and Giuliana Scarpati[2]
[1]*Anestesiologia e Rianimazione, Università Degli Studi di Salerno*
[2]*Anestesiologia e Rianimazione, Università Degli Studi di Napoli Federico II*
Italy

1. Introduction

From single to multicellular organisms, protective mechanisms have evolved against endogenous and exogenous noxious stimuli. Over the past decades numerous signaling pathways by which the brain senses and reacts to such insults as neurotoxins, substrate deprivation and inflammation have been discovered. Research on preconditioning is aimed at understanding endogenous neuroprotection to boost it or to supplement its effectors therapeutically once damage to the brain has occurred, such as after stroke or brain trauma. Another goal of establishing preconditioning protocols is to induce endogenous neuroprotection in anticipation of incipient brain damage. Currently several endogenous neuroprotectants are being investigated in controlled clinical trials. There is consensus that many of the neuroprotectants, which were highly effective in animal models of stroke, but failed in clinical trials, were unsuccessful because of side effects, which in many cases led to premature termination of the trial. Nowadays research aims to overcome this problem by developing compounds which induce, mimic, or boost endogenous protective responses and thus do not interfere with physiological neurotransmission. In the present review we will give a short overview on the signals, sensors, transducers, and effectors of endogenous neuroprotection. We will first focus on common mechanisms, on which pathways of endogenous neuroprotection converge. We will then discuss various applications of endogenous neuroprotectors and explore the prospects of endogenous neuroprotective therapeutic approaches.

2. Phisiopatology of cerebral ischemia

Development of stroke prophylaxis involves the understanding of the mechanisms of damage following cerebral ischemia and elucidation of the endogenous mechanisms that combat further brain injury (FIGURE 1).

The binding of glutamate to its receptors and the activation of voltage-gated Ca^{2+} channels (VGCC) causes calcium to influx into the cell. Calcium is among the mediators that initiate the genomic response to cerebral ischemia. The superoxide dismutase (SOD) gene is upregulated to neutralize the reactive oxygen species (ROS). The generation of nitrous oxide (NO) in the neuron is cytotoxic. The interaction between antiapoptotic genes, such as Bcl-2, and proapoptotic genes, such as Bax, determines whether cytochrome c will be translocated from the mitochondria to the cytosol. In the cytosol, cytochrome c combines with Apaf-1 to activate the caspases. Proinflammatory cytokines, such as interleukin-1 (IL-1) and tumor necrosis factor-a (TNF-a), are generated. Survival pathways involving growth factors (GFs), immediate early genes (IEGs), and heat shock proteins (Hsps) are also stimulated. Ultimately, the activation of these genetic pathways determines the fate of the ischemic cell.

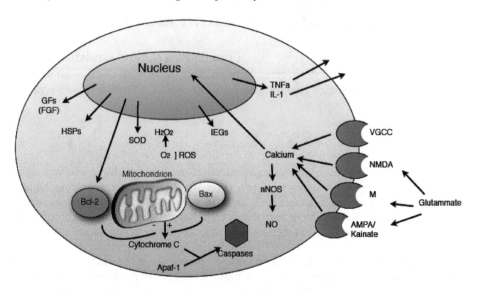

Fig. 1. Phisiopatology of cerebral ischemia

2.1 Excitotoxicity and calcium

Although the brain represents only 2% of body weight, it uses an astonishing 20% of the body's oxygen in adults. The innumerable cells of the brain require an almost continuous flow of oxygen and glucose, making them exquisitely sensitive to any interruption in energy supply. Energy depletion and reduced levels of adenosine triphosphate initiate a series of events that cause cells to die. Glutamate, the main excitatory neurotransmitter of the central nervous system, is a trigger of neuronal loss during stroke. During ischemia, an excess of glutamate is released into the extracellular space. The mechanism to clear glutamate is energy dependent; glutamate quickly builds to toxic levels when energy is depleted. Glutamate causes ionic shifts; Na^+ enters the cell and K^+ exits. Water passively follows the influx of Na^+ leading to cellular swelling and edema. The membrane potential is lost and the cell depolarizes. In the ischemic core, cells undergo anoxic depolarization and never repolarize. However, cells in the penumbra initially retain the ability to repolarize so that they may depolarize again. As cells in the penumbra undergo these peri-infarct depolarizations the energy supply and ionic homeostasis are further compromised, resulting in an increase in the size of the ischemic lesion. Glutamate activates three main families of receptors: N-methyl-d-aspartate (NMDA), a-amino-3-hydroxy-5 methylisoxazole/kainate, and metabotropic glutamate receptors. Activation of these receptors leads to a buildup of Ca^{2+} within the cell. Ischemia therefore triggers glutamate receptor-mediated excitotoxicity and Ca^{2+} overload within the cell. Originally, neuronal death from excitotoxicity was believed to result from depletion of cellular energy stores from overexcited neurons. However, the influx of Ca^{2+} seems to be the major pathogenic event contributing to cell death. This translocation of Ca^{2+} is accomplished through glutamate, particularly through the NMDA receptor, as well as through voltage-gated Ca^{2+} channels that open after cell depolarization. Calcium channel antagonists have displayed neural protection in animal models but have not shown benefit in clinical trials partially because they were administered too late after stroke onset or in insufficient quantity. However, it appears that Ca^{2+} influx into the cell is only the initial step in a complex biochemical cascade.

2.2 Free radicals

Reactive oxygen species are produced after the induction of ischemia and upon reperfusion. The oxidative stress produced by the reactive oxygen species destroys the cell through lipid peroxidation, protein oxidation, and DNA damage. Certain endogenous antioxidants scavenge and neutralize the reactive oxygen species. In particular, the antioxidant superoxide dismutase detoxifies the superoxide ($O2-$) free radical by converting it to hydrogen peroxide ($H2O2$). Glutathione peroxidase can then convert $H2O2$ into oxygen and water. During times of oxidative stress, the superoxide dismutase gene is upregulated. Neural protection strategies have included both the administration of exogenous superoxide dismutase and manipulation of the superoxide dismutase gene family. Nitric oxide (NO) is another free radical that is increased during ischemia due to an increase in intracellular Ca^{2+}. The formation of NO is catalyzed by the enzyme NO synthase (NOS). NOS has several isoforms — a neuronal type (nNOS) located in neurons and an endothelial type (eNOS) in the vascular endothelium. NO is also generated in microglia, astrocytes and invading macrophages after the induction of an inducible isoform (iNOS). Initially after ischemia, the formation of NO in the vascular endothelium by eNOS may improve CBF through vasodilatation offering neuroprotection. However, synthesis of NO by nNOS and iNOS is cytotoxic, leading to an inhibition of mitochondrial respiration, glycolysis, and DNA synthesis. Because of the dual role of NO in cerebral ischemia, neuronal protection strategies need to target the specific isoform of NOS. For instance, deletion of the nNOS or iNOS gene in animal models has provided neuronal protection.

2.3 Apoptosis

After an ischemic event, cells in the penumbra may initiate a program of autodestruction known as apoptosis. Apoptosis occurs in the developing brain. More than half of progenitor neurons undergo this process of programmed cell death while forming neural circuits. During ischemia, cells in the ischemic core undergo necrosis while cells in the ischemic penumbra may actually self destruct through this process of apoptosis. The mitochondria is regarded as the apoptotic headquarters of the cell. One of the key events in apoptosis is the translocation of cytochrome c from the intermembrane of the mitochondria into the cytosol. In the cytosol, cytochrome c combines then with apoptotic activating factor (Apaf-1) to activate a set of proteases known as caspases. These caspases actually dismantle the cell during apoptosis. A family of death-promoting genes, known as the Bcl-2 family, determines whether a cell will undergo apoptosis. The Bcl-2 gene is antiapoptotic and prevents the translocation of cytochrome c and activation of caspases. However, the Bax gene (one of the members of the Bcl-2 family) is proapoptotic, facilitating the translocation of cytochrome c and apoptosis. During ischemia, proapoptotic genes such as Bax are activated, resulting in the autodestruction of the cell. Thus, neuronal protection may be gained through blocking these death-promoting genes. Other strategies include giving caspase antagonists or preventing the translocation of cytochrome c from the mitochondria. Preventing apoptosis in the penumbra is another effective technique in animal models for neuronal protection.

2.4 Inflammation

The inflammatory response may be an important part of the ischemic cascade. Soon after the onset of stroke, leukocytes invade the ischemic zone. The mechanisms by which these inflammatory cells contribute to the evolution of ischemia include microvascular occlusion by adherence to the endothelium, producing cytotoxic enzymes and generating injurious free radicals. Cytokines are intracellular messengers that mediate the recruitment of the leukocytes and the induction of adhesion molecules. The two main proinflammatory cytokines are interleukin-1 (IL-1) and tumor necrosis factor-a (TNF-a). The adhesion molecules that facilitate the movement of leukocytes along the surface of the endothelium are the E and P selectins, whereas intracellular adhesion molecules attach the leukocytes to the endothelium so that they may leave the vascular space and enter the site of injury. Research has been focusing on the manipulation of these proinflammatory cytokines and adhesion molecules to provide neuronal protection.

2.4.1 Survival pathways

The cytokines that are activated during ischemia also include growth factors that actually promote neuronal survival and, in some cases, neuronal outgrowth and synapse formation. Fibroblast growth factor is the most extensively studied growth factor. Although the exact mechanism of neuroprotection of fibroblast growth factor is not fully understood, it includes upregulation of free radical scavenging enzymes and Ca^{2+} binding proteins, downregulation of the NMDA receptor and vasodilatation. The administration of growth factors has provided cerebral protection in animal models. Because they exert both protective and trophic influences on neurons, growth factors remain an exciting prospect in drug development for stroke. Other gene families and proteins are activated during ischemia. Immediate early genes, such as those of the Fos and Jun families, are activated soon after ischemia. It is believed that Ca^{2+} and reactive oxygen species are involved in the expression of immediate early genes. Although the exact role of each of the immediate early genes in ischemia is not yet understood, they are known to participate in apoptosis. Some immediate early genes may even afford neuronal protection. Ischemia also induces the expression of molecular chaperones known as heat shock proteins, which maintain protein function and assist in protein transport in response to injury. Increasing the expression of heat shock proteins to combat ischemia has been attempted.

3. Erythropoietin

The hormone erythropoietin (Epo) is a 165-amino acid (~30 kDa) glycoprotein that belongs to the cytokine type I superfamily. Originally, it was believed that the only role of Epo was the regulation of erythropoiesis. This role is attributed to the ability of Epo to inhibit programmed cell death (apoptosis) in erythroid cells and thus allow the maturation of erythrocytes. Since blood oxygen availability is the main regulator of erythropoiesis, hypoxia induces the gene expression of Epo in the kidney, the main site for Epo production, and in the liver (Cotena et al, 2008) in a negative feedback system between the kidney and the bone marrow. Research performed in the last decade has shown that Epo and its receptor (EpoR) are expressed in tissues other than those involved in erythropoiesis. These include the brain, the reproductive tract (Kobayashi et al, 2002; Marti et al, 1996; Masuda et al, 2000), the lung, the spleen, and the heart (Fandrey and Bunn, 1993). Accordingly, a novel cytoprotective effect of Epo was established in several organs. For example, Epo reduced injury and dysfunction after ischemia-reperfusion in the mouse kidney (Patel et al, 2004), and it showed protection in various myocardial ischemia models (Bogoyevith,2004; Cai et al, 2003; Parsa et al, 2003).

3.1 Epo/EpoR expression and regulation

Epo is mainly produced in the interstitial fibroblasts in the adult kidney and the hepatocytes of the fetus, whereas EpoR is normally expressed in erythroid precursor cells in the bone marrow (Marti, 2004). However, recent data have shown that the expression of Epo and its receptor, EpoR (both mRNA and protein), coincides in the same organ and even within the same cell. Epo and EpoR expression are widely distributed in the mammalian brain (Genc *et al*, 2004; Marti, 2004), albeit at lower levels than in the kidney (Brines and Cerami, 2005). Epo thus has to be added to the growing list of hematopoietic growth factors found to be expressed and act in the central nervous system (CNS).

3.2 Expression of Epo/EpoR in the brain

Epo/EpoR mRNA and protein were detected is several regions of the murine and primate brain, including cortex, hippocampus and amygdale, cerebellum, hypothalamus, and caudate nucleus (Siren et al, 2001). With respect to the type of cells in the brain that express Epo, astrocytes are the main source of Epo in the brain (Masuda et al, 1994). Moreover, it has been shown in vitro and in vivo that neurons express Epo (Bernaudin et al, 1999, 2000). Similarly, EpoR is expressed on neurons and astrocytes. In addition, primary cultures of human neurons, astrocytes, and microglia express EpoR mRNA (Nagai et al, 2001), and EpoR expression was also detected in primary cultures of rat oligodendrocytes (Genc et al, 2006). In addition to neurons, oligodendrocytes, and glial cells, a strong immunoreactivity for EpoR was found to be associated with brain vascular endothelial cells, showing that these cells also express EpoR (Brines et al, 2000). These findings implicate a broad spectrum of actions of Epo in the brain.

3.3 Regulation of Epo/EpoR expression

As mentioned above, Epo is upregulated in response to hypoxia. As, for many of the hypoxic adaptation processes in the body, the regulation of Epo expression is based on the transcriptional regulation of two hypoxia-inducible factors HIF-1 and HIF-2 (Wenger, 2000). HIFs are heterodimers composed of an α- and a β -subunit. Two forms of the oxygen-labile α exist, 1α and 2α. The α-subunit is stabilized under hypoxic conditions leading to the binding of the heterodimer HIF-1 or HIF-2 to specific DNA sequences located in the hypoxia response elements of target genes such as Epo or vascular endothelial growth factor (VEGF) (Wenger, 2002). Although HIF-1α was originally identified as the transcription factor responsible for Epo expression (Semenza et al, 1991), more recent evidence suggests that Epo is a target of HIF-2 (Eckardt and Kurtz, 2005). The stability of HIF-α is regulated by enzymatic hydroxylation of specific amino acids on the α subunit by a group of oxygenases (FIGURE 2). Under normoxic conditions, a specific prolyl hydroxylation within the oxygen-dependent degradation domain of HIF-α takes place. This prolyl hydroxylation allows binding of the von Hippel-Lindau protein (pVHL), leading to ubiquitylation and proteasomal degradation of the HIF-α subunit (Ivan et al, 2001; Jaakkola et al, 2001). The enzymes responsible for this hydroxylation are termed prolyl hydroxylase domain enzymes (PHD1-3) (Bruick and McKnight, 2001; Epstein et al, 2001) and are widely expressed. Furthermore, in the presence of oxygen, another hydroxylation reaction takes place on an asparaginyl group in the COOH-terminal transactivation domain of HIF-α, blocking its binding to the transcriptional coactivators (Lando et al, 2002a). This process is governed by a specific asparaginyl hydroxylase termed factor-inhibiting HIF (FIH) (Hewitson et al, 2002; Lando et al, 2002b). So, under normoxia, FIH and PHD(s) are active, leading to transcriptional inactivation and degradation of HIF-α, whereas under hypoxic conditions both enzymes are inactive. HIF is then stabilized and able to induce the expression of target genes, including Epo.

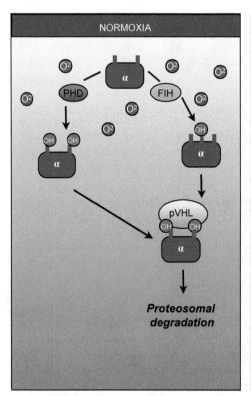 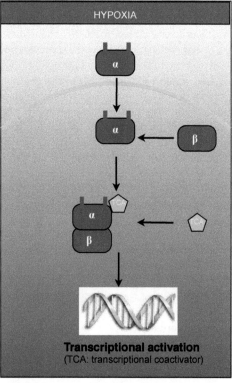

Fig. 2. Under normoxic conditions, specific prolyl hydroxylation within the oxygen-dependent degradation domain of HIF- α takes place. By contrast, under hypoxic conditions, FIH and PHD(s) are both inactive, and HIF is stabilized and able to induce the expression of target genes including Epo.

This basic mechanism of regulation seems to be of relevance for brain-expressed Epo, since in several experimental systems Epo was upregulated under hypoxic conditions in the brain of several mammalian species including mouse, rat, monkey, and human (Marti et al, 1996, 2000; Siren et al, 2001). However, depending on the severity of hypoxia, Epo mRNA level can increase 3- to 20-fold in the brain in contrast to 200-fold in the kidney. Moreover, although the increase in Epo expression in the kidney seems to be transient with a decrease after 8 h of continuous hypoxia, the level of Epo in the brain remains high for at least 24 h (Chikuma et al, 2000). This indicates a tissue-specific degree of regulation. Indeed, although HIF-1α levels in the kidney under systemic hypoxia peak after 1 h and again reach basal levels 4 h thereafter, in the brain the HIF-1α peak level is reached after only 5 h and returns to the basal level not before 12 h (Stroka et al, 2001). A possible explanation for the different time course in the brain might be an altered composition of the various PHD forms. It has to be noted that hypoxia is not the only factor activating HIF. Several studies have shown that pro-inflammatory mediators such as tumor necrosis factor-α (TNF-α), interleukin-1β (IL-1β) or lipopolysaccharide (LPS) induce the expression of HIF (Frede et al, 2007). With regard to the EpoR, it is regulated by pro-inflammatory cytokines (Nagai et al, 2001), such as TNF-α, IL-1β, and Epo itself (Chin et al, 2000). The role of hypoxia in the regulation of EpoR expression is controversial. Whereas we did not observe hypoxic induction of EpoR expression in neurons or astrocytes (Bernaudin et al, 2000), anemic stress induced EpoR expression in the brain of human EpoR transgenic mice (Chin et al, 2000). Moreover, in the same study, hypoxia increased EpoR expression in neuronal cells in vitro. The mechanism of hypoxic EpoR regulation remains to be established, since EpoR has not been identified as HIF target gene so far.

3.4 Epo signaling
Epo promotes cell survival through inhibiting apoptosis (FIGURE 3).
In erythroid cells, after binding of Epo to its receptor (EpoR), Janus tyrosine kinase 2 (JAK2) is phosphorylated and thus activated. This leads to engaging secondary signaling molecules such as signal transducer and activator of transcription 5 (STAT5), followed by the activation of Ras mitogen-activated protein kinase (MAPK), ERK-1/-2, and PI3K/Akt (22). Moreover, Epo induced the upregulation of the anti-apoptotic protein BCL-XL (Kilic et al, 2005). The functional significance of these signaling molecules in erythropoiesis is not absolutely clear though. For instance, whereas in one study STAT5 knockout adult mice were largely unaffected in their erythroid lineage (Teglund et al, 1998), in another study STAT5 knockout embryos suffered from severe anemia, showed a reduced number of erythroid progenitors cells, and had higher numbers of apoptotic cells (Socolovsky et al, 1999). Most of these pathways seem also to be functional in the brain (Brines and Cerami, 2005; Kilic et al, 2005). In vitro, inhibition of MAPK and PI3K blocked Epo-mediated protection of rat hippocampal neurons against hypoxia (Siren et al, 2001b). Moreover, using ERK-1/-2 and Akt inhibitors, Kilic et al. showed that activation of these proteins is essential for Epo-mediated neuroprotection in an animal model of focal cerebral ischemia. The role of STAT5 in Epo-induced neuroprotection is, however, controversial. STAT5 phosphorylation has been shown to occur in hippocampal CA1 neurons after transient global cerebral ischemia in rats (Zhang et al, 2007). Therefore, the authors concluded that STAT5 plays a role in Epo-mediated neuroprotection. However, in a very recent study, in an in vitro model of glutamate toxicity using hippocampal neuronal culture from STAT5 knockout mouse

fetuses, STAT5 was not required for Epo-mediated neuroprotection (Byts et al, 2008). However, STAT5 was indispensable for the neurotrophic function of Epo. A unique pathway for the brain seems to be that activation of EpoR induces nuclear factor- κB (NF-κB) translocation into the nucleus and that this effect is important for Epo-mediated neuroprotection (Digicaylioglu and Lipton, 2001). Interestingly, Epo-induced NF-κB translocation was observed only in neuronal cells and not in astrocytes. Thus it appears likely that NF-κB, in the nucleus, induces the expression of neuroprotective and anti-apoptotic proteins. However, some differences exist between the signaling cascade activated by Epo in the CNS and in erythroid cells. For instance, in one study, BCL-XL has been found to be important in Epo-mediated protection of erythroid but not neuronal cells (Rischer et al, 2002). Additionally, Epo has been found to activate phospholipase C-gamma (PLCγ) (Marreo et al, 1998) and thus can directly influence neuronal activity (Koshimura et al, 1999) and neurotransmitter release (Kawakami et al, 2000) by modulating intracellular calcium concentrations in neurons.

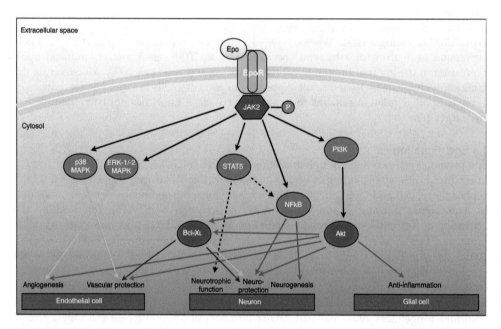

Fig. 3. Epo Signaling

3.5 Epo function in the CNS

For almost a century, Epo was thought to be involved in the process of erythropoiesis only. Through its antiapoptotic action, it enables committed erythroid progenitor cells to survive and mature (Jelkmann, 1992). However, during the last decade, it became evident that Epo is implicated in other processes such as neuroprotection, neurogenesis, and angiogenesis, and plays an important role as neurotrophic as well as immunomodulatory factor. The important role of Epo in the CNS is also evident from studies with EpoR knockout mice. As a result of EpoR deficiency, these mice show massive apoptosis and a reduction in the number of neuronal progenitor cells (Yu et al, 2002). A comprehensive description of the role of the Epo/EpoR system in development is found elsewhere (Arcasoy, 2008; Dame et al, 2001).

3.5.1 Neuroprotection

For a long time, Epo has been used clinically in patients suffering from anemia due to end-stage renal failure. In addition to the correction of anemia, these patients showed improved cognitive abilities (Siren and Ehrenreich, 2001). Initially, since it was believed that systemic Epo cannot pass through the blood-brain-barrier due to its large size (Recny et al, 1987) and brain-derived Epo production and expression of EpoR in the CNS were not yet discovered, the positive effect on cognition was attributed to the improved oxygen-carrying capacity of the blood after Epo-induced erythropoiesis. However, since later studies have shown that both Epo and its receptor are expressed in different regions of the brain by different cell types (Genc et al, 2004; Marti, 2004), the hypothesis was established that locally produced as well as exogenously added Epo could directly influence cognitive function. Interestingly, the expression level of Epo and EpoR is especially high in regions of the brain known to be particularly sensitive to acute hypoxia (Lipton, 1999), the hippocampus and the telencephalon (Digicaylioglu et al, 1995), suggesting that Epo might act as a protective agent against hypoxia. Indeed, infusion of soluble EpoR (capable of binding with endogenous EPO, thus sequestering it) into the brain of gerbils, which were subjected to a mild form of ischemia that normally does not cause neuronal damage, resulted in neuronal death in the hippocampus, clearly showing that endogenous Epo has a neuroprotective effect (Sakanaka et al, 1998).

3.5.2 Neurotrophic function and neurogenesis

Besides neuroprotection under hypoxic conditions, Epo also has a neurotrophic function in normoxic neurons. This was first demonstrated by Konishi and co-workers showing that Epo augments the activity of choline acetyltransferase in primary cultured mouse septal neurons (Konishi et al, 1993). Epo promoted the regeneration of septal cholinergic neurons in adult rats that had undergone fimbria-fornix transections. In addition and similar to its anti-apoptotic role in erythropoiesis, Epo promoted the survival and differentiation of dopaminergic precursor neurons in vitro (Studer et al, 2000). Moreover, hypoxia-induced Epo production appeared to directly act on neuronal stem cells in the forebrain, showing that Epo plays a direct role in neurogenesis after hypoxia (Shingo et al, 2001). In addition, Epo also acts indirectly by inducing brain-derived neurotrophic factor (BDNF) expression (Wang et al, 2004), which in turn augmented the effect of Epo on neurogenesis. These data show that Epo is not only involved in neuroprotection, but also in neuronal survival, differentiation, and neurogenesis.

3.5.3 Angiogenesis and vascular permeability

Besides its direct effects on neurons, Epo-induced neuroprotection may be attributed to an improvement in brain perfusion by promoting new vessel growth. Anagnostou et al demonstrated mitogenic and chemotactic effects of Epo on human umbilical vein and bovine adrenal capillary endothelial cells (Anagnostou et al, 1990). Moreover, Epo stimulated vessel outgrowth of rat aortic rings (Carlini et al, 1995), suggesting that Epo has angiogenic effects. This was further supported by the observation that Epo injection into the mouse uterine cavity stimulated neovascularization in the endometrium (Yasuda et al, 1998). Similarly, neovascularization was stimulated in the chick embryo chorioallantonic membrane upon Epo administration (Ribatti et al, 1999a). The angiogenic effect of Epo was also found in the brain, since capillary endothelial cells express two forms of EpoR mRNA and Epo showed a dose-dependent mitogenic activity on brain capillary endothelial cells (Yamaji et al, 1996). This angiogenic effect was finally confirmed in mice genetically engineered to lack either Epo or its receptor (EpoR) where mutant embryos suffer from severe defects in angiogenesis (Kertesz et al, 2004). In addition to its angiogenic effect, Epo is involved in the regulation of vascular permeability. In an in vitro model of the blood-brain barrier (BBB), Epo treatment protected bovine brain endothelial cells against VEGF-induced increase in vascular permeability (Martinez-Estrada et al, 2003). This suggests that the protective effect of Epo on the brain could be mediated by stimulating angiogenesis as well as by protecting the BBB.

3.5.4 Anti-inflammation

Inflammatory processes play a major role in the pathogenesis of cerebral ischemia, where Epo is protective. Inflammation results in influx of leukocytes from the blood into the brain and in activation of resident microglial cells (Dirnagl et al, 1999). These cells produce inflammatory mediators and cytokines leading to barrier damage, microvascular occlusion, and thus the aggravation of the injury (Witko-Sarsat et al, 2000). In an animal model of cerebral ischemia, administration of Epo resulted in the reduction of the local production of TNF, IL-6, and the chemokine MCP-1, all markers of inflammation, subsequently leading to a marked reduction of infarct size. These results indicate that Epo has an anti-inflammatory effect that contributes to its direct neuroprotective effect during cerebral ischemia (Villa et al, 2003). Since Epo did not reduce cytokine production in response to LPS applied directly in vivo and in vitro, the authors concluded that the observed antiinflammatory effect is due to inhibiting neuronal apoptosis and not to a direct effect on inflammatory cells. Epo might reduce leukocyte transmigration through endothelial cells, since Epo enhances the resistance of endothelial cells toward ischemia (Chong et al, 2002). The protective effect of Epo on oligodendrocytes against cytotoxicity induced by inflammatory stimuli (Genc et al, 2006) could explain the beneficial effect of Epo in case of MS where oligodendrocytes play a crucial role in the pathogenesis of the disease.

3.5.5 Transport through BBB

An important prerequisite for considering Epo as a therapeutic agent in CNS diseases is to answer the question as of whether Epo, administered systemically, is able to cross the BBB. Brines et al. (Brines et al, 2000) injected mice with biotinylated Epo and subsequently visualized brain section with peroxidase-labeled streptavidin. Indeed, a signal for biotin was detected in a region surrounding the capillaries extending into brain parenchyma. The authors concluded that Epo crosses the BBB. However, biotin might not be an ideal tool to study BBB permeability since it is rapidly transported across the BBB (Shi et al, 1993; Spector and Mock, 1987), and, therefore, even a small amount of free biotin in the blood will cross the BBB leading to false results. Since the authors detected EpoR in the brain capillaries, they attributed Epo transport through BBB to transcytosis. This hypothesis was later challenged by the observation that radiolabeled Epo and albumin crossed the BBB and entered the brain parenchyma in similar kinetics, showing that the transport of Epo across BBB is rather mediated by the extracellular pathways (Banks et al, 2004). However, variations in physiological serum Epo level may not result in significant changes of Epo levels within the brain, since no correlation between serum and liquor Epo concentrations was found when the BBB is intact (Marti et al, 1997). In summary, one can conclude that endogenously produced Epo (by kidney or liver) has only a marginal influence on brain Epo availability, whereas high dosages of therapeutically administered r-hu Epo can penetrate even the intact BBB (Marti et al, 1997). Accordingly, many studies are currently ongoing to test the therapeutic potential of Epo in many CNS diseases.

3.6 Epo in stroke

The first hint came from the observation that the expression of Epo and its receptor in the brain is upregulated upon cerebral ischemia (Bernaudin et al, 1999; Siren et al, 2001). Several in vivo experiments confirmed this hypothesis. Intracerebroventricular injection of Epo 24 h before permanent occlusion of the MCA in mice reduced infarct volume significantly. Similarly, infusion of Epo in the lateral ventricles of gerbils in a global ischemia model rescued hippocampal CA1 neurons and increased the number of synapses in the same region (Sakanaka et al, 1998). Moreover, in another experimental rodent model of cerebral ischemia where the MCA is transiently occluded, systemic administration of Epo also reduced the infarct size (Brines et al, 2000). Significantly, this protective effect of Epo was retained even when Epo was applied 6 h after the onset of the cerebral ischemia. In addition, brain-specific overexpression of Epo reduced infarct size in mice subjected to transient cerebral ischemia (Kilic et al, 2005). Other studies, where the functional outcome of Epo treatment was investigated, have shown that Epo not only reduces infarct volume but also improves the learning ability in gerbils and reduces the navigation disability in rats (Sadamoto et al, 1998; Sakanaka et al, 1998). Epo has also been shown to be protective in models of hemorrhagic stroke where the interruption of the cerebral blood flow is due to subarachnoid or cerebral hemorrhage (Alafaci et al, 2000; Grasso et al, 2002). The above-mentioned studies prompted the initiation of clinical trials in stroke patients. The safety and proof-of-concept phases of the Göttingen-Epo-Stroke Study have shown Epo to be safe and to improve the patient functional outcome after stroke (Ehrenreich et al, 2002). Although good evidence for direct neuroprotection exists, the observed brain-protective effect of Epo could also be attributed to its effect on astrocytes. Astrocytes protect neurons from oxidative stress by neutralizing reactive oxygen species (Dringen and Hirrlinger, 2003). It has been reported that activated astrocytes in ischemic human brain express increased levels of EpoR (Siren et al, 2001). Since Epo enhances brain glutathione peroxidase activity (Kumral et al, 2005), Epo, by binding to EpoR on the surface of activated astrocytes, might contribute to the astrocyte-mediated neuroprotective effect against ischemia-induced free-radical formation.

3.7 Safety concerns with the clinical use of EPO

Clinical studies are ongoing to test the safety and efficacy of EPO for the treatment of different neurological diseases. In the recent multicenter Epo stroke trial (Ehreich et al, 2009), adult stroke patients receiving Epo after tissue-plasminogen activator (t-PA)-induced thrombolysis reported increased mortality, intra-cerebral hemorrhage, brain edema, and thromboembolic events. The increased death rate in the rtPA population is still unexplained and may result from a combinant of factors and/or potential rtPA-EPO interactions. In contrast, in non rtPA population, the tendency toward a higher death rate in the EPO group might be explained by higher stroke severity of dead patients on inclusion (before any study medication was applied). Moreover, the mechanism of action of EPO is different from the clot-dissolving strategy pursued by thrombolysis. It would, therefore, have been most attractive to see that the neuroprotective approach using EPO, aimed at salvaging potentially viable brain tissue from spreading of death signals, and thrombolysis, targeting reopening of the feeding artery, had provided additive beneficial outcome. However, the unexpected observation that a combination of EPO and rtPA is not advantageous, and can even be detrimental, poses at present a contraindication for acute EPO treatment in patients receiving rtPA.

4. Albumin

Albumin is the most abundant plasma protein synthesized mainly in the liver. Albumin is also a major component of most extracellular fluids including cerebrospinal fluid (CSF), interstitial fluid (ISF) and lymph. It is a non-glycosylated and negatively charged protein with high ligand binding and transport capacity. It has multifunctional properties which include the maintenance of colloid osmotic pressure of plasma, transportation of hormones, fatty acids, drugs and metabolites, regulation of microvascular permeability, antioxidant activity, anti-thrombotic activity and anti-inflammatory activity (Evans, 2002; Garcovich et al, 2009). Owing to its multifunctional properties it has been widely used in therapeutics related to hepatology. The volumeexpanding property of albumin, in combination with other therapeutic approaches, has been used for the clinical benefit of patients with liver cirrhosis. Also, human serum albumin (HSA) as an iso-oncotic (4-5%) solution has been used to combat blood volume deficits and as a hyperoncotic (20-25%) solution has been used for restoration of oncotic deficits (Arroyo, 2002; Garcovich et al, 2009). Albumin has been shown to play a crucial role in the microcirculation of many organs including brain. Owing to its strong hemodynamic and binding capacity, it has been implicated in physiological and many disease conditions of the brain. Albumin has been implicated in neurological diseases such as ischemic stroke, Alzheimer's disease and epilepsy. High-dose human albumin is robustly neuroprotective in preclinical ischemia models and it is currently in Phase III clinical trials for acute ischemic stroke (Ginsberg, 2008). Albumin also has the potential to produce direct neuroprotective action on neuronal and glial cells.

4.1 Albumin synthesis and distribution
Albumin protein contains a single polypeptide chain of 585 amino acids with a molecular mass of approximately 67 kDa.
In the mouse liver, the albumin gene becomes active during early foetal stages and the transcript levels gradually increase after birth until high levels are reached in the adult animal (Tilghman and Belayew, 1982). Albumin is synthesized as preproalbumin in the liver, which has an N-terminal peptide that is removed before the nascent protein is released from the rough endoplasmic reticulum. The product, proalbumin, is in turn cleaved in the Golgi vesicles to produce albumin. Albumin synthesis predominantly occurs in the liver at the rate of 10-15 g/day. In healthy human adults, total albumin content is approximately 250-300 g/70 kg of the body weight and the majority of synthesized albumin (40-45 %) is maintained in the plasma. A very small amount of albumin is stored in liver (< 2 g) and the remaining amount is located in the muscle and skin (Quinlan et al, 2005). Albumin synthesis

is regulated at both the transcriptional and post-transcriptional levels and this regulation is important to meet the demands of plasma, because albumin is not stored in the liver in large amounts. The rate of albumin transcription is affected by several conditions such as trauma, sepsis, hepatic diseases, diabetes and fasting. The change in interstitial colloid oncotic pressure is thought to be the predominant factor for regulation of albumin synthesis. Albumin homeostasis is maintained by balanced catabolism occurring in all tissues but most of the albumin (40-60 %) is degraded in the muscle and skin. However, the liver (15 %), kidney (10 %) and gastro-intestinal tract (10 %) are also responsible for albumin degradation. Albumin leaks from plasma at a rate of 5 % per hour and is returned to the vascular space at an equivalent rate through the lymphatic system. Albumin is also diffused into CSF and ISF compartments of the central nervous system (CNS) from blood circulation of the brain (Nicholson et al, 2000). Blood derived albumin in CSF and interstitial fluid (ISF is implicated in normal as well as many pathophysiological conditions of the brain.

4.2 Albumin in the CSF

CSF originates from choroid plexus in the ventricles. CSF flows through cisternae and subarachnoid space and finally drains through the arachnoid villi into venous blood. CSF has several important functions; it mainly helps to provide mechanical support for the brain. CSF also acts as a drainage pathway for the brain, by providing a ' sink ' into which products of metabolism or synaptic activity are diluted and subsequently removed. Also, it acts as a route of communication within the CNS, i.e., it carries hormones, nutrients and transmitters between different areas of the brain. CSF albumin is predominantly a blood derived protein and it is mainly entered from the leptomeningeal blood CSF barrier (BCSFB) or from choroid plexus BCSFB (Johanson et al, 2008). The albumin quotient (Q alb) in the CSF is approximately 30-80 % of the total protein. The altered Albumin CSF/serum ratio (QAlb) is the indicator of the dysfunction of the BCSFB. CSF serum Q alb, along with other blood derived proteins in CSF, is widely used in the diagnosis of neurological diseases (Reiber, 1998, 2003; Reiber and Peter, 2001). The exact role of albumin in CSF is not fully known, but it is proposed that albumin could be involved in the maintenance of CSF oncotic pressure, delivery of a wide range of molecules that are important for normal brain function and in the removal of some of the harmful molecules from the brain. The exact roles of albumin in CSF and in the brain function are not fully understood. However, many recent studies indicate that albumin might have a neuroprotective role via multiple mechanisms in different pathophysiological conditions.

4.3 Albumin induced neuroprotection in experimental stroke

Ischemic stroke is an acute cerebrovascular disease resulting from a transient or permanent reduction in the cerebral blood flow (CBF). It mainly occurs due to blockade of the major cerebral blood vessels by a local thrombus or an embolus. Ischemia causes reduction in the oxygen and nutrient supply to the brain areas which leads to neuronal cell damage or cell death. It can cause long-term disabilities such as muscle paralysis, cognitive deficits, language deficits, emotional deficits and even coma or death. Stroke is the third leading cause of death worldwide after coronary heart disease and cancer (Lloyd-Jones et al, 2009) and ischemic stroke comprises approximately 87 % of all types of brain strokes. The only approved treatment with intravenous fibrinolytic such as tissue plasminogen activator (tPA) within 3 h of stroke onset yields reperfusion and clinical benefits (rt -PA Stroke Study

Group, 1995; Hacke et al, 2004; Juttler et al, 2006). However, the goal is to discover a neuroprotective drug which can inhibit reperfusion injury and provide neuroprotection within a wide therapeutic window. Hemodilution is an old approach which has been investigated for many decades as a potential therapy for ischemic stroke. Infusion of dextran has been shown to increase CBF of both the normal and ischemic brain, either by decreasing blood viscosity or by vasodilation in response to diminished oxygen delivery (Wood and Kee, 1985; Korosue and Heros, 1992). Despite neuroprotective benefi ts in experimental set-ups, several clinical trials of hemodilution in ischemic stroke have nonetheless proven negative or inconclusive (Scandinavian Stroke Study Group, 1987; Italian Acute Stroke Study Group, 1988; The Hemodilution in Stroke Study Group,1989). Subsequently, albumin has emerged as an alternative hemodiluting agent to dextran owing to its volume expanding properties (Sundt et al, 1967; Little et al, 1981; Emerson, 1989). However, only recently it has been rigorously evaluated for its anti-ischemic neuroprotective efficacy. Transient focal cerebral ischemia induced by middle cerebral artery occlusion (MCAO) is the most widely used model to study molecular mechanisms of cerebral ischemia-reperfusion injury and to screen neuroprotective drugs. It is less invasive with a low rate of mortality and a low coefficient of variation in lesion size (Longa et al, 1989; Belayev et al, 1997b). In the rat MCAO model, Cole et al. reported that 5 % albumin administration at the onset of ischemia reduced ischemic brain injury as evidenced by reduced hematocrit, infarct volume and cerebral edema (Cole et al, 1990). In another study, administration of concentrated (20%) HSA (1% body weight, intravenously) to rats at the onset of recirculation induced substantial diminution of infarct volume together with a marked reduction of brain edema. Thus, it is proposed that albumin might modify water homeostasis and ultimately reduce edema of the ischemic brain (Belayev et al, 1997a). These two initial studies suggested that albumin therapy at the onset of ischemia or reperfusion induces neuroprotection.In a detailed study using magnetic resonance imaging, by means of diffusion-weighted magnetic resonance imaging (DWI), 25% Human Serum Albumin (HSA) solution (1% by body weight) administered immediately after reperfusion was associated with DWI normalization and a mitigation of pannecrotic changes within zones of residual injury at 24 h of injury. Albumin therapy lowered the hematocrit on average by 37% and raised plasma colloid oncotic pressure by 56%, improved the neurological score and reduced brain swelling throughout the 3-day survival period (Belayev et al, 1998). Similar treatment also improved local CBF as measured autoradiographically with 14C-iodoantipyrine after 1 h of recirculation (Huh et al, 1998). Using laser scanning confocal microscopy and laser Doppler perfusion imaging, it was found that a beneficial effect of albumin therapy was attributed to reversal of stagnation, thrombosis and corpuscular adherence within cortical venules in the reperfusion phase after focal ischemia (Belayev et al, 2002). It was also reported that after 1 h of reperfusion, 1.25 g/kg intravenous HSA administration increased replenishment of polyunsaturated fatty acid (PUFA) lost from cellular membranes during ischemia (Rodriguez de Turco et al, 2002). These studies collectively indicate that albumin induced neuroprotection is attributed to properties such as reversal of thrombosis, improvement in microvascular blood perfusion, reduction in brain swelling and replenishment of PUFA in brain. All these actions could indicate that actions of albumin are confined in vascular space. However, it has been shown that treatment with human albumin following 2 h of MCAO also leads to albumin extravasations and subsequently cellular uptake. It has been observed that cortical neurons with preserved structural features had taken up human albumin. Thus, it is reasonable to speculate that treatment with human albumin could also provide direct neuronal protection (Remmers et al, 1999). For the effective treatment of ischemic stroke, treatment should be started within a narrow therapeutic window of 3 h. Moderate-dose albumin therapy (1.25 g/kg intravenously) markedly provides neuroprotection even when treatment is delayed up to 4 h after onset of ischemia (Belayev et al, 2001). Albumin treatment has also been found to be neuroprotective in other models of focal ischemia. Prompt albumin therapy improved neurological function and blood-brain barrier integrity after acute intracortical hematoma (ICH) (Belayev et al, 2005). In a model of laser-induced cortical arteriolar thrombosis, high-dose albumin therapy induced a prompt, sustained improvement in microvascular hemodynamics distal to a cortical arteriolar thrombosis (Nimmagadda et al, 2008). In acute ischemic stroke, albumin combination therapy can attenuate the deleterious effects of tPA (Tang et al, 2009). Furthermore, albumin (1.25 g/kg) treatment maintains serum albumin at a higher level and attenuates cortex and hippocampus vascular endothelial growth factor (VEGF) expression at 6 h and 1 day after MCAO. This could partially contribute to the protective effects of albumin on reduction of brain edema and infarct size in the early stage of ischemia (Yao et al, 2010). The above mentioned studies prove that in experimental transient ischemia albumin provides neuroprotection via different indirect and direct mechanisms. Albumin has been found to be effective in other models of stroke such as permanent MCAO, global ischemia induced by bilateral common carotid occlusion (BCCO) and traumatic brain injury (TBI). In permanent MCAO, rats treated with 2 g/kg/day concentrated (25%) albumin begun after 30 min of ischemia showed diminished brain edema and infarct volume up to 6 days (Matsui et al, 1993). Furthermore, albumin (1.25 and 2.5 g/kg) significantly reduced cortical and striatal infarct areas and increased cortical perfusion in the permanent ischemia model (Liu et al, 2001). In transient global ischemia, HSA-treated rats showed signifi cantly improved neurological deficits throughout a 7-day survival period along with increases in numbers of surviving CA1 hippocampal pyramidal neurons compared to saline-treated animals (Belayev et al, 1999b). In TBI, 15 min after trauma, HSA administration signifi cantly improved neurological defi cits and also significantly reduced total contusion area (Belayev et al, 1999a). These experimental trials altogether indicated significant neuroprotective roles of albumin in different models of ischemic stroke and encouraged the further development of this important molecule for possible treatment of ischemic stroke in humans.

4.4 Albumin in clinical trials for ischemic stroke

The Albumin In Acute Stroke (ALIAS) Pilot Clinical Trial was conducted during 2001 – 2005 at two clinical sites (Universities of Calgary and Miami). This study was designed to investigate the safety and tolerability of albumin therapy in acute ischemic stroke. The ALIAS Pilot Clinical Trial used a multiple-tier, open-label, dose-escalation design. Human albumin (25%) in doses ranging up to 2.05 g/kg was well tolerated by patients with acute ischemic stroke without major dose-limiting complications. Concurrent tPA therapy did not affect the safety profile of albumin (Ginsberg et al, 2006a). Also, in this pilot trial the neuroprotective efficacy of albumin was evaluated and was found to be neuroprotective after ischemic stroke (Palesch et al, 2006). Based on the encouraging results of pilot trials of albumin, the National Institutes of Health has funded a randomized multicenter placebo-controlled effi cacy trial – the ALIAS Phase III Trial. A randomised, multicenter, double-blind, placebo controlled trial (ALIAS Phase III Trial, www.clinicaltrials. gov; NCT00235495) is currently being conducted at approximately 70 clinical sites in North America (Ginsberg et al, 2006b; Hill et al, 2011).

4.5 Direct neuroprotection by albumin: Mechanisms

The neuroprotective mechanisms of albumin in ischemic stroke and AD are largely attributed to its hemodynamic properties and binding properties. However, in different in vitro systems, albumin has been reported to possess several direct neuroprotective actions. (Figure 4)

Albumin could produce various neuroprotective actions in the intravascular compartment, cerebrospinal fluid-interstitial fluid compartment and intracellular compartment.

HSA and its N-terminal tetrapeptide DAHK can block oxidant-driven cultured neuronal injury produced by hydrogen peroxide and copper/ascorbic acid (Gum et al, 2004). Furthermore, bovine serum albumin has been found to be neuroprotective by reducing both the DNA damage and apoptosis rates in cultured cortical neurons and these effects are probably due to its antioxidant activity (Baltanas et al, 2009). Albumin has been reported to play an important role in astrocyte functions. It is shown that albumin affects metabolism of cultured astrocytes (Tabernero et al, 1999). Albumin up on transcytosis into cultured astrocytes stimulates the synthesis of neurotrophic factor oleic acid which promotes neuronal differentiation (Tabernero et al, 2002). Megalin is a receptor for albumin in astrocytes and is required for the synthesis of the neurotrophic factor oleic acid (Bento - Abreu et al, 2008). Also, this megalin induced albumin transcytosis and synthesis of

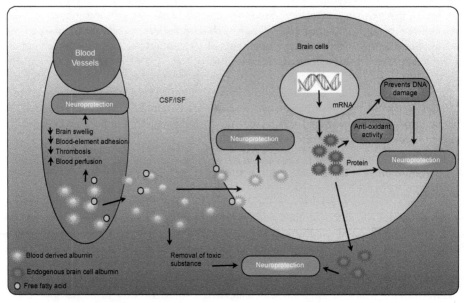

Fig. 4. Overview of possible neuroprotective mechanisms of albumin.

neurotrophic factor is dependent on caveola and the adaptor protein cytosolic adaptor protein disabled (Dab-1) in cultured astrocytes (Bento -Abreu et al, 2009). These studies indicate that albumin could play a role in neuronal differentiation and development. Albumin also induces calcium mobilisation in cultured as well as brain astrocytes (Manning and Sontheimer, 1997; Nadal et al, 1998; Hooper et al, 2005). Albumin elicits calcium entry in the microglia which promotes proliferation of the microglia (Hooper et al, 2005). Astrocyte calcium signalling caused by albumin could have important physiological and pathophysiological consequences when the blood-brain barrier breaks down and allows albumin to enter the CNS. It is reported that albumin leakage induced by blood-brain barrier breaks is followed by albumin uptake into astrocytes which is responsible for epileptogenesis in rats (Ivens et al, 2007; van Vliet et al, 2007). Albumin causes downregulation of Kir current which results in the abnormal accumulation of $[K^+]$ o and consequent NMDA-receptor dependent pathological plasticity which isresponsible for epileptogenesis (Ivens et al, 2007). Recently, it was shown that albumin activates astrocytes and microglia producing infl ammatory responses via the mitogen-activated protein kinase pathway and these effects could be involved both in the mechanism of cellular injury and repair (Ralay Ranaivo and Wainwright, 2010). Altogether these fi ndings suggest that the majority of the effects of albumin on astrocytes, microglia and neuronal cells seem to be benefi cial; however, at augmented levels it could contribute towards astrocyte dysfunction. The direct effects of albumin on neuronal and glial cells necessitate further detailed investigation in individual pathological conditions.

4.6 Endogenous albumin and neuroprotection: possible new paradigm

Although albumin is mainly synthesized in the liver, mRNA expression level of albumin has been found in many non-hepatic rat tissues such as lungs, heart, kidney and pancreas, but not in the brain (Nahon et al, 1988). Also, non-hepatic albumin expression at the protein level is rarely confirmed. A recent study suggests that human brain microglia cells can express albumin both at mRNA and protein levels; furthermore, this expression is increased by amyloid beta (Aβ) and lipopolysaccharide treatment (Ahn et al, 2008). It is suggested that enhanced levels of albumin and subsequent secretion by microglia could be implicated in A β removal from the brain (Ahn et al, 2008). We have also found upregulation of albumin at both mRNA and protein levels in ischemic rat brain. Upregulation of albumin in ischemic brain could play a neuroprotective role against altered brain functions (Prajapati et al, 2010). These results indicate that de novo synthesis of albumin also occurs in the brain tissue. However, possible intracellular and extracellular neuroprotective actions of endogenously synthesized albumin is an unexplored area and warrants further investigations.

5. Antithrombin III

Antithrombin III (ATIII) is a single-chain glycoprotein in plasma and belongs to the family of the serpins. It is synthesized in liver parenchymal cells, and it plays a central role in regulating haemostasis. When bound to glycosaminoglycans, it is an important inhibitor of several serine protease, including factors Xa, IXa, XIa, and thrombin (Bauer and Rosenberg, 1991), wich are involved in blood coagulation. Equimolar, irreversible complexes are formed between ATIII and the enzymes. Heparin and heparan sulfate glycoproteins (HSPGs) bind to multiple sites of the ATIII molecule resulting in a steric reconfiguration, thereby increasing the interaction between ATIII and the activated enzymes. It is believed that much of the physiological inactivation of enzymes by ATIII occurs in the endothelium, mediated by heparan sulfate (Figure 5) (Mammen, 1998).

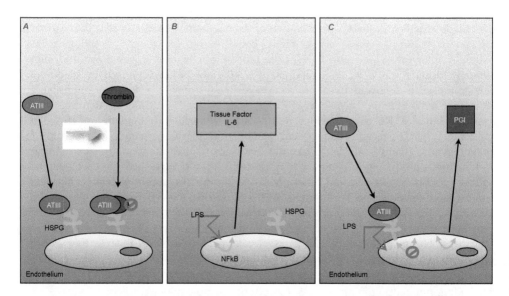

Fig. 5. Role of heparan sulfate proteoglycan (HSPG) in inhibition of thrombin, in induction of prostacyclin, and inhibition of cytokine and tissue factor release from endothelial cells by antithrombin III.

A large number of recent studies have shown that ATIII has anti-inflammatory actions, (Cuomo et al, 2007) which are independent of its effects on coagulation. These effects include the heterologous deactivation of activated leukocytes and the interaction with the endothelium, thereby reducing vessel wall transmigration and subsequent tissue and organ damage. Thus, ATIII may have two distinct and indipendent actions in patients with cerebral ischemia: (1) interference with pathologic coagulation, and (2) inhibition of inflammation.

5.1 Effects of ATIII on abnormal coagulation
The prothrombotic, proinflammatory state of stroke results in a promotion of thrombin formation and fibrin deposition at the vascular wall, as well as in the formetion of platelet-leukocyte coaggregates, leading to severe disturbance of the microcirculation, capillary leakage and tissue damage (Piazza et al, 2010). Many of the events involved in this proinflammatory state have been shown to be inhibited by ATIII. The inhibition of factor Xa by ATIII may be particularly important for protection against, and treatment of, inflammation. This activated clotting factor has a number of proinflammatory effects, including stimulation if the production of IL-6, IL-8, MCP-1, E-selectin, and the soluble adhesion molecules ICAM-1 and vascular cell adhesion molecule (VCAM)-1, wich can be experimentally blocked by ATIII (Senden et al, 1998). The proinflammatory functions of

thrombin include stimulation of neutrophil/monocyte adhesion, action as a chemotactic factor for polymorphonuclear leukocytes (Esmon, 2000), and increased expression of the recently discovered inhibitor of fibrinolysis, thrombin-activable fibrinolysis inhibitor (TAFI) (Opal, 2000). Thrombin also stimulates the increased expression of IL-8 and plays an important role in ischemia-induced leukocyte rolling and adhesion (Kaur et al, 2001; Ludwicka-Bradley et al, 2000; Rabiet et al, 1994). Thus, the ability of ATIII to inhibit the actions of both factor Xa and thrombin gives it the potential to block, in part or fully, a wide range of proinflammatory events (Seegers, 1978).

5.2 Coagulation-indipendent anti-inflammatory effects of ATIII
In the late 1980s, initial publications reported on the property of ATIII to stimulate prostacyclin release from endothelial cells independent of thrombin interaction. Although some recent studies question such a mechanism, at least in vitro, a number of papers make an in vivo contribution of prostacyclin release as part of the ATIII anti-inflammatory properties likely (Uchiba and Okajima, 2001). Independent of ATIII's anticoagulatory activities at multiple points of action, a variety of studies provide evidence for a potent anti-inflammatory ATIII effect, wich can only be induced by high ATIII plasma activities in the range of 150%-200% (Harada et al, 1999; Hoffmann et al, 2000; Okajiama and Uchiba, 1998; Uchiba et al, 1996, 1998). These anti-inflammatory ATIII actions may be mainly mediated by an interaction of ATIII with the endothelium (Hoffmann et al, 2002), thereby producing a profound increase in endothelial prostacyclin production (Figure 5C) (Yamauchi et al, 1989).

5.3 Effects of ATIII on leukocyte-endothelium interactions
ATIII expresses the ability to inhibit leukocyte rolling and adhesion, wich are hallmarks of inflammatory reactions, and have explored the mechanisms underlying these effects. Ostrovsky et al (Ostrovsky et al, 1997) showed that ATIII administration significantly reduced neutrophil rolling and adhesion to pretreatment levels in a feline mesentery ischaemia-reperfusion model. Nevière et al (Nevière et al, 2001) and Hoffmann et al (Hoffmann et al, 2000) showed that the beneficial effects resulting from ATIII's blocking of leukocyte-endothelium interactions were eliminated when indomethacin, a cyclo-oxygenase inhibitor that blocks prostacyclin production, was added to the treatment. The administration of recombinant hirudin did not result in comparable beneficial effects, supporting the thrombin-indipendent mode of action of ATIII. As a consequence of the limited activated leukocyte-endothelium interaction, the severity of subsequent capillary leakage, disturbance of microcirculation, and organ damage were significantly reduced. A report by Yamashiro et al (Yamashiro et al, 2001) suggests direct affects of ATIII on leukocytes and endothelium by demonstrating the downmodulation of P-selectin by ATIII in the LPS-stimulated endothelium, thereby diminishing leukocyte rolling and subsequent transmigration. Support of this hypothesis has also been provided by the work of Souter et al (Souter et al, 2001) showing that the addition of ATIII to LPS-treated whole blood, HUVEC, and mononuclear cells inhibited production of both IL-6 and tissue factor; recombinant hirudin, a specific thrombin inhibitor, did not reduce the production of IL-6 or tissue factor, again suggesting that the observed inhibition by ATIII was not due solely to its ability ti inhibit thrombin (figure 5B and C).

5.4 Direct effect of ATIII on leukocytes

Dunzendorfer et al (Dunzendorfer et al, 2000, 2001) have uncovered a second mechanism by which ATIII may inhibit neutrophil migration and adhesion to the endothelium; namely, heterologous deactivation of activated leukocytes by ATIII. These investigators noted that signaling in ATIII-induced neutrophil chemotaxis mimics an IL-8-induced response, ATIII inhibited migration of neutrophils towards IL-8, GRO-alpha, and fMLP; staurosporine, bisindolylmaleimide I, pertussis toxin, and an anti-CXCR1 monoclonal antibody all blocked ATIII-induced neutrophil chemotaxis. However, additional assays did not reveal binding of ATIII to CXCR1. Thus, the results of these studies are generally consistent with the conclusion that the effect of ATIII in neutrophil migration appear to involve a CXCR1-related signaling pathway, its G-proteins, and protein kinase C. Recent findings have shown that the signalling pathway activated by ATIII in leukocytes are different in neutrophils, monocytes, and lymphocytes (Dunzendorfer et al, 2001; Kaneider et al, 2001, 2002). All togheter, these experiments led to the conclusion that ATIII in circulation protects leukocytes from premature activation.

5.5 ATIII and nuclear factor-kappaB

Oelschager et al (Oelshager et al, 2001) showed that ATIII produces a dose-dependent reduction in both LPS and tissue necrosis factor (TNF)-α activation of nuclear factor-kappaB (NF-κB) in cultured monocytes and endothelial cells. Results reported by this working group and by Iampietro et al (Iampietro et al, 2000) indicate that these actions of ATIII block the increase in IL-6, IL-8, TNF, and tissue factor mRNA expression (figure 5B and C). Beyond control of coagulation, ATIII displays anti-inflammatory properties through an interaction with cells, reducing the synthesis and release of proinflammatory mediators, thereby modulating leukocyte activation and their interaction with the vessel wall. As a consequence, tissue damage and organ failure are reduced.

6. Toll-like receptors

The TLRs, so-called because of their homology to the Drosophila Toll receptor, were first characterized in mammals by their ability to recognize pathogen-associated molecular patterns such as those found in the bacterial cell wall components peptidoglycan (TLR2) and lipopolysaccharide (LPS) (TLR4), as well as viral dsRNA (TLR3), ssRNA (TLR7), and nonmethylated cytosine-guanine (CpG) DNA (TLR9). Recently it has been found that in addition to their role in pathogen detection and defense, TLRs act as sentinels of tissue damage and mediate inflammatory responses to aseptic tissue injury. Surfactant, HSP60, components of the extracellular matrix, and fibrinogen have all been shown to activate TLR4, while host HMGB1 and host mRNA and DNA are endogenous ligands of TLR2 (and TLR4), TLR3 and TLR9, respectively. TLRs, upon activation by either pathogen- or host-derived ligands, induce downstream signals that lead to cytokine and chemokine production and thereby initiate inflammatory responses. TLRs are located on antigen presenting cells such as B cells, dendritic cells, monocytes/macrophages and microglia. In addition, these receptors can be expressed by the cerebral endothelium and by cells within the brain parenchyma such as astrocytes, oligodendrocytes, and neurons (Bsibsi et al., 2002; Singh and Jiang, 2004; Jack et al., 2005; Bsibsi et al., 2006). The TLRs signal through common intracellular pathways leading to transcription factor activation and the generation of cytokines and chemokines (Figure 6) (Vogel et al., 2003; Takeda and Akira, 2005). Each TLR family member, with the exception of TLR3, initiates intracellular signaling via recruitment of the intracellular Toll-interleukin 1 receptor (TIR)–domain-containing adaptor MyD88. When recruited to plasma membrane-associated TLRs, either directly (TLRs 5 and 11) or via the TIRAP adaptor (TLRs 1, 2, 4, 6), MyD88 enlists members of the IRAK family, including IRAK1, IRAK2, and IRAK4, to begin a process of auto- and cross-phosphorylation among the IRAK molecules. Once phosphorylated, IRAKs dissociate from MyD88 and bind TRAF6, an E3 ligase. TRAF6 in turn activates TAK1 which itself activates the IKK complex and MAPKKs. The IKK complex, composed of IKKα, IKKβ and the regulatory subunit IKKγ/NEMO, phosphorylates IκB proteins. This phosphorylation is necessary for the ubiquitination and proteosomal degradation of IκBs and the subsequent nuclear translocation of the transcription factor NFκB. Members of the MAPK family phosphorylate and activate components of the transcription factor AP-1. Together, these transcription factors induce inflammatory cytokine production (e.g. TNFα, IL1). MyD88 is also recruited to the endosomal receptors TLR7 and TLR9 again enlisting members of the IRAK family. Due to the endosomal location of the complex, the phosphorylated IRAKs are able to bind TRAF3 in addition to TRAF6. Activation of TRAF3 leads to phosphorylation, dimerization, and nuclear localization of the transcription factors IRF3, IRF5, and IRF7 with resultant type I interferon (IFN) production. Hence these endosomal TLRs are capable of signaling to NFκB, AP-1 and IRFs, resulting in a diverse genomic response. Endosomal TLR3 is unique among the TLRs because it does not signal through MyD88 but signals instead via recruitment of the Toll-interleukin 1 receptor domain-containing adaptor inducing interferon β (TRIF). TRIF enlists the non-canonical IKKs, TBK1 and IKKε, which activate IRF3. Further, TRIF recruits TRAF6 and RIP-1, which results in activation of MAPK and IKKα/β. Hence TLR3, like the other endosomal receptors, is capable of activating NFκB, AP-1 and IRFs. Of all the TLRs, only TLR4 can recruit either MyD88 (via TIRAP) or TRIF (via TRAM) and can thus induce either the pro-inflammatory cytokines TNFα and IL1 via NFκB or the anti-viral IFNβ via IRF3. The complement of TLR family members expressed by a cell depends on its identity and its activation status. Constitutive expression of TLRs within the brain occurs in microglia and astrocytes and is largely restricted to the circumventricular organs and meninges—areas with direct access to the circulation (Laflamme and Rivest, 2001; Laflamme et al., 2001; Chakravarty and Herkenham, 2005). Human and murine microglia express TLRs 1–9 and generate cytokine profiles specifically tailored by the TLR stimulated (Bsibsi et al., 2002; Olson and Miller, 2004; Jack et al., 2005). Similarly, human and murine astrocytes express multiple TLRs, with particularly prominent TLR3 expression (Bsibsi et al., 2002, 2006; Carpentier et al., 2005; Jack et al., 2005; McKimmie and Fazakerley, 2005). Microglia and astrocytes respond differently to specific TLR engagement reflective of their distinct roles in the brain. Microglia initiate robust cytokine and chemokine responses to stimulation of TLR2 (TNFα, IL-6, IL-10), TLR3 (TNFα, IL-6, IL-10, IL-12, CXCL-10, IFNβ), and TLR4 (TNFα, IL-6, IL-10, CXCL-10, IFNβ), yet astrocytes initiate only minor IL-6 responses to all but TLR3 stimulation (Jack et al., 2005). Microglia express TLR3 and TLR4 at the cell surface while astrocytes express these receptors intracellularly (Bsibsi et al., 2002). The cellular location of TLRs affects their downstream signaling cascades (Kagan et al., 2008), which may explain the different responses of these cells to TLR stimulation. The

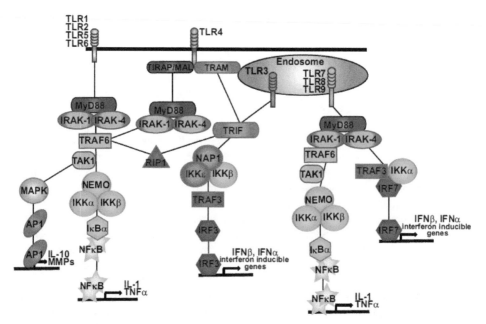

Fig. 6. TLRs signaling

inflammatory milieu also plays a critical role in regulating TLR expression. Microglia stimulated with CpG specifically up-regulate TLR9, whereas those stimulated with a synthetic TLR3 ligand suppress all TLRs except TLR3 (Olson and Miller, 2004). Similarly, astrocytes stimulated with LPS up-regulate TLRs 2 and 3 but suppress TLR4, while astrocytes exposed to RNA viruses up-regulate TLR3 and TLR9 (McKimmie and Fazakerley, 2005). Thus microglia and astrocytes initiate a layered and multifaceted response to TLR engagement. Oligodendrocytes and endothelial cells express a relatively limited repertoire of TLRs. Oligodendrocytes express TLRs 2 and 3 (Bsibsi et al., 2002), while cerebral endothelial cells constitutively express TLRs 2, 4, and 9 (Constantin et al., 2004) and increase their expression of these TLRs in response to stressful stimuli, including systemic LPS and cerebral ischemia (Singh and Jiang, 2004; Zhou et al., 2007; Ziegler et al., 2007). In response to LPS, endothelial cells up-regulate E-selectin, an NFκB-dependent molecule, and IFNβ, an IRF3-dependent molecule, indicating that these cells utilize the TLR–NFκB and the TLR–IRF3 signaling pathways (Lloyd-Jones et al., 2008). Neurons express TLR3 and generate inflammatory cytokines (TNFα, IL-6), chemokines (CCL5, CXCL10) and antiviral molecules (IFNβ) in response to dsRNA (Lafon et al., 2006; Prehaud et al., 2005). Neurons also employ TLRs in their development and differentiation. TLRs 3 and 8 are expressed on murine neurons early in development and inhibit neurite outgrowth in a MyD88- and NFκB-independent manner (Ma et al., 2006). TLR2 and TLR4 have been found on adult neural progenitor cells where they appear to elicit opposing effects. While TLR2 activation stimulates neuronal differentiation of these cells, TLR4 activation decreases proliferation and neuronal differentiation, driving these cells toward an astrocytic fate (Rolls et al., 2007). Curiously, both TLRs exert these endogenous effects in a MyD88-dependent manner, suggesting that these molecules utilize MyD88 in distinct ways. Hence even minor alterations of these fine-tuned endogenous pathways can have profound effects on cellular responses to TLR engagement. Studies with TLR knockout mice illustrate the endogenous function of TLRs in health and disease. TLR2 and TLR4 have been shown to play detrimental roles in the development of congestive heart failure and cardiac hypertrophy, respectively, by signaling through MyD88 and NFκB (Shishido et al., 2003; Ha et al., 2005). TLR2 has additionally been found to be proatherogenic in hyperlipidemic mice (Tobias and Curtiss, 2007), and TLR4 has been shown to produce inflammatory reactions in adipose tissue and thereby mediates obesity and insulin resistance (Tsukumo et al., 2007; Davis et al., 2008). Conversely, TLR2 and TLR4 activation by hyaluronic acid protects lung tissue from non-infectious injury (Jiang et al., 2006), and TLR4 has been shown to help maintain lung integrity, and prevent the development of emphysema, by modulating oxidant generation (Zhang et al., 2006). The effects of endogenous TLR stimulation are clearly varied, depending on the cell and tissue type in which the receptors are found and on the disease process in which they are involved. The overwhelming and generally damaging inflammatory response of TLRs to aseptic tissue injury may be a consequence of TLR evolution in response to pathogens. In the setting of pathogen invasion, an inflammatory deluge may be the most effective means to clear microorganisms. The activation and influx of leukocytes, with the concomitant release of free radicals and tissue-destroying enzymes, assails not only the invading pathogen but any host cells that harbor the pathogen. However, when this same powerful response is co-opted by the host to clear and resolve tissue damage, it can destroy the very cells it is meant to save. This damage promoting characteristic is prominently observed following brain ischemia, where inflammation plays a critical role in both injury progression and resolution.

6.1 TLRS and ischemic damage

A significant portion of the damage associated with stroke injury is due to the resultant inflammatory response. This aspect of the innate immune response is exemplified by the fact that some anti-inflammatory strategies have been shown to ameliorate ischemic damage (Relton et al., 1996; Hara et al., 1997; Spera et al., 1998). The inflammatory response to stroke is initiated by the detection of injury associated molecules by local cells such as microglia and astrocytes. The response is further promoted by infiltrating neutrophils and macrophages, resulting in the production of inflammatory cytokines, proteolytic enzymes, and other cytotoxic mediators. In the mouse, leukocytes and brain cells (microglia, astrocytes and neurons) express TLRs (Zarember and Godowski, 2002; Olson and Miller, 2004). Hence, injury-associated molecules such as HSP60 and HMGB1 may act as endogenous ligands for TLRs, thereby initiating the damaging inflammatory response to stroke. It is increasingly clear that TLRs do in fact play a role in ischemic damage (Fig.). The pathogenic role of TLRs in ischemic processes was first demonstrated in a mouse model myocardial ischemia/reperfusion injury, because mice lacking functional TLR4 incur less damage than wild type mice (Oyama et al., 2004). Since then, TLR2 has also been shown to cause dysfunction following cardiac ischemia and both have been shown to exacerbate renal ischemic damage, in a MyD88-dependent and a MyD88-independent manner (Sakata et al., 2007; Shigeoka et al., 2007). However, the particular pathway responsible for the damaging effects of TLR activation may differ depending on the cell type or organ affected as TLR4 worsens ischemic damage following liver transplant in a MyD88-independent, IRF3 dependent fashion (Zhai et al., 2004; Shen et al., 2005). Importantly, TLR2 and TLR4 have been shown to play a role in cerebral ischemic damage. Mice lacking either functional TLR2 or TLR4 are less susceptible to transient focal cerebral ischemia/reperfusion damage, demonstrating smaller infarcts than wild type controls (Cao et al., 2007; Lehnardt et al., 2007; Ziegler et al., 2007). Further, mice lacking TLR4 incur less damage following global cerebral ischemia and permanent focal ischemia (Caso et al., 2007; Hua et al., 2007). The TLR endogenous ligands HSP 60, HSP70 and HMGB1 are found in the brain following injury (Kinouchi et al., 1993; Faraco et al., 2007; Lehnardt et al., 2008). Hence these molecules may activate TLR2 and TLR4 within the brain itself, leading to the generation of inflammatory mediators such as TNFα, IL1, IL6, and iNOS, all known to be associated with stroke damage.

6.2 TLRS and neuroprotection

In contrast to the detrimental role of TLRs in response to ischemia, stimulation of these receptors prior to ischemia provides robust neuroprotection. TLR4-induced tolerance to cerebral ischemia was first demonstrated with low dose systemic administration of LPS (endotoxin), a cell wall component of gram-negative bacteria, which caused spontaneously hypertensive rats to become tolerant to subsequent ischemic brain damage induced by middle cerebral artery occlusion (MCAO) (Tasaki et al., 1997). Since then, LPS-induced tolerance to brain ischemia has been demonstrated in a mouse model of stroke and in a porcine model of deep hypothermic circulatory arrest (Rosenzweig et al., 2004; Hickey et al., 2007) (for additional information on the dual effects of neuro-immune crosstalk, please refer to Kerschensteiner et al., in this issue). Neuroprotection induced by LPS is time and dose dependent. Tolerance appears by 24 h after LPS administration and extends out to 7 days but is gone by 14 days (Rosenzweig et al., 2007). Protective doses of LPS appear to depend on the animal model of stroke and the route of systemic administration, ranging from 0.02–1 mg/kg (Tasaki et al., 1997; Ahmed et al., 2000; Bordet et al., 2000; Furuya et al., 2005; Hickey et al., 2007; Kunz et al., 2007; Rosenzweig et al., 2007). Tolerance induction has been shown to require new protein synthesis and a modest inflammatory response, as it can be blocked by prior administration of cycloheximide or dexamethasone (Bordet et al., 2000). Specifically, TNFα has been implicated as a mediator of LPS-induced ischemic tolerance because inhibition of TNFα systemically (Tasaki et al., 1997) or within the brain (Rosenzweig et al., 2007) blocks neuroprotection, and mice lacking TNFα fail to be protected by LPS preconditioning (Rosenzweig et al., 2007). In addition to its neuroprotective effects, LPS preconditioning has vasculoprotective efficacy. Nitric oxide appears to play a critical role in the protective effects of LPS. Mice lacking iNOS expression fail to be protected by LPS pretreatment (Kunz et al., 2007), and eNOS expression within the brain is directly correlated to the time window of LPS-induced neuroprotection (Furuya et al., 2005). LPS pretreatment has further been shown to prevent the impairment of endothelial and smooth muscle relaxation normally induced by ischemia/reperfusion injury (Bastide et al., 2003), resulting in normalization of cerebral blood flow in peri-infarct regions lasting out to 24 h after MCAO (Dawson et al., 1999; Furuya et al., 2005). LPS-induced ischemic protection requires an inflammatory response prior to the ischemic event, yet protection occurs through modulation of the inflammatory response following ischemia. Rosenzweig et al. (2004) have shown that LPS preconditioning changes the response of circulating leukocytes to stroke, attenuating stroke-induced neutrophilia, lymphopenia, and monocyte activation. This altered inflammatory response extends into the brain itself. LPS preconditioning attenuates activation of microglia after stroke and reduces neutrophil infiltration into the ischemic hemisphere. Hence, LPS-induced preservation of microvascular function following MCAO may be due to suppressed lymphocyte adhesion to activated endothelium, either by TNFα-induced suppression of endothelial activation and adhesion molecules (Ginis et al., 1999; Ahmed et al., 2000) or by prevention of cellular inflammatory responses to ischemia (Rosenzweig et al., 2004). One hallmark of LPS preconditioning is suppression of cytotoxic TNFα signaling following stroke. Mice that have been preconditioned with LPS prior to ischemia display a pronounced suppression of the TNFα pathway following stroke, as evinced by reduced TNFα in the serum, decreased levels of cellular TNFR1, and enhanced levels of neutralizing soluble-TNFR1. These mice are thus protected from the cytotoxic effects of TNFα after cerebral ischemia (Rosenzweig et al., 2007). Collectively, these mechanisms lead to a muted TNFα response to ischemic injury and increased cell survival. Recently a new TLR ligand has been shown to induce tolerance to brain ischemia. As with TLR4 and LPS, stimulation of TLR9 by systemically administered CpG oligodeoxynucleotides induces robust protection against brain ischemia in a time and dose dependent manner. CpG pretreatment protects neurons in both in vivo and in vitro models of stroke (Stevens et al., 2008). Notably, the protection afforded by CpG depends on TNFα, as systemic CpG administration acutely and significantly increases serum TNFα, and TNFα knockout mice fail to be protected by CpG preconditioning. Similarities among the known TLR signaling pathways and their shared ability to induce TNFα, itself a potent preconditioning stimulus, suggest that stimulation of TLR4 and TLR9 may induce ischemic tolerance by similar means. The neuroprotective potential of other TLRs has yet to be explored, but this family of molecules may be a rich source of therapeutic targets. The finding that TLRs are mediators of ischemic injury provides insight into the potential mechanisms of LPS- and CpG-induced neuroprotection. In fact, TLR-induced tolerance to subsequent ischemia may occur by the same mechanisms that govern a very similar phenomenon — that of LPS-induced tolerance to subsequent LPS exposure. The latter phenomenon is known as "endotoxin tolerance" and occurs when pretreatment with a low dose of LPS renders cells or whole animals tolerant to the normally detrimental effects of a second, higher dose of LPS. Cells that are tolerant to LPS are defined by their inability to generate TNFα in response to TLR4 activation. Upon TLR4 ligation, LPS tolerant cells, unlike naive cells, do not recruit MyD88 to TLR4, and fail to activate IRAK-1 and NFκB (Medvedev et al., 2002). The TLR4–NFκB signaling axis becomes decommissioned following a primary exposure to LPS via an elaborate negative feedback loop that involves known inhibitors of TLR signaling. Among those inhibitors are Ship-1, which prevents TLR4-MyD88 interaction, IRAK-M, a non-functional IRAK decoy, and TRIM30α, which destabilized the TAK1 complex (Kobayashi et al., 2002; Sly et al., 2004; Shi et al., 2008). Thus, subsequent signaling of TLR4 to NFκB is blocked and inflammatory cytokine production is suppressed. Conversely, secondary exposure causes enhanced IFNβ release, suggesting increased signaling via the TLR4-IRF3 axis (Broad et al., 2007). Thus, pretreatment with LPS causes cells to switch their transcriptional response to TLR4 stimulation by enhancing the IRF3- induced cytokine IFNβ and suppressing the NFκB-induced cytokine TNFα. Similar to endotoxin tolerance, priming TLR9 with its ligand, CpG, induces a state of hypo-responsiveness to subsequent challenge with CpGs (Dalpke et al., 2005). Interestingly, cross-tolerance between the two receptors has also been reported, as ligands for TLR9 induce tolerance against a subsequent challenge with a TLR4 ligand (Bagchi et al., 2007; Broad et al., 2007). CpG-pretreated cells not only produce less TNFα when secondarily challenged with LPS, they also produce significantly higher levels of IFNβ (Broad et al., 2007). Together, the aforementioned studies suggest the intriguing possibility that TLR stimulation prior to stroke may reprogram ischemia-induced TLR activation (Fig.). Specifically, administration of LPS or CpG may activate TLR4 and TLR9, respectively, causing a small inflammatory response, with an initial rise in TNFα. Cells would then regulate their inflammatory response through expression of negative feedback inhibitors of the TLR4–NFκB signaling axis that remain present when cells are subsequently exposed to endogenous TLR ligands generated from ischemia-injured tissue. Within this new cellular environment, stimulated TLRs such as TLR2 and TLR4 would be unable to activate NFκB-inducing pathways. Because of this, stroke-induced TLR2 signaling may be blocked completely leading to reduced injury, and stroke-induced TLR4 signaling would shift from NFκB induction to IRF3 induction (Fig.). Suppression of NFκB induction would be expected to protect the brain, as mice lacking the p50 subunit of NFκB suffer less cerebral ischemic damage than wild type mice (Schneider et al., 1999). Enhancement of IRF signaling would also be expected to protect the brain, as IFNβ, a downstream product of IRF3 induction, has been shown to act as an acute neuroprotectant (Liu et al., 2002; Veldhuis et al., 2003a). IFNβ, best known for its anti-viral effects, has potent anti-inflammatory activities as well. Several studies have shown that IFNβ can stabilize the blood–brain barrier, potentially by reducing matrix metalloprotease production by activated glia (Veldhuis et al., 2003b; Kraus et al., 2004; Liuzzi et al., 2004). Similarly, it has been shown to inhibit monocyte migration across human brainderived endothelial cells (Seguin et al., 2003) and reduce cellular infiltration into damaged brain regions (Veldhuis et al., 2003b). On a cellular level, IFNβ has been shown to reduce reactive oxygen species (Lopez-Collazo et al., 1998; Stewart et al., 1998; Hua et al., 2002), suppress inflammatory cytokine production and induce IL-1Ra (Bosca et al., 2000; Palmer et al., 2004), promote nerve growth factor production by astrocytes (Boutros et al., 1997) and protect neurons from toxicity induced by activated microglia (Jin et al., 2007). In addition, systemic administration of IFNβ has been shown to reduce infarct damage in rat and rabbit models of ischemic stroke (Liu et al., 2002; Veldhuis et al., 2003a). Therefore, in the setting of LPS preconditioning, upregulation of this cytokine following stroke would be expected to contribute to neuroprotection. IFNβ may not be the only neuroprotective molecule downstream of IRF signaling. TLR3 signals exclusively through the TRIF-dependent pathway and stimulation of TLR3 in human astrocyte cultures induces the expression of several neuroprotective molecules such as brainderived neurotrophic factor, neurotrophin 4, pleiotrophin, and TGFβ2 (Bsibsi et al., 2006), all of which have been implicated in endogenous neuroprotection (Yeh et al., 1998; Endres et al., 2000; Zhang et al., 2005). Astrocytic TLR3 stimulation also results in production of the anti-inflammatory cytokine IL-10 (Bsibsi et al., 2006). Conditioned media from these cultures enhance neuronal survival and suppress astrocyte growth in slice cultures. Interestingly, LPS stimulation of macrophages has been shown to upregulate TLR3 expression (Nhu et al., 2006), inviting the possibility that LPS preconditioning may upregulate TLR3 in the brain, further enhancing stroke-induced IRF signaling. We suggest that pretreatment with TLR ligands reprograms the brain's response to ischemia and alters endogenous stroke-induced TLR signaling by suppression of the NFκB-inducing pathway and upregulation of the IRF-inducing pathway. Reprogramming causes a finely controlled shift in the balance of proinflammatory and antiinflammatory cytokines, and represents an endogenously orchestrated mechanism that protects the organism from additional damage. We further suggest that reprogramming of endogenous TLR signaling, with the subsequent generation of neuroprotective type I IFNs, is a unifying property of the neuroprotected phenotype. The brain has evolved numerous mechanisms that allow it to withstand the shortage of energy and the oxidative stress caused by ischemia. This tolerant state can be induced by prior exposure to LPS or CpG, or by prior exposure to other non-damaging (i.e. sub-threshold) noxious stimuli. For example, mild exposure to ischemia, excitotoxic stimuli, or inflammatory mediators can precondition the brain to better tolerate a subsequent injurious ischemic event. These mild preconditioning exposures herald impending danger and, as such, induce endogenous protective strategies in anticipation of injury. Though the final outcome of tolerance induction is the same — protection of brain tissue from ischemic injury — the effector mechanisms employed by the brain are as diverse as the preconditioning stimuli that induced them. In fact, the phenotype of neuroprotection may be specifically tailored by the nature of the preconditioning stimulus (Stenzel-Poore et al., 2007). For example, preconditioning events that deprive the brain of oxygen or glucose for a short time lead to conservation of energy regulation and mitochondrial integrity during the injurious ischemic episode (Stenzel-Poore et al., 2003; McFalls et al., 2006). Further, as we have described above, preconditioning events that invoke a small inflammatory response lead to altered inflammatory responses to damaging ischemia (Rosenzweig et al., 2004, 2007). It should be emphasized that although significant overlap exists in the cellular processes induced by these diverse stimuli, the pathways that dominate each response are distinct. The first demonstration that a short period of oxygen deprivation could protect the brain from a subsequent extended period of hypoxia occurred in 1943 (Noble, 1943). Since then, hundreds of studies have been undertaken to better understand the underlying mechanisms of "ischemic preconditioning." Though several endogenously protective pathways are induced by the initiating ischemic event, one particular theme is emerging — that of mitochondrial maintenance and energy conservation (Dirnagl and Meisel, 2008). The priming ischemic episode appears to induce cellular pathways that protect mitochondria against stroke induced deficits in the electron transport chain (Dave et al., 2001). These pathways protect mitochondrial membrane potential (Wu et al., 2004), preserve mitochondrial cytochrome c (Zhan et al., 2002), increase mitochondrial sequestration of Ca^+ and increase Ca^+-ATPase activity. In addition, ischemic preconditioning appears to suppress molecules that regulate ion channels, leading to channel arrest — i.e. reduction in ion permeability through the plasma membrane — which has been shown to reduce the amount of ATP required to maintain ionic homeostasis (Buck and Hochachka, 1993; Stenzel-Poore et al., 2003). Finally, a decrease in the overall cellular metabolic rate limits the stressful effects of oxygen deprivation. The pre preconditioning stimulus suppresses the expression of genes involved in protein turnover, proteasomal degradation, and energy metabolism (Stenzel-Poore et al., 2003). Although ischemic preconditioning has also been shown to help maintain protein structure and function and to suppress the damaging inflammatory response to stroke, it is increasingly clear that sustaining mitochondrial integrity and conserving energy are important mechanisms driving endogenous ischemic tolerance. Several studies have shown that the priming ischemic event induces HSP70 within the brain (Truettner et al., 2002). In addition to its role in stabilizing protein structure, HSP70 acts as an endogenous ligand of TLR4. In fact, extracellular HSP70 has been shown to induce endotoxin tolerance (Aneja et al., 2006). Hence TLRs may be stimulated in the course of ischemic preconditioning, resulting in a reprogrammed TLR response to subsequent injurious ischemia. One of the molecular consequences of reprogrammed TLR signaling is an increase in IFNβ. Notably, IFNβ has been shown to aid in the maintenance of mitochondrial integrity. For example, treatment of astrocytes with IFNβ prevents neuronal mitochondrial respiratory chain damage (Stewart et al., 1998) and reduce IFNβ induced nitric oxide synthase (Stewart et al., 1997). Thus reprogrammed TLR signaling may help shape the phenotype of ischemia-induced tolerance The phenomenon of inflammation-induced cross-tolerance to ischemia is not limited to LPS, but extends to TNFα as well. Nawashiro et al. (1997) were the first to demonstrate that intracisternal administration of TNFα protects the brain from subsequent ischemic challenge. This protection is correlated to a decrease in CD11b immunoreactivity, suggesting a decrease in the inflammatory response to ischemia in the setting of preconditioning. Consistent with this observation, TNFα pretreatment of astrocytes and endothelial cells, through its signaling intermediate ceramide, produces a state of hypo-responsiveness as pretreated cells fail to upregulate ICAM-1 during subsequent hypoxia (Ginis et al., 2002). The decrease in ICAM-1 does not reflect global cellular suppression, but instead signifies a reprogrammed genomic response to stroke, as the hypoxiainduced expression of cytoprotective MnSOD is not affected by preconditioning. Evidence for a reprogrammed genomic response to ischemia is supported by the observation that TNFα preconditioning prevents hypoxia-induced phosphorylation of the proinflammatory transcription factor component NFκBp65, thereby preventing its interaction with the transcriptional activator p300. Taken together, these data indicate that pretreatment with TNFα reprograms the cellular environment and hence alters inflammatory reactions in response to ischemia. Just as TNFα can induce tolerance to subsequent ischemic exposure, it can induce tolerance to subsequent LPS exposure (Porter et al., 1998; Ferlito et al., 2001; Murphey and Traber, 2001). Hence TNFα preconditioning has the potential to induce a state of cross-tolerance to TLR ligands, and thereby reprogram the TLR response to stroke. IFNβ has been shown to cause many of the effects observed in TNFα-induced ischemic tolerance, such as suppression of inflammatory cytokine production, including TNFα itself, and reduction of cellular infiltration into ischemic brain regions (Veldhuis et al., 2003a). Together, these studies suggest that multiple preconditioning stimuli may cause a reprogrammed TLR response to stroke. IFNβ, produced secondary to this reprogrammed response, may aid in maintaining mitochondrial stability and in dampening the inflammatory responses to injurious ischemia.

7. The receptor for Advanced Glycation End Products (RAGE)

Advanced glycation end products (AGEs) are nonenzymatical adducts of proteins, lipids, and nucleic acids which form in a time-dependent manner in a pro-oxidant environment, especially when target molecules turnover slowly and the level of aldoses is elevated

(Schmidt et al, 1995; Vlassara et al, 1994; Bierhaus et al, 1998; Baynes, 2003; Thornalley, 1998; Brownlee, 2000). Glycation of macromolecules was originally thought to mark senescent proteins for subsequent degradation by macrophages. Receptors binding AGEs were regarded as scavenger receptors involved in AGE disposal and cell regeneration, and defective clearance of such modified proteins was believed to be important in aging and diseases with accelerated AGE-formation, such as diabetes or atherosclerosis (Vlassara et al,1994, 1985). However, when the receptor for AGEs (RAGE) was cloned and first characterized (Neeper et al,1992; Schmidt et al,1992, 1994) it turned out that binding of AGEs to RAGE did not accelerate their clearance and degradation. Rather, ligand–receptor interaction induced sustained post-receptor signaling, including activation of p21ras, MAP kinases, and the NF-κB pathway (Lander et al, 1997; Basta et al, 2002; Bucciarelli et al, 2002). Thus, the concept of RAGE as a scavenger/clearance receptor has to be revised and extended.

7.1 RAGE: Structure and ligand recognition

RAGE is a member of the immunoglobulin superfamily of cell surface molecules (Schmidt et al, 1993; Sugaya, 1994). The gene is localized on chromosome 6 near the HLA locus in the vicinity of the MHCIII complex in humans and mice, in close proximity to the homeobox gene HOX12 and the human counterpart of the mouse mammary tumor gene int-3 (Malherbe et al, 1999). The receptor is composed of three immunoglobulin-like regions: one "V"- type domain and two "C"-type-domains, a short transmembrane domain, and a 43-amino acid cytoplasmic tail (Neeper et al, 1992; Schmidt et al, 1994; Lander et al, 1997). While the "V type" domain confers ligand binding, the cytoplasmic tail is critical for intracellular signaling. Shortly after RAGE was recognized as a receptor for AGEs, it became evident that a number of other ligands also interacted with the receptor (Bucciarelli et al, 2002; Schmidt et al, 2001; Du Yan et al, 1997; Yan et al, 1996, 2000). Structural analysis of ligand–RAGE interaction revealed that the receptor recognized three-dimensional structures, such as β-sheets and fibrils, rather than specific amino acid sequences (i.e., primary structure) (Bucciarelli et al, 2002; Schmidt et al, 2001). In addition to AGEs, RAGE binds amyloid-β peptide (accumulating in Alzheimer's disease) (Du Yan et al, 1997; Yan et al, 2000) and amyloid A (accumulating in systemic amyloidosis). Further, ligands of RAGE are S100/calgranulins, a family of closely related calcium-binding polypeptides that accumulate extracellularly at sites of chronic inflammation (Hofmann et al, 1999; Marenholz et al, 2004). Another proinflammatory ligand of RAGE is the DNA binding protein HMGB1 (amphoterin), which is released by cells undergoing necrosis (Hori et al, 1995; Wang et al, 1999; Anderson and Tracey, 2003; Treutiger et al, 2003). Besides binding ligands actively participating in chronic inflammatory and immune responses, RAGE also interacts with surface molecules on bacteria (Chapman et al, 2002), prions (Sasaki et al, 2002), and leukocytes (Chavakis et al, 2003). Thus, RAGE is much more than a receptor for AGEs; it has a broad repertoire of ligands, which share the propensity to accumulate in tissues during aging, chronic degenerative diseases, inflammation and the host response (Tretiger et al,2003). Therefore, RAGE should be considered a pattern recognition receptor (PRR) (Schmidt et al, 2001; Chavakis et al, 2003; Liliensiek et al, 2004; Gordon, 2002), and potential similarities to members of the family of Toll-like receptors should be considered (Akira et al, 2001).

7.2 RAGE-mediated NF-κB activation

Engagement of RAGE results in intracellular signaling which leads to activation of the proinflammatory transcription factor NF-κB, the latter rapidly activated as part of the first line of cellular defense (Bierhaus et al, 2001). In resting cells, NF-κB resides in the cytoplasm in its inactive form bound to the inhibitor molecule IκBα (Barnes and Karin, 1997). Upon activation, IκBα is rapidly phosphorylated and degraded, resulting in release and translocation of NF-κB (preferentially the NF-κB-heterodimer p50/p65) into the nucleus. Subsequent to nuclear translocation, NF-κB binds to decameric DNA sequences and activates transcription of NF-κB regulated target genes, such as cytokines, adhesion molecules, prothrombotic and vasoconstrictive gene products, RAGE itself, and IκBα (Barnes and Karin, 1997; Li and Schmidt, 1997; Bierhaus et al, 2000). A number of anti-apoptotic genes, including Bcl-XL, Bcl-2, and the Bcl-2 homologues A1, are also under control of NF-κB. NF-κB activation therefore provides a rapid and sensitive cellular response in the absence of new protein synthesis, which promotes cellular survival. One unique feature of RAGE-mediated NF-κB activation is the prolonged time course which appears to overwhelm endogenous autoregulatory feedback inhibition loops (Bierhaus et al, 2001). NF-κB activation subsequent to ligation of RAGE is initiated by the degradation of IκBα and IκBβ, followed by new synthesis of NF-κBp65 in the presence of newly synthesized IκBβ. De novo synthesis of p65 mRNA results in a constantly growing pool of excess transcriptionally active NF-κBp65. In contrast, the amount of newly synthesized IκBα is not sufficient to retain NF-κBp65 in the cytoplasm. In addition, newly synthesized IκBβ has been shown to be hyperphosphorylated, thereby sequestering newly synthesized NF-κB from IκBα (Thompson et al, 1995; Johnson et al, 1996)? Thus, new synthesis of IκBβ might further promote RAGEdependent sustained NF-κB activation. Since, in turn, RAGE expression is induced by NF-κB (Li and Schmidt, 1997), sustained activation of NF-κB results in upregulation of the receptor and further ensures maintenance and amplification of the signal.

7.3 AGEs and RAGE affect cellular defense mechanisms

Besides activating proinflammatory responses, RAGE downregulates cellular defense mechanisms. Ligation of RAGE by AGEs results in the suppression of reduced glutathione (GSH) and ascorbic acid levels and thereby contributes to increased intracellular oxidant stress (Lander et al, 1997; Bierhaus et al, 1997). Depletion of glutathione accounts for diminished glyoxalase-1 recycling and decreased in situ activity of glyoxalase-1 (Thornalley,1998). Glyoxalase-1, in turn, is required to catalyze the conversion of reactive, acyclic alpha-oxoaldehydes into the corresponding alpha-hydroxyacids (Degenhard 1998; Thornalley et al,1999). Since alpha-oxoaldehydes, such as methylglyoxal, represent the largest pool of reactive intracellular AGEs, glyoxalase-1 has an important role in reduction of the cellular AGE load. Consistent with this concept, in vitro experiments with cultivated endothelial cells have demonstrated that glyoxalase-1 overexpression prevents intracellular AGE formation (Shinohara et al,1998). Studies in the model organism Caenorhabditis elegans have recently confirmed that overexpression of glyoxalase-1 not only prevents AGE formation, but also protects the animals from deleterious effects of oxidant stress, as evidenced by increased longevity (Morcos et al,2004). These observations imply that engagement of RAGE not only results in increased cellular activation, but also in reduction of AGE detoxifying mechanisms.

7.4 RAGE and neuroprotection

RAGE transcription is controlled by several transcription factors, including SP-1, AP-2, NF-κB, and NF-IL6 (Li and Schmidt, 1997). RAGE expression occurs in both a constitutive and inducible manner, depending on the cell type and developmental stage (Hori et al,1995; Brett et al,1993). Whereas RAGE is constitutively expressed during embryonic development, its expression is downregulated in adult life. However, known exceptions are skin and lung, which constitutively express RAGE throughout life. Most other cells, including monocytes/macrophages, endothelial cells, smooth musclecells, fibroblasts, and neuronal cells, do not express significant amounts of RAGE under physiological conditions but can be induced to express RAGE in situations where either ligands accumulate and/or transcription factors regulating RAGE are activated (Basta et al, 2002; Bucciarelli et al, 2002; Hanford et al, 2004; Akira et al, 2001; Li et al,2004; Sorci et al, 2004a, 2004b; Cortizo et al, 2003; Shanmugam et al, 2003; Ishihara et al, 2003). Due to its ability to sustain cellular activation, RAGE has the potential to function as a master switch capable of converting a transient proinflammatory response, evoked by an inflammatory stimulus into sustained cellular dysfunction (Schmidt et al, 2001; Bierhaus et al, 2001). The majority of cellular stressors induce both the formation of reactive oxygen species (ROS) and transient activation of NF-κB (Yeh et al, 2001; Taguchi et al, 2000; Huttunen et al, 19999; Huang et al, 2001; Wautier et al, 2001). In addition, inflammatory cells directly release RAGE ligands, such as S100/calgranulins and HMGB-1 (Kokkola et al, 2005). The myeloperoxidase system of human phagocytes generates N'' -(carboxymethyl)lysine, a highly reactive AGE and RAGE-ligand, at sites of inflammation (Anderson et al, 1999; Kislinger et al, 1999). High glucose concentrations promote AGE formation inside and outside cells (Brownlee, 2000; Schiekofer et al, 2003). Such time-dependent formation of AGE might also play a role in the expression of binding sites for amyloid peptides (Yan et al, 2000). In turn, RAGE has been shown to mediate transport of pathophysiologically relevant concentrations of amyloid-β peptide into the CNS (Mackic et al, 1998). Thus, stimuli initially inducing oxidant stress and NF-κB activation have the potential to activate RAGE and thereby sustain NF-κB-dependent gene expression. Activation of NF-κB results in increased RAGE expression and increases the number of ligand binding sites, thereby prolonging NF-κB activation (Schmidt et al, 2001; Bierhaus et al, 2001). Frequently, the biology of RAGE coincides with settings in which ligands of the receptor accumulate, especially in a proinflammatory environment such as diabetes mellitus, atherosclerosis, neurodegenerative disorders, rheumatoid arthritis, chronic renal disease, and inflammatory bowl disease (Basta et al, 2002; Schmidt et al, 2001; Lalla et al, 2001; Wendt et al, 2003; Bierhaus et al, 2004; Sakaguchi et al, 2003; Kislinger et al, 2001; Drinda et al, 2004; Chen et al, 2004; Goosa et al, 2001). To better understand the role of RAGE in these pathophysiological situations, interaction of ligands with cell surface RAGE was intercepted using soluble RAGE (sRAGE). Soluble RAGE is a truncated form of the receptor comprising the extracellular domain and thereby functions as a decoy that prevents ligands from interacting with cell surface receptor. Application of sRAGE in vitro and in vivo resulted in an effective blockade of RAGE, according to a decoy mechanism, in a range of animal models (Hudson et al, 2003; Lue et al, 2001; Arancio et al, 2004; Constien et al, 2001). sRAGE prevented development of micro- and macrovascular diseases in rodents, suggesting a key role for RAGE in the development of chronic vascular disorders. Moreover, sRAGE efficiently reduced late complications of experimental diabetes in both autoimmune (Chen et al, 2004) and streptozotocin induced diabetes (Wendt et al, 2003; Bierhaus et al,

2004), restored delayed wound healing (Goosa et al, 2001), protected rodent from tumor metastases and growth of primary tumors (Taguchi et al, 2000), and improved the outcome of experimental colitis (Hofmann et al, 1999). sRAGE and anti-RAGE F(ab')2-fragments suppressed abnormal findings associated with Alzheimer's-like pathology in transgenic rodent models (Lue et al, 2001; Arancio et al, 2004) and reduced the transport of amyloid-β-peptide across the blood-brain barrier (Mackic et al, 1998) . Since most of the data obtained with sRAGE were confirmed by application of neutralizing antibodies to the receptor and/or transfection with plasmids overexpressing dominant negative RAGE, the receptor has been suggested as a potentially effective therapeutic target (Hudson et al, 2003). At the same time, it seemed unlikely that RAGE could mediate so many deleterious effects in such diverse models of disease. Since RAGE has properties of a PRR, binding to a variety of ligands, the promising effects observed with sRAGE might not only result from intercepting the interaction of ligands with cell surface RAGE, but possibly with other receptors. For example, S100 proteins and HMGB1 certainly do not exclusively bind to RAGE. These ligands also recognize other cellular structures (Robinson et al, 2002; Erlandsson et al, 2004). In order to test the potential impact of RAGE blockade and to further define a potential role of RAGE in diabetic complications and chronic inflammatory disease, homozygous RAGE-deficient mice (RAGE−/− mice) and mice with tissue-specific RAGE expression (tie2-RAGE and tie2-RAGE°−RAGE−/−) have been made (Constien et al, 2001). These mice are viable and display normal reproductive fitness without any striking phenotype (Wendt et al, 2003; Bierhaus et al, 2004; Sakaguchi et al, 2003). Induction of diabetes in these mice confirmed that RAGE contributes, at least in part, to the development of diabetic complications. Diabetic nephropathy, characterized by renal enlargement, glomerular hypertrophy, albuminuria, and mesangial expansion, was significantly increased in diabetic mice overexpressing RAGE in the vasculature, but was reduced in RAGE−/−mice (Yamamoto et al, 2001). Similar changes were observed in diabetic neuropathy. Whereas diabetic mice overexpressing RAGE showed an increase in functional deficits, such as delayed motor nerve conduction velocity (Yajima et al, 2004), RAGE−/− mice were partially protected from diabetes-induced loss of neural function (Bierhaus et al, 2004). Neointimal expansion in RAGE−/− mice was significantly suppressed compared with that observed in wildtype littermates using a femoral artery denudation protocol to induce arterial injury (Sakaguchi et al, 2003). Remarkably, in each of these models (diabetic nephropathy, neuropathy, arterial restenosis, etc.), protection from development of pathology was more profound in wild-type mice treated with sRAGE than in RAGE−/− mice. In diabetic neuropathy, for example, administration of sRAGE to diabetic wild-type animals completely restored pain perception, whereas diabetic RAGE−/− mice were only partly protected from loss of pain perception. These observations suggest that ligands sequestered by sRAGE are likely to interact with cellular structures different from RAGE and are also involved in perturbation of pain perception. The absence of a developmental phenotype in RAGE−/− mice and the possibility that RAGE might impact on multiple chronic disease states have largely focussed attention away from physiologic roles of the receptor. So far, only a few reports have suggested that RAGE expression might contribute to developmental paradigms, based on in vitro studies. For example, in axonal sprouting which accompanies neuronal development, RAGE–HMGB1 interaction may contribute (Fages et al, 2000; Hittinen et al, 2000). Huttunen et al. further demonstrated that activation of RAGE by HMGB1 (amphoterin) and S100B can promote cell survival through increased expression of the anti-apoptotic protein Bcl-2. However, whereas nanomolar concentrations of S100B induced trophic effects in RAGEexpressing cells, micromolar concentrations caused apoptosis in a manner that appeared to depend on oxidant stress. For both of these outcomes, the cytoplasmic domain of RAGE was required, as cells expressing a dominant-negative mutant (i.e., lacking the cytosolic tail) are unresponsive to these stimuli. The neurite outgrowth-promoting role of RAGE was recently confirmed in vivo in a unilateral sciatic nerve crush model, in which blockade of RAGE, either by sRAGE or by blocking F(ab')2 fragments of antibodies (raised to either RAGE or to S100/calgranulins or amphoterin) reduced functional regeneration of the peripheral nerve (Rong et al, 2004a). Similar results were observed in transgenic mice overexpressing dominant negative RAGE (Rong et al, 2004b). However, RAGE−/− mice demonstrate neither obvious neuronal deficits nor overt behavior abnormalities, indicating that RAGE may contribute to neuronal development, but that there are redundant systems that substitute for this receptor in its absence. Furthermore, it will be interesting to see if future experiments in RAGE−/− mice confirm a role for RAGE in the repair of peripheral nerve injury. In terms of a contribution for RAGE in development, expression of the receptor in vivo appears to mirror developmental processes. After being highly expressed during embryonic development, RAGE is downregulated in most organs during normal life (Kokkola et al, 2005). Upon aging, RAGE expression increases again, although it is not known whether this is due to accumulation of RAGE ligands (which upregulate receptor expression) or whether this represents a compensatory mechanism protecting aging cells from cell death. Another line of evidence for a role of RAGE in the regulation of differentiation comes from recently published studies showing that non-small cell lung carcinomas are characterized by downregulation of RAGE (Bartling et al, 2004). One reason for this might be that loss of HMGB1(amphoterin)/RAGE-mediated regulation of tumor cell migration and invasive processes results in more aggressive tumor behavior (Huttunen et al, 2002). A COOH-terminal motif in HMGB1 (amino acids 150–183) has recently been identified as responsible for RAGE binding. This portion of HMGB1 efficiently inhibits RAGE-mediated extension of cellular processes and transendothelial migration of tumor cells. This observation leads us to propose that loss of RAGE might promote tumor growth, at least in settings affecting the lung, one of the few tissues in which RAGE is constitutively expressed at high levels. Since this observation contrasts with a previous finding in which sRAGE suppressed tumor growth and metastasis (Taguchi et al, 2000), the latter observations might be due to the ability of sRAGE to intercept the interaction of RAGE ligands with other receptors.

8. Conclusion and prospective

Cell death from ischemia involves a complex biological cascade. Initially, energy failure is followed by glutamate overload and Ca^{2+} influx into the cell. These processes initiate a series of events, including the generation of free radicals, apoptosis, an inflammatory response and generation of growth factors. Many of these processes are the direct result of the up- or downregulation of specific gene families. Thus, a desirable neuroprotectant would, in theory, be one that antagonises multiple injury mechanisms. The studies described above demonstrate an emerging role for endogenous neuroprotectant in ischemic damage and ischemic prophylaxis. Among these, erythropoietin (Epo), has a dominant role for neuroprotection, neurogenesis and act as a neurotrophic factor in the central nervous system. These functions make erythropoietin a good candidate for treating disease associated with neuronal cell death. However, our understanding of the underlying mechanisms is far from being complete and a number of open questions remain to be answered: 1) What is the exact route and mechanism through which Epo passes through the BBB? 2) Which cellular mechanisms govern the immunomodulatory effects of Epo in glial cells? 3) Does Epo activate the same or diverse intracellular signaling pathways in the different cells that express EpoR in the brain, neurons, glial, and endothelial cells? Nevertheless, since the discovery of Epo expression in the brain less than 15 years ago, a tremendous achievement in the understanding of its action in the CNS has been accomplished. Today, Epo is a prominent member of a growing list of hematopoietic and angiogenic factors found to be expressed and acting as protective factors in the CNS. Because of the observed increased death rate, rtPA-treated patients should be excluded from acute poststroke EPO application. In cerebral ischemia, albumin is mainly involved in the improvement of blood microcirculation; however, direct neuroprotection cannot be overlooked. Different in vitro and in vivo studies indicate that albumin has direct neuroprotective effects by acting on astrocytes, microglia and neurons. Altogether albumin can alter brain function by many direct and indirect mechanisms and detailed study of these actions will reveal the role of this multifunctional protein in brain functions. Furthermore, the evidence of de novo synthesis of albumin in microglial cells could encourage the neurologist to investigate newer roles of this multifunctional protein in many neurodegenerative diseases. The prothrombotic, proinflammatory state of stroke results in a promotion of thrombin formation and fibrin deposition at the vascular wall, as well as in the formation of platelet-leukocyte coaggregates, leading to severe disturbance of the microcirculation, capillary leakage and tissue damage. The ability of ATIII to inhibit the actions of both factor Xa and thrombin gives it the potential to block, in part or fully, a wide rage of proinflammatory events. Heparin and heparan sulfate glycoproteins (HSPGs) appear to function as receptors for ATIII on endothelium and leukocytes and can lead to the reduced expression of procoagulatory tissue factor and proinflammatory cytokines as well as heterologous receptor regulatory processes. ATIII has been shown in vitro to increase prostacyclin responses and to inhibit a variety of cell responses including endotoxin-induced nuclear translocation of NF-kB, a key step in the generation of the inflammatory response.

Here, we also discussed the critical role of Toll-like receptors in mediating cerebral ischemic injury and suggested endogenous mechanisms that, when induced, redirect this role from detrimental to beneficial. In fact, many diverse neuroprotective paradigms may redirect TLR signaling as one mechanism of endogenous protection. Paradoxically, TLR ligands administered systemically induce a state of tolerance to subsequent ischemic injury. Herein we suggest that stimulation of TLRs prior to ischemia reprograms TLR signaling that occurs following ischemic injury. Such reprogramming leads to suppressed expression of pro-inflammatory molecules and enhanced expression of numerous anti-inflammatory mediators that collectively confer robust neuroprotection. Research findings indicate that numerous preconditioning stimuli lead to TLR activation, an event that occurs prior to ischemia and ultimately leads to TLR reprogramming. Thus genomic reprogramming of

TLR signaling may be a unifying principle of tolerance to cerebral ischemia. Recent studies have also demonstrated an increased expression of the cell-surface RAGE in dying neurons after hypoxic-ischemic insults and human cerebral ischemia, and suggested that the RAGE-ligand interaction causes neuronal cytotoxicity. RAGE also has a circulating truncated variant isoform, soluble RAGE (sRAGE), which corresponds to its extracellular domain only. Exogenously administered sRAGE has been successfully used to antagonize advanced glycation end products (AGE)-RAGE-mediated vascular damage. Accordingly, sRAGE may compete with cell-surface RAGE for the ligand, thus functioning as a decoy and possibly exerting a cytoprotective effect. Most of the data available so far point to the RAGE/NF-κB axis as an attractive target for future clinical interventions in several chronic disease states. However, until physiologic properties of RAGE have been clearly deciphered, it is most prudent to adopt a cautious approach when future therapeutic strategies involving long-term blockade of RAGE or its ligands are considered. Another important issue to be addressed concerns how studies performed in rodent models will translate to human disease. Alternatively, if RAGE antagonists are eventually used in humans, it will be fascinating to understand the impact of long-term blockade of RAGE in critically ill patients, in view of the likely complex role of RAGE, and other receptors interacting with RAGE ligands, in regulating physiologic and pathophysiologic processes in a wide range of situations.

9. References

Ahmed S, He Y, Nassief A, Xu J, Xu X, Hsu C (2000) Effects of lipopolysaccharide priming on acute ischemic brain injury. Stroke 31:193–199.

Ahn, S.M., Byun, K., Cho, K., Kim, J.Y., Yoo, J.S., Kim, D., Paek, S.H., Kim, S.U., Simpson, R.J., and Lee, B. (2008). Human microglial cells synthesize albumin in brain. PLoS One 3 , e2829.

Akira S, Takeda K, Kaisho T (2001) Toll-like receptors: critical proteins linking innate and acquired immunity. Nat Immunol 1:675–680

Alafaci C, Salpietro F, Grasso G, Sfacteria A, Passalacqua M, Morabito A, Tripodo E, Calapai G, Buemi M, Tomasello F. Effect of recombinant human erythropoietin on cerebral ischemia following experimental subarachnoid hemorrhage. *Eur J Pharmacol* 406: 219–225, 2000.

Anagnostou A, Lee ES, Kessimian N, Levinson R, Steiner M. Erythropoietin has a mitogenic and positive chemotactic effect on endothelial cells. *Proc Natl Acad Sci USA* 87: 5978–5982, 1990.

Anderson MM, Requena JR, Crowley JR, Thorpe SR, Heinecke JW (1999) The myeloperoxidase system of human phagocytes generates Nepsilon-(carboxymethyl)lysine on proteins: a mechanism for producing advanced glycated endproducts at sites of inflammation. J Clin Invest 104:103–113

Andersson U, Tracey KJ (2003) HMGB1 in sepsis. Scand J Infect Dis 35:577–584

Aneja R, Odoms K, Dunsmore K, Shanley TP, Wong HR (2006) Extracellular heat shock protein-70 induces endotoxin tolerance in THP-1 cells. J Immunol 177:7184–7192.

Arancio O, Zhang HP, Chen X, Lin C, Trinchese F, Puzzo D, Liu S, Hegde A, Yan SF, Stern A, Luddy JS, Lue LF, Walker DG, Roher A, Buttini M, Mucke L, Li W, Schmidt AM, Kindy M, Hyslop PA, Stern DM, Du Yan SS (2004) RAGE potentiates Abeta-induced perturbation of neuronal function in transgenic mice. EMBO J 23:4096–4105

Arcasoy MO. The non-haematopoietic biological effects of erythropoietin. *Br J Haematol* 141: 14–31, 2008.

Arroyo, V. (2002). Review article: albumin in the treatment of liver diseases – new features of a classical treatment. Aliment Pharmacol. Ther. *16* (Suppl. 5), 1 – 5.

Bagchi A, Herrup EA, Warren HS, Trigilio J, Shin HS, Valentine C, Hellman J (2007) MyD88-dependent and MyD88- independent pathways in synergy, priming, and tolerance between TLR agonists. J Immunol 178:1164–1171.

Baltanas, F.C., Weruaga, E., Valero, J., Recio, J.S., and Alonso, J.R. (2009). Albumin attenuates DNA damage in primary- cultured neurons. Neurosci. Lett. *450*, 23 – 26.

Banks WA, Jumbe NL, Farrell CL, Niehoff ML, Heatherington AC. Passage of erythropoietic agents across the blood- brain barrier: a comparison of human and murine erythropoietin and the analog darbepoetin alfa. *Eur J Pharmacol* 505: 93–101, 2004

Barnes PJ, Karin M (1997) Nuclear factor-κB-a pivotal transcription factor in chronic inflammatory diseases. N Engl J Med 336:1066–1071

Bartling B, Hofmann HS, Weigle B, Silber RE, Simm A (2004) Down-regulation of the receptor for advanced glycation endproducts (RAGE) supports non-small cell lung carcinoma. Carcinogenesis [Epub ahead of print]

Basta G, Lazzerini G, Massaro M, Simoncini T, Tanganelli P, Fu C, Kislinger T, Stern DM, Schmidt AM, De Caterina R (2002) Advanced glycation end products activate endothelium through signal-transduction receptor RAGE: a mechanism for amplification of inflammatory responses. Circulation 105:816–822

Bastide M, Gele P, Petrault O, Pu Q, Caliz A, Robin E, Deplanque D, Duriez P, Bordet R (2003) Delayed cerebrovascular protective effect of lipopolysaccharide in parallel to brain ischemic tolerance. J Cereb Blood Flow Metab 23:399- 405.

Bauer KA, Rosenberg RD: Role of antithrombin III as a regulator of in vivo coagulation. Semin Hematol 1991;28:10-18.

Baynes JW (2003) Chemical modification of proteins by lipids in diabetes. Clin Chem Lab Med 41:1159–1165

Belayev, L., Alonso, O.F., Huh, P.W., Zhao, W., Busto, R., and Ginsberg, M.D. (1999a). Posttreatment with high-dose albumin reduces histopathological damage and improves neurological deficit following fl uid percussion brain injury in rats. J. Neurotrauma *16*, 445 – 453.

Belayev, L., Busto, R., Zhao, W., Clemens, J.A., and Ginsberg, M.D. (1997a). Effect of delayed albumin hemodilution on infarction volume and brain edema after transient middle cerebral artery occlusion in rats. J. Neurosurg. *87*, 595 – 601.

Belayev, L., Liu, Y., Zhao, W., Busto, R., and Ginsberg, M.D. (2001). Human albumin therapy of acute ischemic stroke: marked neuroprotective efficacy at moderate doses and with a broad therapeutic window. Stroke *32*, 553 – 560.

Belayev, L., Pinard, E., Nallet, H., Seylaz, J., Liu, Y., Riyamongkol, P., Zhao, W., Busto, R., and Ginsberg, M.D. (2002). Albumin therapy of transient focal cerebral ischemia: in vivo analysis of dynamic microvascular responses. Stroke *33*, 1077 – 1084.

Belayev, L., Saul, I., Busto, R., Danielyan, K., Vigdorchik, A., Khoutorova, L., and Ginsberg, M.D. (2005). Albumin treatment reduces neurological defi cit and protects blood-brain barrier integrity after acute intracortical hematoma in the rat. Stroke *36* , 326 – 331.

Belayev, L., Saul, I., Huh, P.W., Finotti, N., Zhao, W., Busto, R., and Ginsberg, M.D. (1999b). Neuroprotective effect of highdose albumin therapy against global ischemic brain injury in rats. Brain Res. *845* , 107 – 111.

Belayev, L., Zhao, W., Busto, R., and Ginsberg, M.D. (1997b). Transient middle cerebral artery occlusion by intraluminal suture: I. Three-dimensional autoradiographic image-analysis of local cerebral glucose metabolism-blood flow interrelationships during ischemia and early recirculation. J. Cereb. Blood Flow Metab. *17* , 1266 – 1280.

Belayev, L., Zhao, W., Pattany, P.M., Weaver, R.G., Huh, P.W., Lin, B., Busto, R., and Ginsberg, M.D. (1998). Diffusion- weighted magnetic resonance imaging confi rms marked neuroprotective efficacy of albumin therapy in focal cerebral ischemia. Stroke *29* , 2587 – 2599.

Bento-Abreu, A., Velasco, A., Polo-Hernandez, E., Lillo, C., Kozyraki, R., Tabernero, A., and Medina, J.M. (2009). Albumin endocytosis via megalin in astrocytes is caveola- and Dab-1 dependent and is required for the synthesis of the neurotrophic factor oleic acid. J. Neurochem. *111* , 49 – 60.

Bento-Abreu, A., Velasco, A., Polo-Hernandez, E., Perez-Reyes, P.L., Tabernero, A., and Medina, J.M. (2008). Megalin is a receptor for albumin in astrocytes and is required for the synthesis of the neurotrophic factor oleic acid. J. Neurochem. *106* , 1149 – 1159.

Bernaudin M, Bellail A, Marti HH, Yvon A, Vivien D, Duchatelle I, MacKenzie ET, Petit E. Neurons and astrocytes express EPO mRNA: oxygen-sensing mechanisms that involve the redox-state of the brain. Glia 30: 271–278, 2000.

Bernaudin M, Marti HH, Roussel S, Divoux D, Nouvelot A, MacKenzie ET, Petit E. A potential role for erythropoietin in focal permanent cerebral ischemia in mice. *J Cereb Blood Flow Metab* 19: 643–651, 1999.

Biere, A.L., Ostaszewski, B., Stimson, E.R., Hyman, B.T., Maggio, J.E., and Selkoe, D.J. (1996). Amyloid beta-peptide is transported on lipoproteins and albumin in human plasma. J. Biol. Chem. *271* , 32916 – 32922.

Bierhaus A, Chen J, Liliensiek B, Nawroth PP (2000) LPS and cytokine activated endothelium. In: Nawroth PP (ed) Seminars in Thrombosis and Hemostasis, vol. 26, pp 571–588

Bierhaus A, Chevion S, Chevion M, Hofmann M, Quehenberger P, Illmer T, Luther T, Wahl P, Tritschler H, Müller M, Ziegler R, Nawroth PP (1997) Advanced glycation endproduct (AGEs) induced activation of NF-κB is suppressed by α-lipoic acid in cultured endothelial cells. Diabetes 46:1481–1490

Bierhaus A, Haslbeck KM, Humpert PM, Liliensiek B, Dehmer T, Morcos M, Sayed AA, Andrassy M, Schiekofer S, Schneider J, Schulz J, Heuss D, Neundörfer B, Dierl S, Huber J, Tritschler H, Schmidt AM, Schwaninger M, Häring HU, Schleicher E, Stern DM, Kasper M, Arnold B, Nawroth PP (2004) Loss of pain perception in diabetic neuropathy is dependent on a receptor of the immune globulin superfamily. J Clin Invest 114:1741-1751

Bierhaus A, Hofmann MA, Ziegler R, Nawroth PP (1998) The AGE/RAGE pathway in vascular disease and diabetes mellitus. Part I: the AGE-concept. Cardiovasc Res 37:586–600

Bierhaus A, Schiekofer S, Schwaninger M, Andrassy M, Humpert P, Chen J, Hong M, Luther T, Henle T, Klöting I, biphasic activation of NF-κB. Cell 80:573–582

Boada, M., Ortiz, P., Anaya, F., Hernandez, I., Munoz, J., Nunez, L., Olazaran, J., Roca, I., Cuberas, G., Tarraga, L., et al. (2009). Amyloid-targeted therapeutics in Alzheimer ' s disease: use of human albumin in plasma exchange as a novel approach for Abeta mobilization. Drug News Perspect. 22 , 325 – 339.

Bogoyevitch MA. An update on the cardiac effects of erythropoietin cardioprotection by erythropoietin and the lessons learnt from studies in neuroprotection. Cardiovasc Res 63: 208–216, 2004.

Bohrmann, B., Tjernberg, L., Kuner, P., Poli, S., Levet-Trafi t, B., Naslund, J., Richards, G., Huber, W., Dobeli, H., and Nordstedt, C. (1999). Endogenous proteins controlling amyloid beta-peptide polymerization. Possible implications for beta-amyloid formation in the central nervous system and in peripheral tissues. J. Biol. Chem. 274 , 15990 – 15995.

Bond R, Rerkasem K, Shearman CP, Rothwell PM (2004) Time trends in the published risks of stroke and death due to endarterectomy for symptomatic carotid stenosis. Cerebrovasc Dis 18:37–46.

Bordet R, Deplanque D, Maboudou P, Puisieux F, Pu Q, Robin E, Martin A, Bastide M, Leys D, Lhermitte M, Dupuis B (2000) Increase in endogenous brain superoxide dismutase as a potential mechanism of lipopolysaccharide- induced brain ischemic tolerance. J Cereb Blood Flow Metab 20:1190–1196.

Bosca L, Bodelon OG, Hortelano S, Casellas A, Bosch F (2000) Anti-inflammatory action of type I interferons deduced from mice expressing interferon beta. Gene Ther 7:817–825.

Boutros T, Croze E, Yong VW (1997) Interferon-beta is a potent promoter of nerve growth factor production by astrocytes. J Neurochem 69:939–946.

Brett J, Schmidt AM, Yan SD, Zhou YS, Weidmann E, Pinsky D, Nowygrod R, Neeper M, Przysiecki C, Dhaw A, Migheli A, Stern DM (1993) Survey of the distribution of a newly characterized receptor for advanced glycation end products in tissue. Am J Pathol 143:1699–1712

Brines M, Cerami A. Emerging biological roles for erythropoietin in the nervous system. Nat Rev Neurosci 6: 484–494, 2005.

Brines ML, Ghezzi P, Keenan S, Agnello D, de Lanerolle NC, Cerami C, Itri LM, Cerami A. Erythropoietin crosses the blood-brain barrier to protect against experimental brain injury. Proc Natl Acad Sci USA 97: 10526–10531, 2000.

Broad A, Kirby JA, Jones DE (2007) Toll-like receptor interactions: tolerance of MyD88-dependent cytokines but enhancement of MyD88-independent interferon-beta production. Immunology 120:103–111.

Brownlee M (2000) Negative consequences of glycation. Metabolism 49:9–13

Bruick RK, McKnight SL. A conserved family of prolyl-4- hydroxylases that modify HIF. Science 294: 1337–1340, 2001.

Bsibsi M, Persoon-Deen C, Verwer RW, Meeuwsen S, Ravid R, Van Noort JM (2006) Toll-like receptor 3 on adult human astrocytes triggers production of neuroprotective mediators. Glia 53:688–695.

Bsibsi M, Ravid R, Gveric D, van Noort JM (2002) Broad expression of Toll-like receptors in the human central nervous system. J Neuropathol Exp Neurol 61:1013–1021.

Bucciarelli LG, Wendt T, Rong L, Lalla E, Hofmann MA, Goova MT, Taguchi A, Yan SF, Yan SD, Stern DM, Schmidt AM (2002) RAGE is a multiligand receptor of the immunoglobulin superfamily: implications for homeostasis and chronic disease.Cell Mol Life Sci 59:1117–1128

Bucerius J, Gummert JF, Borger MA, Walther T, Doll N, Onnasch JF, Metz S, Falk V, Mohr FW (2003) Stroke after cardiac surgery: a risk factor analysis of 16,184 consecutive adult patients. Ann Thorac Surg 75:472–478.

Buck LT, Hochachka PW (1993) Anoxic suppression of Na^+-K^+-ATPase and constant membrane potential in hepatocytes: support for channel arrest. Am J Physiol 265:R1020–R1025.

Byts N, Samoylenko A, Fasshauer T, Ivanisevic M, Hennighausen L, Ehrenreich H, Siren AL. Essential role for Stat5 in the neurotrophic but not in the neuroprotective effect of erythropoietin. *Cell Death Differ* 15: 783–792, 2008.

Cai Z, Manalo DJ, Wei G, Rodriguez ER, Fox-Talbot K, Lu H, Zweier JL, Semenza GL. Hearts from rodents exposed to intermittent hypoxia or erythropoietin are protected against ischemiareperfusion injury. *Circulation* 108: 79–85, 2003.

Candelario-Jalil E, Yang Y, Rosenberg GA (2009) Diverse roles of matrix metalloproteinases and tissue inhibitors of metalloproteinases in neuroinflammation and cerebral ischemia. Neuroscience 158:983–994.

Cao CX, Yang QW, Lv FL, Cui J, Fu HB, Wang JZ (2007) Reduced cerebral ischemia-reperfusion injury in Toll-like receptor 4 deficient mice. Biochem Biophys Res Comm 353:509–514.

Carlini RG, Reyes AA, Rothstein M. Recombinant human erythropoietin stimulates angiogenesis in vitro. *Kidney Int* 47: 740–745, 1995.

Carpentier PA, Begolka WS, Olson JK, Elhofy A, Karpus WJ, Miller SD (2005) Differential activation of astrocytes by innate and adaptive immune stimuli. Glia 49:360–374.

Caso JR, Pradillo JM, Hurtado O, Lorenzo P, Moro MA, Lizasoain I (2007) Toll-like receptor 4 is involved in brain damage and inflammation after experimental stroke. Circulation 115:1599–1608.

Chakravarty S, Herkenham M (2005) Toll-like receptor 4 on nonhematopoietic cells sustains CNS inflammation during endotoxemia, independent of systemic cytokines. J Neurosci 25:1788–1796.

Chapman MR, Robinson LS, Pinkner JS, Roth R, Heuser J, Hammar M, Normark S, Hultgren SJ (2002) Role of Escherichia coli curli operons in directing amyloid fiber formation. Science 5556:851–855

Chavakis T, Bierhaus A, Schneider D, Linn T, Nagashima K, Arnold B, Preissner KT, Nawroth PP (2003) The pattern recognition receptor (RAGE) is a counter receptor for leukocyte integrins: a novel pathway for inflammatory cell recruitment. J Exp Med 198:1507–1515

Chen Y, Yan SS, Colgan J, Zhang HP, Luban J, Schmidt AM, Stern D, Herold KC (2004) Blockade of late stages of autoimmune diabetes by inhibition of the receptor for advanced glycation end products. J Immunol 173:1399– 1405

Chikuma M, Masuda S, Kobayashi T, Nagao M, Sasaki R. Tissue-specific regulation of erythropoietin production in the murine kidney, brain, and uterus. *Am J Physiol Endocrinol Metab* 279: E1242–E1248, 2000.

Chin K, Yu X, Beleslin-Cokic B, Liu C, Shen K, Mohrenweiser HW, Noguchi CT. Production and processing of erythropoietin receptor transcripts in brain. *Brain Res Mol Brain Res* 81: 29–42, 2000.

Chong ZZ, Kang JQ, Maiese K. Erythropoietin is a novel vascular protectant through activation of Akt1 and mitochondrial modulation of cysteine proteases. *Circulation* 106: 2973–2979, 2002.

Cole, D.J., Drummond, J.C., Osborne, T.N., and Matsumura, J. (1990). Hypertension and hemodilution during cerebral ischemia reduce brain injury and edema. Am. J. Physiol. *259* , H211 – H217.

Constantin D, Cordenier A, Robinson K, Ala'Aldeen DA, Murphy S (2004) Neisseria meningitidis-induced death of cerebrovascular endothelium: mechanisms triggering transcriptional activation of inducible nitric oxide synthase. J Neurochem 89:1166–1174.

Constien R, Forde A, Liliensiek B, Grone HJ, Nawroth PP, Hammerling G, Arnold B (2001) Characterization of a novel EGFP reporter mouse to monitor Cre recombination as demonstrated by a Tie2 Cre mouse line. Genesis 30:36– 44

Cortizo AM, Lettieri MG, Barrio DA, Mercer N, Etcheverry SB, McCarthy AD (2003) Advanced glycation end-products (AGEs) induce concerted changes in the osteoblastic expression of their receptor RAGE and in the activation of extracellular signal-regulated kinases (ERK). Mol Cell Biochem 250:1–10

Cotena S, Piazza O, Tufano R: The use of erythtropoietin in cerebral diseases. Panminerva Medica 2008;50(2):185-92.

Cuomo O, Pignataro G, Gala R, Scorziello A, Gravino E, Piazza O, Tufano R, Di Renzo G, Annunziato L. Antithrombin reduces ischemic volume, ameliorates neurologic deficits, and prolongs animal survival in both transient and permanent focal ischemia. Stroke. 2007 Dec;38(12):3272-9. Epub 2007 Nov 1.

Dalpke AH, Lehner MD, Hartung T, Heeg K (2005) Differential effects of CpG-DNA in Toll-like receptor-2/-4/-9 tolerance and cross-tolerance. Immunology 116:203–212.

Dame C, Juul SE, Christensen RD. The biology of erythropoietin in the central nervous system and its neurotrophic and neuroprotective potential. *Biol Neonate* 79: 228–235, 2001.

Dave KR, Saul I, Busto R, Ginsberg MD, Sick TJ, Perez-Pinzon MA (2001) Ischemic preconditioning preserves mitochondrial function after global cerebral ischemia in rat hippocampus. J Cereb Blood Flow Metab 21:1401– 1410.

Davis JE, Gabler NK, Walker-Daniels J, Spurlock ME (2008) Tlr-4 deficiency selectively protects against obesity induced by diets high in saturated fat. Obesity 16:1248-1255.

Dawson DA, Furuya K, Gotoh J, Nakao Y, Hallenbeck JM (1999) Cerebrovascular hemodynamics and ischemic tolerance: lipopolysaccharide-induced resistance to focal cerebral ischemia is not due to changes in severity of the initial ischemic insult, but is associated with preservation of microvascular perfusion. J Cereb Blood Flow Metab 19:616–623.

Degenhard TP, Thorpe SR, Baynes J (1988) Chemical modification of proteins by methylglyoxal. Cell Mol Biol (Noisy- legrand) 44:1139–1145

Digicaylioglu M, Bichet S, Marti HH, Wenger RH, Rivas LA, Bauer C, Gassmann M. Localization of specific erythropoietin binding sites in defined areas of the mouse brain. Proc Natl Acad Sci USA 92: 3717–3720, 1995.

Digicaylioglu M, Lipton SA. Erythropoietin-mediated neuroprotection involves cross-talk between Jak2 and NF-kappaB signalling cascades. Nature 412: 641–647, 2001.

Dirnagl U, Iadecola C, Moskowitz MA. Pathobiology of ischaemic stroke: an integrated view. Trends Neurosci 22: 391– 397, 1999.

Dirnagl U, Meisel A (2008) Endogenous neuroprotection: mitochondria as gateways to cerebral preconditioning? Neuropharmacology 55:334–344.

Drinda S, Franke S, Ruster M, Petrow P, Pullig O, Stein G, Hein G (2004) Identification of the receptor for advanced glycation end products in synovial tissue of patients with rheumatoid arthritis. Rheumatol Int [Epub ahead of print]

Dringen R, Hirrlinger J. Glutathione pathways in the brain. Biol Chem 384: 505–516, 2003.

Du Yan S, Zhu H, Fu J, Yan SF, Roher A, Tourtellotte WW, Rajavashisth T, Chen X, Godman GC, Stern D, Schmidt A (1997) Amyloid-beta peptide-receptor for advanced glycation endproduct interaction elicits neuronal expression of macrophage-colony stimulating factor: a proinflammatory pathway in Alzheimer disease. Proc Natl Acad Sci U S A 94:5296–5301

Dunzendorfer S, Kaneider N, Rabensteiner A, Meierhofer C, Reinisch C, Romisch J, Wiedermann CJ: Cell-surface heparan sulfate proteoglycan-mediated regulation of neutrophil migration by the serpin antithrombin III. Blood 2001;97:1079-1085.

Dunzendorfer S, Rabensteiner A, Kaneider N, Meierhofer C, Romisch J, Wiedermann CJ: Involvement of CXC-receptor-1 in antithrombin-induced neutrophil migration. In: Faist E (ed): Proceedings of the 5th World Congress on Trauma, Shock, Inflammation and Sepsis, Munich, Germany, 29 February-4 March 2000. Monduzzi Editore, Italy, 2000, pp 703-706.

Eckardt KU, Kurtz A. Regulation of erythropoietin production. Eur J Clin Invest 35, Suppl 3: 13–19, 2005.

Ehrenreich H, Hasselblatt M, Dembowski C, Cepek L, Lewczuk P, Stiefel M, Rustenbeck HH, Breiter N, Jacob S, Knerlich F, Bohn M, Poser W, Ruther E, Kochen M, Gefeller O, Gleiter C, Wessel TC, De Ryck M, Itri L, Prange H, Cerami A, Brines M, Siren AL. Erythropoietin therapy for acute stroke is both safe and beneficial. Mol Med 8: 495–505, 2002.

Ehrenreich H, Weissenborn K, Prage H et al: Epo Stroke Trial Group. Recombinant human erythropoietin in the treatment of acute ischemic stroke. Stroke.2009 Dec;40(12):e647-56.

Ekdahl CT, Kokaia Z, Lindvall O (2009) Brain inflammation and adult neurogenesis: the dual role of microglia. Neuroscience 158: 1021–1029.

Emerson, T.E., Jr. (1989). Unique features of albumin: a brief review. Crit. Care Med. 17 , 690 – 694.

Endres M, Fan G, Hirt L, Fujii M, Matsushita K, Liu X, Jaenisch R, Moskowitz MA (2000) Ischemic brain damage in mice after selectively modifying BDNF or NT4 gene expression. J Cereb Blood Flow Metab 20:139–144.

Epstein AC, Gleadle JM, McNeill LA, Hewitson KS, O'Rourke J, Mole DR, Mukherji M, Metzen E, Wilson MI, Dhanda A, Tian YM, Masson N, Hamilton DL, Jaakkola P, Barstead R, Hodgkin J, Maxwell PH, Pugh CW, Schofield CJ, Ratcliffe PJ. *C. elegans* EGL-9 and mammalian homologs define a family of dioxygenases that regulate HIF by prolyl hydroxylation. *Cell* 107: 43–54, 2001.

Erlandsson Harris H, Andersson U (2004) Mini-review: the nuclear protein HMGB1 as a proinflammatory mediator. Eur J Immunol 34:1503–1512

Esmon C: The protein C pathway. Crit Care Med 2000;28(Suppl):44–48.

Evans, T.W. (2002). Review article: albumin as a drug – biological effects of albumin unrelated to oncotic pressure. Aliment Pharmacol. Ther. *16* (Suppl. 5), 6 – 11.

Fages C, Nolo R, Huttunen HJ, Eskelinen E, Rauvala H (2000) Regulation of cell migration by amphoterin. J Cell Sci 113:611–620

Fandrey J, Bunn HF. In vivo and in vitro regulation of erythropoietin mRNA: measurement by competitive polymerase chain reaction. *Blood* 81: 617–623, 1993.

Faraco G, Fossati S, Bianchi ME, Patrone M, Pedrazzi M, Sparatore B, Moroni F, Chiarugi A (2007) High mobility group box 1 protein is released by neural cells upon different stresses and worsens ischemic neurodegeneration in vitro and in vivo. J Neurochem 103:590–603.

Ferlito M, Romanenko OG, Ashton S, Squadrito F, Halushka PV, Cook JA (2001) Effect of cross-tolerance between endotoxin and TNFalpha or IL-1beta on cellular signaling and mediator production. J Leukoc Biol 70:821–829.

Frede S, Berchner-Pfannschmidt U, Fandrey J. Regulation of hypoxia-inducible factors during inflammation. *Methods Enzymol* 435: 405–419, 2007.

Furuya K, Zhu L, Kawahara N, Abe O, Kirino T (2005) Differences in infarct evolution between lipopolysaccharide- induced tolerant and nontolerant conditions to focal cerebral ischemia. J Neurosurg 103:715–723.

Garcovich, M., Zocco, M.A., and Gasbarrini, A. (2009). Clinical use of albumin in hepatology. Blood Transfus. *7* , 268 – 277.

Genc K, Genc S, Baskin H, Semin I. Erythropoietin decreases cytotoxicity and nitric oxide formation induced by inflammatory stimuli in rat oligodendrocytes. *Physiol Res* 55: 33–38, 2006.

Genc S, Koroglu TF, Genc K. Erythropoietin and the nervous system. *Brain Res* 1000: 19–31, 2004.

Ginis I, Jaiswal R, Klimanis D, Liu J, Greenspon J, Hallenbeck J (2002) TNFa induced tolerance to ischemic injury involves differential control of NF-kB transactivation: the role of NF-kB association with p300 adaptor. J Cereb Blood Flow Metab 22:142–152.

Ginis I, Schweizer U, Brenner M, Liu J, Azzam N, Spatz M, Hallenbeck J (1999) TNF-alpha pretreatment prevents subsequent activation of cultured brain cells with TNF-alpha and hypoxia via ceramide. Am J Physiol 276:C1171.

Ginsberg, M.D. (2008). Neuroprotection for ischemic stroke: past, present and future. Neuropharmacology *55* , 363 – 389.

Ginsberg, M.D., Hill, M.D., Palesch, Y.Y., Ryckborst, K.J., and Tamariz, D. (2006a). The ALIAS Pilot Trial: a dose escalation and safety study of albumin therapy for acute ischemic stroke– I: Physiological responses and safety results. Stroke *37* , 2100 – 2106.

Ginsberg, M.D., Palesch, Y.Y., and Hill, M.D. (2006b). The ALIAS (ALbumin In Acute Stroke) Phase III randomized multicentre clinical trial: design and progress report. Biochem. Soc. Trans. *34* , 1323 – 1326.

Ginsberg, M.D., Palesch, Y.Y., Martin, R.H., Hill, M.D., Moy, C.S., Waldman, B.D., Yeatts, S.D., Tamariz, D., and Ryckborst, K. (2011). The Albumin In Acute Stroke (ALIAS) Multicenter Clinical Trial: safety analysis of part 1 and rationale and design of part 2. Stroke *42* , 119 – 127.

Goosa MT, Li J, Kislinger T, Qu W, Lu Y, Bucciarelli LG, Nowgrod S, Wolf BM, Calistle X, Yan SD, Stern DM, Schmidt AM (2001) Blockade of receptor for Advanced Glycation Endproducts restores effective wound healing in diabetic mice. Am J Pathol 159:513–525

Gordon S (2002) Pattern recognition receptors: doubling up for the innate immune response. Cell 111:927–930

Grasso G, Buemi M, Alafaci C, Sfacteria A, Passalacqua M, Sturiale A, Calapai G, De Vico G, Piedimonte G, Salpietro FM, Tomasello F. Beneficial effects of systemic administration of recombinant human erythropoietin in rabbits subjected to subarachnoid hemorrhage. *Proc Natl Acad Sci USA* 99: 5627–5631, 2002.

Gum, E.T., Swanson, R.A., Alano, C., Liu, J., Hong, S., Weinstein, P.R., and Panter, S.S. (2004). Human serum albumin and its N-terminal tetrapeptide (DAHK) block oxidant-induced neuronal death. Stroke *35* , 590 – 595.

Ha T, Li Y, Hua F, Ma J, Gao X, Kelley J, Zhao A, Haddad GE, Williams DL, William Browder I, Kao RL, Li C (2005) Reduced cardiac hypertrophy in toll-like receptor 4-deficient mice following pressure overload. Cardiovasc Res 68:224–234.

Hacke, W., Donnan, G., Fieschi, C., Kaste, M., von Kummer, R., Broderick, J.P., Brott, T., Frankel, M., Grotta, J.C., Haley, E.C., Jr., et al. (2004). Association of outcome with early stroke treatment: pooled analysis of ATLANTIS, ECASS, and NINDS rt-PA stroke trials. Lancet *363* , 768 – 774.

Hanford LE, Enghild JJ, Valnickova Z, Petersen SV, Schaefer LM, Schaefer TM, Reinhart TA, Oury TD (2004) Purification and characterization of mouse soluble Receptor for Advanced Glycation End Products (sRAGE). J Biol Chem 279:50019–50024

Hara H, Friedlander RM, Gagliardini V, Ayata C, Fink K, Huang Z, Shimizu-Sasamata M, Yuan J, Moskowitz MA (1997) Inhibition of interleukin 1beta converting enzyme family proteases reduces ischemic and excitotoxic neuronal damage. Proc Natl Acad Sci U S A 94:2007–2012.

Harada N, Okajima K, Kushimoto S, Isobe H, Tanaka K: Antithrombin reduces ischemia/reperfusion injury of rat liver by increasing the hepatic level of prostacyclin. Blood 1999;93:157-164.

Hasselblatt M, Ehrenreich H, Siren AL. The brain erythropoietin system and its potential for therapeutic exploitation in brain disease. *J Neurosurg Anesthesiol* 18: 132–138, 2006.

Hewitson KS, McNeill LA, Riordan MV, Tian YM, Bullock AN, Welford RW, Elkins JM, Oldham NJ, Bhattacharya S, Gleadle JM, Ratcliffe PJ, Pugh CW, Schofield CJ. Hypoxia-inducible factor (HIF) asparagine hydroxylase is identical to factor inhibiting HIF (FIH) and is related to the cupin structural family. *J Biol Chem* 277: 26351– 26355, 2002.

Hickey EJ, You X, Kaimaktchiev V, Stenzel-Poore M, Ungerleider RM (2007) Lipopolysaccharide preconditioning induces robust protection against brain injury resulting from deep hypothermic circulatory arrest. J Thorac Cardiovasc Surg 133:1588–1596.

Hill MD, Martin RH, Palesh YY, Tamariz D, Waldman BD, Ryckborst KJ, May CS, Barsan WG, Ginsberg MD; ALIAS Investigators; Neurological Emergencies Treatment trials Network. The Albumin in acute Stroke Part 1 Trial: an exploratory efficacy analysis. Stroke 2001Jun;42(6):1621-5.

Hoffmann JN, Vollmar B, Roemisch J, Inthorn D, Schildberg FW, Menger MD: Antithrombin effects on endotoxin- induced microcirculatory disorders are mainly mediated by its interaction with microvascular endothelium. Crit Care Med, Jan 2002-30(1):218- 225.

Hofmann MA, Drury S, Fu C, Wu Q, Taguchi A, Lu Y, Avila C, Kambham N, Slattery T, Beach D, McClary J, Nagashima M, Morser J, Bierhaus A, Neurath M, Nawroth P, Stern D, Schmidt AM (1999) RAGE mediates a novel proinflammatory axis: the cell surface receptor for S100/calgranulin polypeptides. Cell 97:889–901

Hooper, C., Taylor, D.L., and Pocock, J.M. (2005). Pure albumin is a potent trigger of calcium signalling and proliferation in microglia but not macrophages or astrocytes. J. Neurochem. *92* , 1363 – 1376.

Hori O, Brett J, Slattery T, Cao R, Zhang J, Chen JX, Nagashima M, Lundh ER, Vijay S, Nitecki D, Morser J, Stern D, Schmidt AM (1995) The receptor for advanced glycation end products (RAGE) is a cellular binding site for amphoterin. Mediation of neurite outgrowth and co-expression of rage and amphoterin in the developing nervous system. J Biol Chem 270:25752–25761

Hua F, Ma J, Ha T, Xia Y, Kelley J, Williams DL, Kao RL, Browder IW, Schweitzer JB, Kalbfleisch JH, Li C (2007) Activation of Toll-like receptor 4 signaling contributes to hippocampal neuronal death following global cerebral ischemia/reperfusion. J Neuroimmunol 190:101–111.

Hua L, Kim M, Brosnan C, Lee S (2002) Modulation of astrocyte inducible nitric oxide synthase and cytokine expression by interferon beta is associated with induction and inhibition of interferon gamma-activated sequence binding activity. J Neurochem 83:1120–1128.

Huang JS, Guh JY, Chen HC, Hung WC, Lai YH, Chuang LY (2001) Role of receptor for advanced glycation end-product (RAGE) and the JAK/STAT-signaling pathway in AGE-induced collagen production in NRK-49F cells. J Cell Biochem 81:102–113

Hudson BI, Bucciarelli LG, Wendt T et al (2003) Blockade of receptor for advanced glycation endproducs: a new target for therapeutic intervention in diabetic complications and inflammatory disorders. Arch Biochem Biophys 419:80–88

Huh, P.W., Belayev, L., Zhao, W., Busto, R., Saul, I., and Ginsberg, M.D. (1998). The effect of high-dose albumin therapy on local cerebral perfusion after transient focal cerebral ischemia in rats. Brain Res. *804* , 105 – 113.

Huttunen HJ, Fages C, Kuja-Panula J, Ridley AJ, Rauvala H (2002) Receptor for advanced glycation end products- binding COOH-terminal motif of amphoterin inhibits invasive migration and metastasis. Cancer Res 62:4805– 4811

Huttunen HJ, Fages C, Rauvala H (1999) Receptor for advanced glycation end products (RAGE)-mediated neurite outgrowth and activation of NF-kappaB require the cytoplasmic domain of the receptor but different downstream signaling pathways. J Biol Chem 274:19919–19924

Huttunen HJ, Kuja-Panula J, Sorci G, Agneletti AL, Donato R, Rauvala H (2000) Coregulation of neurite outgrowth and cell survival by amphoterin and S100 proteins through receptor for advanced glycation end products (RAGE) activation. J Biol Chem 275:40096–40105

Iampietro R, Souter P, Romisch J, Poole S, Gray E: Antithrombin inhibits in vitro lipopolysaccharide induced interleukin- 6 production by suppression of mRNA. Intensive Care Med 2000;26(Suppl 3):302.

Ishihara K, Tsutsumi K, Kawane S, Nakajima M, Kasaoka T (2003) The receptor for advanced glycation end-products (RAGE) directly binds to ERK by a D-domain-like docking site. FEBS Lett 550:107–113

Italian Acute Stroke Study Group. (1988). Haemodilution in acute stroke: results of the Italian Haemodilution Trial. Lancet *i* , 318 – 321.

Ivan M, Kondo K, Yang H, Kim W, Valiando J, Ohh M, Salic A, Asara JM, Lane WS, Kaelin, WG Jr. HIFalpha targeted for VHL-mediated destruction by proline hydroxylation: implications for O2 sensing. *Science* 292: 464–468, 2001.

Ivens, S., Kaufer, D., Flores, L.P., Bechmann, I., Zumsteg, D., Tomkins, O., Seiffert, E., Heinemann, U., and Friedman, A. (2007). TGF-beta receptor-mediated albumin uptake into astrocytes is involved in neocortical epileptogenesis. Brain *130* , 535 – 547.

Jaakkola P, Mole DR, Tian YM, Wilson MI, Gielbert J, Gaskell SJ, Kriegsheim A, Hebestreit HF, Mukherji M, Schofield CJ, Maxwell PH, Pugh CW, Ratcliffe PJ. Targeting of HIF-alpha to the von Hippel-Lindau ubiquitylation complex by O2-regulated prolyl hydroxylation. *Science* 292: 468–472, 2001.

Jack CS, Arbour N, Manusow J, Montgrain V, Blain M, McCrea E, Shapiro A, Antel JP (2005) TLR signaling tailors innate immune responses in human microglia and astrocytes. J Immunol 175: 4320–4330.

Jelkmann W. Erythropoietin: structure, control of production, and function. *Physiol Rev* 72: 449–489, 1992.

Jiang D, Liang J, Li Y, Noble PW (2006) The role of Toll-like receptors in non-infectious lung injury. Cell Res 16:693–701.

Jin S, Kawanokuchi J, Mizuno T, Wang J, Sonobe Y, Takeuchi H, Suzumura A (2007) Interferon-beta is neuroprotective against the toxicity induced by activated microglia. Brain Res 1179:140–146.

Johanson, C.E., Duncan, J.A., 3rd, Klinge, P.M., Brinker, T., Stopa, E.G., and Silverberg, G.D. (2008). Multiplicity of cerebrospinal fluid functions: new challenges in health and disease. Cerebrospinal Fluid Res. *5* , 10.

Johnson DR, Douglas I, Jahnke A, Ghosh S, Pober JS (1996) A sustained reduction in IκB-β may contribute to persistent NF-κB activation in human endothelial cells. J Biol Chem 271:16317–16322

Juttler, E., Kohrmann, M., and Schellinger, P.D. (2006). Therapy for early reperfusion after stroke. Nat. Clin. Pract. Cardiovasc. Med. *3* , 656 – 663.

Kagan JC, Su T, Horng T, Chow A, Akira S, Medzhitov R (2008) TRAM couples endocytosis of Toll-like receptor 4 to the induction of interferon-beta. Nat Immunol 9:361–368.

Kaneider NC, Egger P, Dunzendorfer S, Wiedermann CJ: Syndecan-4 as antithrombin receptor of human neutrophils. Biochem Biophys Res Commun 2001;287:42-46.

Kaneider NC, Reinisch CM, Dunzendorfer S, Romisch J, Wiedermann CJ: Syndecan-4 on huan peripheral blood lymphocytes and monocytes mediates effects of antithrombin on chemotaxis. J Cell Sci 2002

Kaur J, Woodman RC, Ostrovsky L, Kubes P: Selective recruitment of neutrophils and lymphocytes by thrombin: a role for NF-kappaB. Am J Physiol Heart Circ Physiol 2001; 281:784-795.

Kawakami M, Iwasaki S, Sato K, Takahashi M. Erythropoietin inhibits calcium-induced neurotransmitter release from clonal neuronal cells. *Biochem Biophys Res Commun* 279: 293–297, 2000.

Kerschensteiner M, Meinal E, Hohlfeld R (2009) Neuro-immune crosstalk in CNS diseases. Neuroscience 158:1122–1132.

Kertesz N, Wu J, Chen TH, Sucov HM, Wu H. The role of erythropoietin in regulating angiogenesis. *Dev Biol* 276: 101– 110, 2004.

Kilic E, Kilic U, Soliz J, Bassetti CL, Gassmann M, Hermann DM. Brain-derived erythropoietin protects from focal cerebral ischemia by dual activation of ERK-1/-2 and Akt pathways. *FASEB J* 19: 2026–2028, 2005.

Kinouchi H, Sharp FR, Hill MP, Koistinaho J, Sagar SM, Chan PH (1993) Induction of 70-kDa heat shock protein and hsp70 mRNA following transient focal cerebral ischemia in the rat. J Cereb Blood Flow Metab 13:105–115.

Kislinger T, Fu C, Huber B, Qu W, Taguchi A, Du Yan S, Hofmann M, Yan SF, Pischetsrieder M, Stern D, Schmidt AM (1999) N(epsilon)-(carboxymethyl)lysine adducts of proteins are ligands for receptor for advanced glycation end products that activate cell signaling pathways and modulate gene expression. J Biol Chem 274:31740–31749

Kislinger T, Tanji N, Wendt T, Qu W, Lu Y, Ferran LJ Jr, Taguchi A, Olson K, Bucciarelli L, Goova M, Hofmann MA, Cataldegirmen G, D'Agati V, Pischetsrieder M, Stern DM, Schmidt AM (2001) Receptor for advanced glycation end products mediates inflammation and enhanced expression of tissue factor in vasculature of diabetic apolipoprotein E-Null mice. Arterioscl Thromb Vasc Biol 21:905–910

Kobayashi K, Hernandex L, Galan J, Janeway J, Medzhitov R, Flavell R (2002) IRAK-M is a negative regulator of Toll-like receptor signaling. Cell 110:191–202.

Kobayashi T, Yanase H, Iwanaga T, Sasaki R, Nagao M. Epididymis is a novel site of erythropoietin production in mouse reproductive organs. *Biochem Biophys Res Commun* 296: 145-151, 2002.

Kokkola R, Andersson A, Mullins G, Ostberg T, Treutiger CJ, Arnold B, Nawroth P, Andersson U, Harris RA, Harris HE (2005) RAGE is the major receptor for the proinflammatory activity of HMGB1 in rodent macrophages. Scand J Immunol 61:1–9

Konishi Y, Chui DH, Hirose H, Kunishita T, Tabira T. Trophic effect of erythropoietin and other hematopoietic factors on central cholinergic neurons in vitro and in vivo. *Brain Res* 609: 29–35, 1993.

Korosue, K. and Heros, R.C. (1992). Mechanism of cerebral blood flow augmentation by hemodilution in rabbits. Stroke 23 , 1487 – 1492; discussion 1492 – 1493.

Koshimura K, Murakami Y, Sohmiya M, Tanaka J, Kato Y. Effects of erythropoietin on neuronal activity. J Neurochem 72: 2565–2572, 1999.

Kraus J, Ling AK, Hamm S, Voigt K, Oschmann P, Engelhardt B (2004) Interferon-beta stabilizes barrier characteristics of brain endothelial cells in vitro. Ann Neurol 56:192–205.

Kumral A, Gonenc S, Acikgoz O, Sonmez A, Genc K, Yilmaz O, Gokmen N, Duman N, Ozkan H. Erythropoietin increases glutathione peroxidase enzyme activity and decreases lipid peroxidation levels in hypoxic-ischemic brain injury in neonatal rats. Biol Neonate 87: 15–18, 2005.

Kunz A, Park L, Abe T, Gallo EF, Anrather J, Zhou P, Iadecola C (2007) Neurovascular protection by ischemic tolerance: role of nitric oxide and reactive oxygen species. J Neurosci 27:7083–7093.

Laflamme N, Rivest S (2001) Toll-like receptor 4: the missing link of the cerebral innate immune response triggered by circulating gramnegative bacterial cell wall components. FASEB J 15:155–163.

Laflamme N, Soucy G, Rivest S (2001) Circulating cell wall components derived from gram-negative, not gram-positive, bacteria cause a profound induction of the gene-encoding Toll-like receptor 2 in the CNS. J Neurochem 79:648– 657.

Lafon M, Megret F, Lafage M, Prehaud C (2006) The innate immune facet of brain: human neurons express TLR-3 and sense viral dsRNA. J Mol Neurosci 29:185–194.

Lalla F, Lamster IB, Stern DM, Schmidt AM (2001) Receptor for advanced glycation end products, inflammation, and accelerated periodontal disease in diabetes: mechanisms and insights into therapeutic modalities. Ann Periodontol 6:113–118

Lander HM, Taurus JM, Ogiste JS, Hori O, Moss RA, Schmidt AM(1997) Activation of the receptor for advanced glycation end products triggers a p21(ras)-dependent mitogen-activated protein kinase pathway regulated by oxidant stress. J Biol Chem 272:17810–17814

Lando D, Peet DJ, Gorman JJ, Whelan DA, Whitelaw ML, Bruick RK. FIH-1 is an asparaginyl hydroxylase enzyme that regulates the transcriptional activity of hypoxia-inducible factor. Genes Dev 16: 1466–1471, 2002b.

Lando D, Peet DJ, Whelan DA, Gorman JJ, Whitelaw ML. Asparagine hydroxylation of the HIF transactivation domain a hypoxic switch. Science 295: 858–861, 2002a.

Lehnardt S, Lehmann S, Kaul D, Tschimmel K, Hoffmann O, Cho S, Krueger C, Nitsch R, Meisel A, Weber JR (2007) Toll- like receptor 2 mediates CNS injury in focal cerebral ischemia. J Neuroimmunol 190:28–33.

Lehnardt S, Schott E, Trimbuch T, Laubisch D, Krueger C, Wulczyn G, Nitsch R, Weber JR (2008) A vicious cycle involving release of heat shock protein 60 from injured cells and activation of toll-like receptor 4 mediates neurodegeneration in the CNS. J Neurosci 28: 2320–2331.

Li J, Schmidt AM (1997) Characterization and functional analysis of the promoter of RAGE, the receptor for advanced glycation end products. J Biol Chem 272(1):6498–6506

Li JH, Wang W, Huang XR, Oldfield M, Schmidt AM, Cooper ME, Lan HY (2004) Advanced glycation end products induce tubular epithelial-myofibroblast transition through the RAGEERK1/2 MAP kinase signaling pathway. Am J Pathol 164: 1389–1397

Liliensiek B, Weigand MA, Bierhaus A, Nicklas W, Kasper M, Hofer S, Plaschky J, Gröne HJ, Kurschus FJ, Schmidt AM, Yan SD, Martin E, Schleicher E, Stern DM, Hämmerling GJ, Nawroth PP, Arnold B (2004) Receptor for advanced glycation end products (RAGE) regulates sepsis, but not the adaptive immune response. J Clin Invest 113:1641–1650

Lipton P. Ischemic cell death in brain neurons. *Physiol Rev* 79: 1431–1568, 1999.

Little, J.R., Slugg, R.M., Latchaw, J.P., Jr., and Lesser, R.P. (1981). Treatment of acute focal cerebral ischemia with concentrated albumin. Neurosurgery 9 , 552 – 558.

Liu H, Xin L, Chan BPL, Teoh R, Tang BL, Tan YH (2002) Interferon beta administration confers a beneficial outcome in a rabbit model of thromboembolic cerebral ischemia. Neurosci Lett 327:146–148.

Liu, Y., Belayev, L., Zhao, W., Busto, R., Belayev, A., and Ginsberg, M.D. (2001). Neuroprotective effect of treatment with human albumin in permanent focal cerebral ischemia: histopathology and cortical perfusion studies. Eur. J. Pharmacol. 428 , 193 – 201.

Liuzzi GM, Latronico T, Fasano A, Carlone G, Riccio P (2004) Interferon-beta inhibits the expression of metalloproteinases in rat glial cell cultures: implications for multiple sclerosis pathogenesis and treatment. Mult Scler 10:290–297.

Lloyd-Jones KL, Kelly MM, Kubes P (2008) Varying importance of soluble and membrane CD14 in endothelial detection of lipopolysaccharide. J Immunol 181:1446–1453.

Lloyd-Jones, D., Adams, R., Carnethon, M., De Simone, G., Ferguson, T.B., Flegal, K., Ford, E., Furie, K., Go, A., Greenlund, K., et al. (2009). Heart disease and stroke statistics – 2009 update: a report from the American Heart Association Statistics Committee and Stroke Statistics Subcommittee. Circulation 119 , e21 – e181.

Longa, E.Z., Weinstein, P.R., Carlson, S., and Cummins, R. (1989). Reversible middle cerebral artery occlusion without craniectomy in rats. Stroke 20 , 84 – 91.

Lopez-Collazo E, Hortelano S, Rojas A, Bosca L (1998) Triggering of peritoneal macrophages with IFN-alpha/beta attenuates the expression of inducible nitric oxide synthase through a decrease in NF-kappaB activation. J Immunol 160:2889–2895.

Ludwicka-Bradley A, Tourkina E, Suzuki S, Tyson E, Bonner M, Fenton JW II, Hoffman S, Silver RM: Thrombin upregulates interleukin-8 in lung fibroblasts via cleavage of proteolytically activated receptor-I and protein kinase C-gamma activation. Am J Respir Cell Mol Biol 2000;22:235-243.

Lue LF, Walker DG, Brachova L, Beach TG, Rogers J, Schmidt AM, Stern DM, Yan SD (2001) Involvement of microglial receptor for advanced glycation endproducts (RAGE) in Alzheimer's disease: identification of a cellular activation mechanism. Exp Neurol 171:29-45

Ma Y, Li J, Chiu I, Wang Y, Sloane JA, Lu J, Kosaras B, Sidman RL, Volpe JJ, Vartanian T (2006) Toll-like receptor 8 functions as a negative regulator of neurite outgrowth and inducer of neuronal apoptosis. J Cell Biol 175:209– 215.

Mackic JB, Stins M, McComb JG, Calero M, Ghiso J, Kim KS, Yan SD, Stern D, Schmidt AM, Frangione B, Zlokovic BV (1998) Human blood-brain barrier receptors for Alzheimer's amyloid-beta 1–40. Asymmetrical binding, endocytosis, and transcytosis at the apical side of brain microvascular endothelial cell monolayer. J Clin Invest 102:734–743

Malherbe R, Richards JG, Gaillard H, Thompson A, Diener C, Schuler A, Huber G (1999) cDNA cloning of a novel secreted isoform of the human receptor for advanced glycation end products and characterisation of cells co- expresing cell-surface scavenger receptors and Swedish mutant amyloid precursor protein. Mol Brain Res 71:159–170

Mammen EF: Antithrombin: its physiological importance and role in DIC. Semin Thromb Hemost 1998;24:19-25.

Manning, T.J., Jr. and Sontheimer, H. (1997). Bovine serum albumin and lysophosphatidic acid stimulate calcium mobilization and reversal of cAMP-induced stellation in rat spinal cord astrocytes. Glia 20 , 163 – 172.

Marenholz I, Heizmann CW, Fritz G (2004) S100 proteins in mouse and man: from evolution to function and pathology (including an update of the nomenclature). Biochem Biophys Res Commun 322:1111–1122

Marrero MB, Venema RC, Ma H, Ling BN, Eaton DC. Erythropoietin receptor-operated Ca2+ channels: activation by phospholipase C-gamma 1. *Kidney Int* 53: 1259–1268, 1998.

Marti HH, Bernaudin M, Petit E, Bauer C. Neuroprotection and angiogenesis: dual role of erythropoietin in brain ischemia. *News Physiol Sci* 15: 225–229, 2000.

Marti HH, Gassmann M, Wenger RH, Kvietikova I, Morganti-Kossmann MC, Kossmann T, Trentz O, Bauer C. Detection of erythropoietin in human liquor: intrinsic erythropoietin production in the brain. *Kidney Int* 51: 416–418, 1997.

Marti HH, Wenger RH, Rivas LA, Straumann U, Digicaylioglu M, Henn V, Yonekawa Y, Bauer C, Gassmann M. Erythropoietin gene expression in human, monkey and murine brain. *Eur J Neurosci* 8: 666–676, 1996.

Marti HH. Erythropoietin and the hypoxic brain. *J Exp Biol* 207: 3233–3242, 2004.

Martinez-Estrada OM, Rodriguez-Millan E, Gonzalez-De Vicente E, Reina M, Vilaro S, Fabre M. Erythropoietin protects the in vitro blood-brain barrier against VEGF-induced permeability. *Eur J Neurosci* 18: 2538–2544, 2003.

Masuda S, Kobayashi T, Chikuma M, Nagao M, Sasaki R. The oviduct produces erythropoietin in an estrogen- and oxygen-dependent manner. *Am J Physiol Endocrinol Metab* 278: E1038–E1044, 2000.

Masuda S, Okano M, Yamagishi K, Nagao M, Ueda M, Sasaki R. A novel site of erythropoietin production. Oxygen- dependent production in cultured rat astrocytes. *J Biol Chem* 269: 19488–19493, 1994.

Matsui, T., Sinyama, H., and Asano, T. (1993). Benefi cial effect of prolonged administration of albumin on ischemic cerebral edema and infarction after occlusion of middle cerebral artery in rats. Neurosurgery 33 , 293 – 300; comment 300.

McFalls EO, Sluiter W, Schoonderwoerd K, Manintveld OC, Lamers JM, Bezstarosti K, van Beusekom HM, Sikora J, Ward HB, Merkus D, Duncker DJ (2006) Mitochondrial adaptations within chronically ischemic swine myocardium. J Mol Cell Cardiol 41:980–988.

McKhann GM, Grega MA, Borowicz LM Jr, Baumgartner WA, Selnes OA (2006) Stroke and encephalopathy after cardiac surgery: an update. Stroke 37:562–571.

McKimmie CS, Fazakerley JK (2005) In response to pathogens, glial cells dynamically and differentially regulate Toll-like receptor gene expression. J Neuroimmunol 169:116–125.

Medvedev AE, Lentschat A, Wahl LM, Golenbock DT, Vogel SN (2002) Dysregulation of LPS-induced Toll-like receptor 4-MyD88 complex formation and IL-1 receptor-associated kinase1 activation in endotoxin-tolerant cells. J Immunol 169:5209-5216.

Morcos M, Hofmann M, Tritschler H, Weigle B, Kasper M, Smith MA, Perry G, Schmidt AM, Stern DM, Häring HU, Schleicher E, Nawroth PP (2001) Diabetes-associated sustained activation of the transcription factor NF-κB. Diabetes 50:2792-2809

Morcos M, Sayed A, Pfisterer F, Hutter H, Thornalley P, Ahmed N, Miftari N, Mörlen F, Hamann A, Bierhaus A,

Murphey ED, Traber DL (2001) Protective effect of tumor necrosis factor-alpha against subsequent endotoxemia in mice is mediated, in part, by interleukin-10. Crit Care Med 29:1761-1766.

Murphy, M.P. and LeVine, H., 3rd. (2010). Alzheimer's disease and the amyloid-beta peptide. J. Alzheimers Dis. *19*, 311 - 323.

Murray CJ, Lopez AD (1997) Alternative projections of mortality and disability by cause 1990-2020: Global Burden of Disease Study. Lancet 349:1498-1504.

Nadal, A., Sul, J.Y., Valdeolmillos, M., and McNaughton, P.A. (1998). Albumin elicits calcium signals from astrocytes in brain slices from neonatal rat cortex. J. Physiol. *509*, 711 - 716.

Nagai A, Nakagawa E, Choi HB, Hatori K, Kobayashi S, Kim SU. Erythropoietin and erythropoietin receptors in human CNS neurons, astrocytes, microglia, and oligodendrocytes grown in culture. *J Neuropathol Exp Neurol* 60: 386- 392, 2001.

Nahon, J.L., Tratner, I., Poliard, A., Presse, F., Poiret, M., Gal, A., Sala-Trepat, J.M., Legres, L., Feldmann, G., and Bernuau, D. (1988). Albumin and alpha-fetoprotein gene expression in various nonhepatic rat tissues. J. Biol. Chem. *263*, 11436 - 11442.

Nawashiro H, Tasaki K, Ruetzler CA, Hallenbeck JM (1997) TNFalpha pretreatment induces protective effects against focal cerebral ischemia in mice. J Cereb Blood Flow Metab 17:483-490.

Nawroth PP (2004) Glyoxalase I als endogener Schutz vor Advanced Glycation Endproducts (AGE)-formation und oxidativem stress in Caenorhabditis elegans. Diab Stoffw 13 (Supplementheft 1):33 V-70

Neeper M, Schmidt AM, Brett J, Yan SD, Wang F, Pa YCE, Elliston K, Stern DM, Shaw A (1992) Cloning and Expression of a cell surface receptor for advanced glycosylation end products of proteins. J Biol Chem 267:14998-15004

Neugroschl, J. and Sano, M. (2010). Current treatment and recent clinical research in Alzheimer's disease. Mt. Sinai J. Med. *77*, 3 - 16.

Neviere R, Tournoys A, Mordon S, Marechal X, Song FL, Jourdain M, Fourrier F: Antithrombin reduces mesenteric venular leukocyte interactions and small intestine injury in endotoxemic rats. Shock 2001;15:220-225.

Nhu QM, Cuesta N, Vogel SN (2006) Transcriptional regulation of lipopolysaccharide (LPS)-induced Toll-like receptor (TLR) expression in murine macrophages: role of interferon regulatory factors 1 (IRF-1) and 2 (IRF-2). J Endotoxin Res 12:285-295.

Nicholson, J.P., Wolmarans, M.R., and Park, G.R. (2000). The role of albumin in critical illness. Br. J. Anaesth. *85*, 599 - 610.

Nimmagadda, A., Park, H.P., Prado, R., and Ginsberg, M.D. (2008). Albumin therapy improves local vascular dynamics in a rat model of primary microvascular thrombosis: a two-photon laserscanning microscopy study. Stroke *39*, 198 - 204.

Noble R (1943) The development of resistance by rats and guinea pigs to amounts of trauma usually fatal. Am J Physiol 38:346–351.

Oelschlager C, Leithauser B, Romisch J, Tillmanns H, Holschermann H: Antithrombin inhibits NF-KB signaling pathways in monocytes and endothelial cells in vitro. Ann Hematol 2001;80(Suppl 1):A51.

Okajima K, Uchiba M: The anti-inflammatory properties of antithrombin III:new therapeutic implications. Semin Thromb Hemost 1998;24:27-32.

Olson JK, Miller SD (2004) Microglia initiate central nervous system innate and adaptive immune responses through multiple TLRs. J Immunol 173:3916–3924.

Opal SM: Phylogenetic and functional relationship between coagulation and the innate immune response. Crit Care Med 2000;28(Suppl):77-80.

Ostrovsky L, Woodman RC, Payne D, Teoh D, Kubes P: Antithrombin III prevents and rapidly reverse leukocyte recruitment in ischemia/reperfusion. Circulation 1997;96:2302-2310.

Oyama J, Blais C Jr, Liu X, Pu M, Kobzik L, Kelly RA, Bourcier T (2004) Reduced myocardial ischemia-reperfusion injury in toll-like receptor 4-deficient mice. Circulation 109:784–789.

Palesch, Y.Y., Hill, M.D., Ryckborst, K.J., Tamariz, D., and Ginsberg, M.D. (2006). The ALIAS Pilot Trial: a dose escalation and safety study of albumin therapy for acute ischemic stroke – II: neurologic outcome and effi cacy analysis. Stroke *37* , 2107 – 2114.

Palmer G, Mezin F, Juge-Aubry CE, Plater-Zyberk C, Gabay C, Guerne PA (2004) Interferon beta stimulates interleukin 1 receptor antagonist production in human articular chondrocytes and synovial fibroblasts. Ann Rheum Dis 63:43–49.

Parsa CJ, Matsumoto A, Kim J, Riel RU, Pascal LS, Walton GB, Thompson RB, Petrofski JA, Annex BH, Stamler JS, Koch WJ. A novel protective effect of erythropoietin in the infarcted heart. *J Clin Invest* 112: 999–1007, 2003.

Patel NS, Sharples EJ, Cuzzocrea S, Chatterjee PK, Britti D, Yaqoob MM, Thiemermann C. Pretreatment with EPO reduces the injury and dysfunction caused by ischemia/reperfusion in the mouse kidney in vivo. *Kidney Int* 66: 983–989, 2004.

Piazza O, Scarpati G, Cotena S, Lonardo M, Tufano R:Thrombin antithrombin complex and IL-18 serum levels in stroke patients. Neurol Int. 2010 Jun 21;2(1):e1.

Porter MH, Arnold M, Langhans W (1998) TNF-alpha tolerance blocks LPS-induced hypophagia but LPS tolerance fails to prevent TNFalpha- induced hypophagia. Am J Physiol 274:R741–R745.

Prajapati, K.D., Sharma, S.S., and Roy, N. (2010). Upregulation of albumin expression in focal ischemic rat brain. Brain Res. *1327* , 118 – 124.

Prehaud C, Megret F, Lafage M, Lafon M (2005) Virus infection switches TLR-3-positive human neurons to become strong producers of beta interferon. J Virol 79:12893–12904.

Quinlan, G.J., Martin, G.S., and Evans, T.W. (2005). Albumin: biochemical properties and therapeutic potential. Hepatology *41* , 1211 – 1219.

Rabiet MJ, Plantier JL, Dejana E: Thrombin-induced endothelial cell dysfunction. Br Med Bull 1994;50:936-945.

Ralay Ranaivo, H. and Wainwright, M.S. (2010). Albumin activates astrocytes and microglia through mitogen-activated protein kinase pathways. Brain Res. *1313* , 222 – 231.

Recny MA, Scoble HA, Kim Y. Structural characterization of natural human urinary and recombinant DNA-derived erythropoietin. Identification of des-arginine 166 erythropoietin. *J Biol Chem* 262: 17156–17163, 1987.

Reiber, H. (1998). Cerebrospinal fl uid – physiology, analysis and interpretation of protein patterns for diagnosis of neurological diseases. Mult. Scler. *4* , 99 – 107.

Reiber, H. (2003). Proteins in cerebrospinal fl uid and blood: barriers, CSF fl ow rate and source-related dynamics. Restor. Neurol. Neurosci. *21* , 79 – 96.

Reiber, H. and Peter, J.B. (2001). Cerebrospinal fl uid analysis: disease- related data patterns and evaluation programs. J. Neurol. Sci. *184* , 101 – 122.

Relton JK, Martin D, Thompson RC, Russell DA (1996) Peripheral administration of interleukin-1 receptor antagonist inhibits brain damage after focal cerebral ischemia in the rat. Exp Neurol 138:206–213.

Remmers, M., Schmidt-Kastner, R., Belayev, L., Lin, B., Busto, R., and Ginsberg, M.D. (1999). Protein extravasation and cellular uptake after high-dose human-albumin treatment of transient focal cerebral ischemia in rats. Brain Res. *827* , 237 – 242.

Ribatti D, Presta M, Vacca A, Ria R, Giuliani R, Dell'Era P, Nico B, Roncali L, Dammacco F. Human erythropoietin induces a pro-angiogenic phenotype in cultured endothelial cells and stimulates neovascularization in vivo. *Blood* 93: 2627–2636, 1999.

Robinson MJ, Tessier P, Poulsom R, Hogg N (2002) The S100 family heterodimer, MRP-8/14, binds with high affinity to heparin and heparan sulfate glycosaminoglycans on endothelial cells. J Biol Chem 277:3658–3665

Rodriguez de Turco, E.B., Belayev, L., Liu, Y., Busto, R., Parkins, N., Bazan, N.G., and Ginsberg, M.D. (2002). Systemic fatty acid responses to transient focal cerebral ischemia: infl uence of neuroprotectant therapy with human albumin. J. Neurochem. *83* , 515– 524.

Rolls A, Shechter R, London A, Ziv Y, Ronen A, Levy R, Schwartz M (2007) Toll-like receptors modulate adult hippocampal neurogenesis. Nat Cell Biol 9:1081–1088.

Rong LL, Trojaborg W, Qu W, Kostov K, Yan SD, Gooch C, Szabolcs M, Hays AP, Schmidt AM (2004) Antagonism of RAGE suppresses peripheral nerve regeneration. FASEB J 18: 1812–1817

Rong LL, Yan SF, Wendt T, Hans D, Pachydaki S, Bucciarelli LG, Adebayo A, Qu W, Lu Y, Kostov K, Lalla E, Yan SD, Gooch C, Szabolcs M, Trojaborg W, Hays AP, Schmidt AM (2004) RAGE modulates peripheral nerve regeneration via recruitment of both inflammatory and axonal outgrowth pathways. FASEB J 18:1818–1825

Rosenzweig HL, Lessov NS, Henshall DC, Minami M, Simon RP, Stenzel-Poore MP (2004) Endotoxin preconditioning prevents the cellular inflammatory response during ischemic neuroprotection in mice. Stroke 35:2576–2581.

Rosenzweig HL, Minami M, Lessov NS, Coste SC, Stevens SL, Henshall DC, Meller R, Simon RP, Stenzel-Poore MP (2007) Endotoxin preconditioning protects against the cytotoxic effects of TNFa after stroke: a novel role for TNFa in LPS-ischemic tolerance. J Cereb Blood Flow Metab 27:1663–1674.

rt-PA Stroke Study Group. (1995). Tissue plasminogen activator for acute ischemic stroke. The National Institute of Neurological Disorders and Stroke rt-PA Stroke Study Group. N. Engl. J. Med. *333* , 1581 – 1587.

Ruscher K, Freyer D, Karsch M, Isaev N, Megow D, Sawitzki B, Priller J, Dirnagl U, Meisel A. Erythropoietin is a paracrine mediator of ischemic tolerance in the brain: evidence from an in vitro model. *J Neurosci* 22: 10291– 10301, 2002.

Sadamoto Y, Igase K, Sakanaka M, Sato K, Otsuka H, Sakaki S, Masuda S, Sasaki R. Erythropoietin prevents place navigation disability and cortical infarction in rats with permanent occlusion of the middle cerebral artery. *Biochem Biophys Res Commun* 253: 26–32, 1998.

Sakaguchi T, Yan SF, Yan SD, Belov D, Rong LL, Sousa M, Andrassy M, Marso SP, Duda S, Arnold B, Liliensiek B, Nawroth PP, Stern DM, Schmidt AM, Naka Y (2003) Central role of RAGE-dependent neointimal expansion in arterial restenosis. J Clin Invest 111:959-972

Sakanaka M, Wen TC, Matsuda S, Masuda S, Morishita E, Nagao M, Sasaki R. In vivo evidence that erythropoietin protects neurons from ischemic damage. *Proc Natl Acad Sci USA* 95: 4635–4640, 1998.

Sakata Y, Dong JW, Vallejo JG, Huang CH, Baker JS, Tracey KJ, Tacheuchi O, Akira S, Mann DL (2007) Toll-like receptor 2 modulates left ventricular function following ischemia-reperfusion injury. Am J Physiol Heart Circ Physiol 292:H503-H509.

Sasaki N, Takeuchi M, Chowei H, Kikuchi S, Hayashi Y, Nakano N, Ikeda H, Yamagishi S, Kitamoto T, Saito T, Makita Z (2002) Advanced glycation end products (AGE) and their receptor (RAGE) in the brain of patients with Creutzfeldt-Jakob disease with prion plaques. Neurosci Lett 326:117-120

Scandinavian Stroke Study Group. (1987). Multicenter trial of hemodilution in acute ischemic stroke. I. Results in the total patient population. Stroke *18* , 691 – 699.

Schiekofer S, Andrassy M, Schneider J, Fritsche A, Chen J, Humpert P, Stumvoll M, Schleicher E, Häring HU, Nawroth PP, Bierhaus A (2003) Acute (2 h) hyperglycemic clamp causes intracellular formation of carboxymethyllysine, activation of Ras, p42/p44 MAPK and NF-κB in peripheral blood mononuclear cells. Diabetes 52:621-633

Schmidt AM, Mora R, Cap R, Yan SD, Brett J, Ramakrishnan R, Tsang TC, Simionescu M, Stern D (1994) The endothelial cell binding site for advanced glycation end products consists of a complex: an integral membrane protein and a lactoferrin-like polypeptide. J Biol Chem 269:9882-9888

Schmidt AM, Vianna M, Gerlach M, Brett J, Ryan J, Kao Jm Esposito C, Hegarty H, Hurley W, Clauss M, Wang F, Pan YE, Tsang C, Stern D (1992) Isolation and characterisation of two binding proteins gor advanced glycosylation end products from bovine lung which are present on the endothelial cell surface. J Biol Chem 267:14987-14997

Schmidt AM, Yan SD, Brett J, Mora R, Nowygrod R, Stern D (1993) Regulation of human mononuclear phagocyte migration by cell surface-binding proteins for advanced glycation end products. J Clin Invest 91:2155-2168

Schmidt AM, Yan SD, Stern DM (1995) The dark side of glucose. Nat Med 1:1002-1004

Schmidt AM, Yan SD, Yan SF, Stern DM (2001) The multiligand receptor RAGE is a progression factor amplifying immune and inflammatory responses. J Clin Invest 108:949-955

Schneider A, Martin-Villalba A, Weih F, Vogel J, Wirth T, Schwaninger M (1999) NF-kappaB is activated and promotes cell death in focal cerebral ischemia. Nat Med 5:554-559.

Seegers WH: Antithrombin III: theory and clinical applications: H.P. Smith Memorial Lecture. Am J Clin Pathol 1978;69:299-359.

Seguin R, Moditi Z, Rotondo R, Biernacki K, Wosik K, Prat A, Antel JP (2003) Human brain endothelial cells supply support for monocyte immunoregulatory functions. J Neuroimmunol 135:96-106.

Selkoe, D.J. (1991). The molecular pathology of Alzheimer ' s disease. Neuron 6 , 487 - 498.

Semenza GL, Nejfelt MK, Chi SM, Antonarakis SE. Hypoxia-inducible nuclear factors bind to an enhancer element located 3' to the human erythropoietin gene. *Proc Natl Acad Sci USA* 88: 5680-5684, 1991.

Senden NH, Jeunhomme TM, Heemskerk JW, Wagen voord R, van't Veer C, Hemker HC, Buurman WA: Factor Xa induces cytokine production and expression of adhesion molecules by human umbilical vein endothelial cells. J Immunol 1998;161:4318-4324.

Shanmugam N, Kim YS, Lanting L, Natarajan R (2003) Regulation of cyclooxygenase-2 expression in monocytes by ligation of the receptor for advanced glycation end products. J Biol Chem 278:34834-34844

Shen XD, Ke B, Zhai Y, Gao F, Busuttil RW, Cheng G, Kupiec- Weglinski JW (2005) Toll-like receptor and heme oxygenase-1 signaling in hepatic ischemia/reperfusion injury. Am J Transplant 5:1793-1800.

Shi F, Bailey C, Malick AW, Audus KL. Biotin uptake and transport across bovine brain microvessel endothelial cell monolayers. *Pharm Res* 10: 282-288, 1993.

Shi M, Deng W, Bi E, Mao K, Ji Y, Lin G, Wu X, Tao Z, Li Z, Cai X, Sun S, Xiang C, Sun B (2008) TRIM30 alpha negatively regulates TLR-mediated NF-kappa B activation by targeting TAB2 and TAB3 for degradation. Nat Immunol 9:369-377.

Shigeoka AA, Holscher TD, King AJ, Hall FW, Kiosses WB, Tobias PS, Mackman N, McKay DB (2007) TLR2 is constitutively expressed within the kidney and participates in ischemic renal injury through both MyD88- dependent and -independent pathways. J Immunol 178:6252-6258.

Shingo T, Sorokan ST, Shimazaki T, Weiss S. Erythropoietin regulates the in vitro and in vivo production of neuronal progenitors by mammalian forebrain neural stem cells. *J Neurosci* 21: 9733-9743, 2001.

Shinohara M, Thornalley PJ, Giardino I, Beisswenger P, Thorpe SR, Onorato J, Brownlee M (1998) Overexpression of glyoxalase-I in bovine endothelial cells inhibits intracellular advanced glycation endproduct formation and prevents hyperglycemia- induced increases in macromolecule endocytosis. J Clin Invest 101:1142-1147

Shishido T, Nozaki N, Yamaguchi S, Shibata Y, Nitobe J, Miyamoto T, Takahashi H, Arimoto T, Maeda K, Yamakawa M, Takeuchi O, Akira S, Takeishi Y, Kubota I (2003) Toll-like receptor-2 modulates ventricular remodeling after myocardial infarction. Circulation 108: 2905-2910.

Singh AK, Jiang Y (2004) How does peripheral lipopolysaccharide induce gene expression in the brain of rats? Toxicology 201: 197-207.

Siren AL, Ehrenreich H. Erythropoietin: a novel concept for neuroprotection. *Eur Arch Psychiatry Clin Neurosci* 251: 179- 184, 2001.

Siren AL, Fratelli M, Brines M, Goemans C, Casagrande S, Lewczuk P, Keenan S, Gleiter C, Pasquali C, Capobianco A, Mennini T, Heumann R, Cerami A, Ehrenreich H,

Ghezzi P. Erythropoietin prevents neuronal apoptosis after cerebral ischemia and metabolic stress. *Proc Natl Acad Sci USA* 98: 4044–4049, 2001b.

Siren AL, Knerlich F, Poser W, Gleiter CH, Bruck W, Ehrenreich H. Erythropoietin and erythropoietin receptor in human ischemic/hypoxic brain. *Acta Neuropathol (Berl)* 101: 271–276, 2001a.

Sly LM, Rauh MJ, Kalesnikoff J, Song CH, Krystal G (2004) LPSinduced upregulation of SHIP is essential for endotoxin tolerance. Immunity 21:227–239.

Socolovsky M, Fallon AE, Wang S, Brugnara C, Lodish HF. Fetal anemia and apoptosis of red cell progenitors in Stat5a- /-5b-/- mice: a direct role for Stat5 in Bcl-X(L) induction. *Cell* 98: 181–191, 1999.

Sorci G, Riuzzi F, Agneletti AL, Marchetti C, Donato R (2004) S100B causes apoptosis in a myoblast cell line in a RAGEindependent manner. J Cell Physiol 199:274–283

Sorci G, Riuzzi F, Arcuri C, Giambanco I, Donato R (2004) Amphoterin stimulates myogenesis and counteracts the antimyogenic factors basic fibroblast growth factor and S100B via RAGE binding. Mol Cell Biol 24:4880–4894

Souter PJ, Thomas S, Hubbard AR, Poole S, Romish J, Gray E: Antithrombin inhibits lipoopolysaccharide-induced tissue factor and interleukin-6 production by mononuclear cells, human umbilical vein endothelial cells, and whole blood. Crit Care Med 2001;29:134-139.

Spector R, Mock D. Biotin transport through the blood-brain barrier. *J Neurochem* 48: 400–404, 1987.

Spera PA, Ellison JA, Feuerstein GZ, Barone FC (1998) IL-10 reduces rat brain injury following focal stroke. Neurosci Lett 251:189–192.

Stenzel-Poore MP, Stevens SL, King JS, Simon RP (2007) Preconditioning reprograms the response to ischemic injury and primes the emergence of unique endogenous neuroprotective phenotypes: a speculative synthesis. Stroke 38:680–685.

Stenzel-Poore MP, Stevens SL, Xiong Z, Lessov NS, Harrington CA, Mori M, Meller R, Rosenzweig HL, Tobar E, Shaw TE, Chu X, Simon RP (2003) Effect of ischemic preconditioning on genomic response to cerebral ischemia: similarity to neuroprotective strategies in hibernation and hypoxia-tolerant states. Lancet 362:1028–1037.

Stevens SL, Ciesielski TM, Marsh BJ, Yang T, Homen DS, Boule JL, Lessov NS, Simon RP, Stenzel-Poore MP (2008) Toll- like receptor 9: a new target of ischemic preconditioning in the brain. J Cereb Blood Flow Metab 28:1040–1047.

Stewart VC, Giovannoni G, Land JM, McDonald WI, Clark JB, Heales SJ (1997) Pretreatment of astrocytes with interferon-alpha/beta impairs interferon-gamma induction of nitric oxide synthase. J Neurochem 68:2547–2551.

Stewart VC, Land JM, Clark JB, Heales SJ (1998) Pretreatment of astrocytes with interferon-alpha/beta prevents neuronal mitochondrial respiratory chain damage. J Neurochem 70:432–434.

Stroka DM, Burkhardt T, Desbaillets I, Wenger RH, Neil DA, Bauer C, Gassmann M, Candinas D. HIF-1 is expressed in normoxic tissue and displays an organ-specific regulation under systemic hypoxia. *FASEB J* 15: 2445–2453, 2001.

Studer L, Csete M, Lee SH, Kabbani N, Walikonis J, Wold B, McKay R. Enhanced proliferation, survival, and dopaminergic differentiation of CNS precursors in lowered oxygen. *J Neurosci* 20: 7377–7383, 2000.

Sugaya K, Fukagawa T, Matsumoto K, Mita K, Takahashi E, Ando A, Inoko H, Ikemura T (1994) Three genes in the human MHC class III region near the junction with the class II: gene for receptor of advanced glycosylation end products, PBX2 homeobox gene and a notch homolog, human counterpart of mouse mammary tumor gene int- 3. Genomics 23:408–419

Sundt, T.M., Jr., Waltz, A.G., and Sayre, G.P. (1967). Experimental cerebral infarction: modifi cation by treatment with hemodiluting, hemoconcentrating, and dehydrating agents. J. Neurosurg. *26* , 46 – 56.

Swerdlow, R.H., Burns, J.M., and Khan, S.M. (2010). The Alzheimer ' s disease mitochondrial cascade hypothesis. J. Alzheimers Dis. *20* (Suppl. 2), S265 – S279.

Tabernero, A., Medina, A., Sanchez-Abarca, L.I., Lavado, E., and Medina, J.M. (1999). The effect of albumin on astrocyte energy metabolism is not brought about through the control of cytosolic $Ca2+$ concentrations but by free-fatty acid sequestration. Glia *25* , 1 – 9.

Tabernero, A., Velasco, A., Granda, B., Lavado, E.M., and Medina, J.M. (2002). Transcytosis of albumin in astrocytes activates the sterol regulatory element-binding protein-1, which promotes the synthesis of the neurotrophic factor oleic acid. J. Biol. Chem. *277* , 4240 – 4246.

Taguchi A, Blood DC, del Toro G, Canet A, Lee DC, Qu W, Tanji N, Lu Y, Lalla E, Fu C, Hofmann MA, Kislinger T, Ingram M, Lu A, Tanaka H, Hori O, Ogawa S, Stern DM, Schmidt AM (2000) Blockade of RAGE-amphoterin signaling suppresses tumour growth and metastases. Nature 405:354– 360

Takeda K, Akira S (2005) Toll-like receptors in innate immunity. Int Immunol 17:1–14.

Tang, J., Li, Y.J., Mu, J., Li, Q., Yang, D.Y., and Xie, P. (2009). Albumin ameliorates tissue plasminogen activator-mediated blood-brain barrier permeability and ischemic brain injury in rats. Neurol. Res. *31* , 189 – 194.

Tasaki K, Ruetzler CA, Ohtsuki T, Martin D, Nawashiro H, Hallenbeck JM (1997) Lipopolysaccharide pre-treatment induces resistance against subsequent focal cerebral ischemic damage in spontaneously hypertensive rats. Brain Res 748:267– 270.

Teglund S, McKay C, Schuetz E, van Deursen JM, Stravopodis D, Wang D, Brown M, Bodner S, Grosveld G, Ihle JN. Stat5a and Stat5b proteins have essential and nonessential, or redundant, roles in cytokine responses. *Cell* 93: 841–850, 1998.

The Hemodilution in Stroke Study Group. (1989). Hypervolemic hemodilution treatment of acute stroke. Results of a randomized multicenter trial using pentastarch. Stroke *20* , 317 – 323.

Thompson JE, Phillips RJ, Erdjument-Bromage H, Tempst P, Ghosh S (1995) IκB-β regulates the persistent response in a

Thornalley PJ (1998) Cell activation by glycated proteins. AGE receptors, receptor recognition factors and functional classification of AGEs. Cell Mol Biol (Noisy-le-grand) 44:1013–1023

Thornalley PJ (1998) Glutathione-dependent detoxification of alpha-oxoaldehydes by the glyoxalase system: involvement in disease mechanisms and antiproliferative activity of glyoxalase I inhibitors. Chem Biol Interact 111:137–151

Thornalley PJ, Langborg A, Minhas HS (1999) Formation of glyoxal, methylglyoxal and 3-deoxyglucosone in the glycation of proteins by glucose. Biochem J 344(Pt 1):109–116

Tilghman, S.M. and Belayew, A. (1982). Transcriptional control of the murine albumin/alpha-fetoprotein locus during development. Proc. Natl. Acad. Sci. USA 79 , 5254 – 5257.

Tobias PS, Curtiss LK (2007) Toll-like receptors in atherosclerosis. Biochem Soc Trans 35:1453–1455.

Tracey KJ, Andersson J, Palmblad JE (2003) High mobility group 1 B-box mediates activation of human endothelium. J Intern Med 254:375–385

Treutiger CJ, Mullins GE, Johansson AS, Rouhiainen A, Rauvala HM, Erlandsson-Harris H, Andersson U, Yang H,

Truettner J, Busto R, Zhao W, Ginsberg MD, Perez-Pinzon MA (2002) Effect of ischemic preconditioning on the expression of putative neuroprotective genes in the rat brain. Brain Res Mol Brain Res 103:106–115.

Tsukumo DM, Carvalho-Filho MA, Carvalheira JB, Prada PO, Hirabara SM, Schenka AA, Araujo EP, Vassallo J, Curi R, Velloso LA, Saad MJ (2007) Loss-of-function mutation in Toll-like receptor 4 prevents dietinduced obesity and insulin resistance. Diabetes 56:1986–1998.

Uchiba M, Okajima K, Murakami K, Okabe H, Takatsuki K: Attenuation of endotoxin-induced pulmonary vascular injury by antithrombin III. Am J Physiol 1996;270:L921-L930.

Uchiba M, Okajima K, Murakami K: Effects of various doses of antithrombin on endotoxin-induced endothelial cell injury and coagulation abnormalities in rats. Thromb Res 1998;89:233-241.

van Vliet, E.A., da Costa Araujo, S., Redeker, S., van Schaik, R., Aronica, E., and Gorter, J.A. (2007). Blood-brain barrier leakage may lead to progression of temporal lobe epilepsy. Brain 130, 521 – 534.

Veldhuis W, Derksen J, Floris S, van der Meide P, de Vries H, Schepers J, Vos I, Dijkstra C, Kappelle L, Nicolay K, Bar P (2003a) Interferon-beta blocks infiltration of inflammatory cells and reduces infarct volume after ischemic stroke in the rat. J Cereb Blood Flow Metab 23:1029–1039.

Veldhuis WB, Floris S, van der Meide PH, Vos IM, de Vries HE, Dijkstra CD, Bar PR, Nicolay K (2003b) Interferon-beta prevents cytokine-induced neutrophil infiltration and attenuates blood-brain barrier disruption. J Cereb Blood Flow Metab 23:1060–1069.

Villa P, Bigini P, Mennini T, Agnello D, Laragione T, Cagnotto A, Viviani B, Marinovich M, Cerami A, Coleman TR, Brines M, Ghezzi P. Erythropoietin selectively attenuates cytokine production and inflammation in cerebral ischemia by targeting neuronal apoptosis. J Exp Med 198: 971–975, 2003.

Vlassara H, Brownlee M, Cerami A (1985) High affinity receptor mediated uptake and degradation of glucose modified proteins: a potential mechanism for the removal of senescent macromolecules. Proc Natl Acad Sci U S A 82:5588–5592

Vlassara H, Bucala R, Striker L (1994) Pathogenetic effects of advanced glycosylation: biochemical, biologic and clinical implications for diabetes and aging. Lab Invest 70:138–151

Vogel SN, Fitzgerald KA, Fenton MJ (2003) TLRs: differential adapter utilization by toll-like receptors mediates TLR- specific patterns of gene expression. Mol Intervent 3:466–477.

174 Preclinical Aspects of Ischemic Stroke

Wang H, Bloom O, Zhang M, Vishnubhakat JM, Ombellino M, Che J, Frazier A, Yang H,
    Ivanova S, Borovikova L, Manogue KR, Faist E, Abraham E, Andersson J,
    Andersson U, Molina PE., Abumrad NN, Sama A, Tracey KJ (1999) HMG-1 as a late
    mediator of endotoxin lethality in mice. Science 285:248–251
Wang L, Zhang Z, Wang Y, Zhang R, Chopp M. Treatment of stroke with erythropoietin
    enhances neurogenesis and angiogenesis and improves neurological function in
    rats. Stroke 35: 1732–1737, 2004.
Wautier MP, Chappey O, Corda S, Stern DM, Schmidt AM, Wautier JL (2001) Activation of
    NADPH oxidase by AGE links oxidant stress to altered gene expression via RAGE.
    Am J Physiol Endocrinol Metab 280:E685–E694
Wendt TM, Tanji N, Kislinger TR, Qu W, Lu Y, Bucciarelli LG, Rong L, Bierhaus A, Nawroth
    PP, Moser B, Markowitz GS, Stein G, Dágati V, Stern DM, Schmidt AM (2003)
    RAGE drives the development of glomerulosclerosis and implicates podocyte
    activation in the pathogenesis of diabetic nephropathy. Am J Pathol 162:1123–1137
Wenger RH. Cellular adaptation to hypoxia: O2-sensing protein hydroxylases, hypoxia-
    inducible transcription factors, and O2-regulated gene expression. FASEB J 16:
    1151–1162, 2002.
Wenger RH. Mammalian oxygen sensing, signalling and gene regulation. J Exp Biol 203:
    1253–1263, 2000.
Witko-Sarsat V, Rieu P, Descamps-Latscha B, Lesavre P, Halbwachs-Mecarelli L.
    Neutrophils: molecules, functions and pathophysiological aspects. Lab Invest 80:
    617–653, 2000.
Wood, J.H. and Kee, D.B., Jr. (1985). Hemorheology of the cerebral circulation in stroke.
    Stroke 16 , 765 – 772.
Wu LY, Ding AS, Zhao T, Ma ZM, Wang FZ, Fan M (2004) Involvement of increased
    stability of mitochondrial membrane potential and overexpression of Bcl-2 in
    enhanced anoxic tolerance induced by hypoxic preconditioning in cultured
    hypothalamic neurons. Brain Res 999:149–154.
Yadav JS, Wholey MH, Kuntz RE, Fayad P, Katzen BT, Mishkel GJ, Bajwa TK, Whitlow P,
    Strickman NE, Jaff MR, Popma JJ, Snead DB, Cutlip DE, Firth BG, Ouriel K (2004)
    Protected carotid-artery stenting versus endarterectomy in high-risk patients. N
    Engl J Med 351:1493–1501.
Yajima N, Yamamoto Y, Yamamoto H, Takeuchi M, Yaghihashi S (2004) Peripheral
    neuropathy in diabetic mice overexpressing receptor for advanced glycation
    endproducts (RAGE). Collected abstracts of the 8th International Symposium on
    the Maillard reaction (Charleston, SC): no. SXI-7; 55
Yamaji R, Okada T, Moriya M, Naito M, Tsuruo T, Miyatake K, Nakano Y. Brain capillary
    endothelial cells express two forms of erythropoietin receptor mRNA. Eur J Biochem
    239: 494–500, 1996.
Yamamoto Y, Kazio I, Doi T et al (2001) Development and prevention of advanced diabetic
    nephropathy in RAGE- overexpressing mice. J Clin Invest 108:261–268
Yamashiro K, Kiryu J, Tsujikawa A, Honjo M, Nonaka A, Miyamoto K, Honda Y, Tanihara
    H, Ogura Y: Inhibitory effects of antithrombin III against leukocyte rolling and
    infiltration during endotoxin-induced uveitis in rats. Invest Ophthalmol Vis Sci
    2001;42:1553-1560.

Yamauchi T, Umeda F, Inoguchi T, Nawata H: Antithrombin III stimulates prostecyclin production by cultured aortic endothelial cells. Biochem Biophys Res Commun 1989;163:1404-1411.

Yan SD, Chen X, Fu J, Chen M, Zhu H, Roher A, Slattery T, Zhao L, Nagashima M, Morser J, Migheli A, Nawroth P, Stern D, Schmidt AM (1996) RAGE and amyloid-beta peptide neurotoxicity in Alzheimer's disease. Nature 382:685-691

Yan SD, Zhu H, Zhu A, Golabek A, Du H, Roher A, Yu J, Soto C, Schmidt AM, Stern D, Kindy M (2000) Receptor dependent cell stress and amyloid accumulation in systemic amyloidosis. Nat Med 6:643-651

Yao, X., Miao, W., Li, M., Wang, M., Ma, J., Wang, Y., Miao, L., and Feng, H. (2010). Protective effect of albumin on VEGF and brain edema in acute ischemia in rats. Neurosci. Lett. 472 , 179 -183.

Yasuda Y, Masuda S, Chikuma M, Inoue K, Nagao M, Sasaki R. Estrogen-dependent production of erythropoietin in uterus and its implication in uterine angiogenesis. J Biol Chem 273: 25381-25387, 1998.

Yeh CH, Sturgis L, Haidacher J, Zhang XN, Sherwood SJ, Bjercke RJ, Juhasz O, Crow MT, Tilton RG, Denner L (2001) Requirement for p38 and p44/p42 mitogen-activated protein kinases in RAGE-mediated nuclear factor-kappaB transcriptional activation and cytokine secretion. Diabetes 50:1495-1504

Yeh HJ, He YY, Xu J, Hsu CY, Deuel TF (1998) Upregulation of pleiotrophin gene expression in developing microvasculature, macrophages, and astrocytes after acute ischemic brain injury. J Neurosci 18:3699-3707.

Yu X, Shacka JJ, Eells JB, Suarez-Quian C, Przygodzki RM, Beleslin-Cokic B, Lin CS, Nikodem VM, Hempstead B, Flanders KC, Costantini F, Noguchi CT. Erythropoietin receptor signalling is required for normal brain development. Development 129: 505-516, 2002.

Yusuf S, Reddy S, Ounpuu S, Anand S (2001a) Global burden of cardiovascular diseases: part I: general considerations, the epidemiologic transition, risk factors, and impact of urbanization. Circulation 104:2746-2753.

Yusuf S, Reddy S, Ounpuu S, Anand S (2001b) Global burden of cardiovascular diseases: part II: variations in cardiovascular disease by specific ethnic groups and geographic regions and prevention strategies. Circulation 104:2855-2864.

Zarember KA, Godowski PJ (2002) Tissue expression of human Toll-like receptors and differential regulation of Toll-like receptor mRNAs in leukocytes in response to microbes, their products, and cytokines. J Immunol 168:554-561.

Zhai Y, Shen XD, O'Connell R, Gao F, Lassman C, Busuttil RW, Cheng G, Kupiec-Weglinski JW (2004) Cutting edge: TLR4 activation mediates liver ischemia/reperfusion inflammatory response via IFN regulatory factor 3- dependent MyD88-independent pathway. J Immunol 173:7115-7119.

Zhan RZ, Fujihara H, Baba H, Yamakura T, Shimoji K (2002) Ischemic preconditioning is capable of inducing mitochondrial tolerance in the rat brain. Anesthesiology 97:896-901.

Zhang F, Wang S, Cao G, Gao Y, Chen J. Signal transducers and activators of transcription 5 contributes to erythropoietin-mediated neuroprotection against hippocampal neuronal death after transient global cerebral ischemia. Neurobiol Dis 25: 45-53, 2007.

Zhang W, Potrovita I, Tarabin V, Herrmann O, Beer V, Weih F, Schneider A, Schwaninger M (2005) Neuronal activation of NFkappaB contributes to cell death in cerebral ischemia. J Cereb Blood Flow Metab 25:30–40.

Zhang X, Shan P, Jiang G, Cohn L, Lee PJ (2006) Toll-like receptor 4 deficiency causes pulmonary emphysema. J Clin Invest 116: 3050–3059.

Zhou ML, Shi JX, Hang CH, Zhang FF, Gao J, Yin HX (2007) Expression of Toll-like receptor 4 in the brain in a rabbit experimental subarachnoid haemorrhage model. Inflamm Res 56:93–97.

Ziegler G, Harhausen D, Schepers C, Hoffmann O, Rohr C, Prinz V, Konig J, Lehrach H, Nietfeld W, Trendelenburg G (2007) TLR2 has a detrimental role in mouse transient focal cerebral ischemia. Biochem Biophys Res Comm 359:574–579.

7

The Na$^+$/H$^+$ Exchanger-1 as a New Molecular Target in Stroke Interventions

Vishal Chanana[1], Dandan Sun[2] and Peter Ferrazzano[1,3]
[1]Waisman Center, University of Wisconsin, Madison, WI
[2]Dept. of Neurology, University of Pittsburgh, Pittsburgh, PA
[3]Dept. of Pediatrics, University of Wisconsin, Madison, WI
USA

1. Introduction

Loss of ion homeostasis plays an important role in the pathogenesis of ischemic cell damage. Ischemia induces accumulation of intracellular Na$^+$ ([Na$^+$]$_i$) and Ca^{2+} ([Ca^{2+}]$_i$), and subsequent activation of proteases, phospholipases, and formation of oxygen and nitrogen free radicals. The Na$^+$/H$^+$ exchanger (NHEs) family is a group of secondary active membrane transport proteins that catalyze the electroneutral exchange of Na$^+$ for H$^+$ and is important in restoring intracellular pH (pH$_i$) after ischemia-induced intracellular acidosis. Nine isoforms of NHE (NHE1-9) have been identified in mammalian tissues (Orlowski & Grinstein, 2004). These isoforms differ in their tissue expression, subcellular distribution, kinetic properties, inhibitor sensitivity, and physiological functions. NHE-1 is ubiquitously expressed on the plasma membrane of virtually all mammalian cell types (Sardet et al., 1989). NHE-2-4 are expressed on the plasma membrane, predominantly in the epithelia of the kidney and gastrointestinal tract (Orlowski & Grinstein, 2004). NHE-3 is the only isoform known to recycle between the plasma membrane and the endosomal compartment (D'Souza et al., 1998). NHE-5 expression is concentrated in neurons (Attaphitaya et al., 1999) and may modulate the pH of synaptic vesicles (Szaszi et al., 2002). NHE-6 and NHE-9 are expressed predominantly in endosomal vesicles (Nakamura et al., 2005) and NHE-7 localizes to the trans-Golgi network and associated endosomes (Numata & Orlowski, 2001). NHE-8 has been localized to the plasma membrane of renal proximal tubule epithelial cells, and to endosomal vesicles and the trans-Golgi network (Goyal et al., 2003; Nakamura et al., 2005).

NHE-1 is the most extensively studied isoform, and the most abundant isoform in the CNS (Ma & Haddad, 1997; Orlowski et al., 1992). Research over the past two decades has expanded our understanding of the role of NHE-1 beyond that of simply maintenance of ion homeostasis and cell volume, to an emerging picture of a regulator of many cell functions. NHE-1 plays a role in regulation of cell proliferation, migration (Bussolino et al., 1989), and the microglial respiratory burst (Liu et al., 2010). NHE-1 protein consists of 815 amino acids with a calculated molecular weight of 85 kDa. However, NHE-1 has an apparent size of ~110 kDa due to its N- and O- linked glycosylation in the extracellular loop 1. NHE-1 has two large functional domains, the highly conserved amphipathic N-terminal domain (~500 amino acids), which is responsible for cation translocation, and a less conserved hydrophilic cytoplasmic C-terminal domain (~315 amino acids), which is crucial for modulating NHE-1 activity (Putney et al., 2002). Activation of NHE-1 has been shown to be a pivotal event in cell damage induced by ischemia and reperfusion in the brain (Horikawa et al., 2001; Hwang et al., 2008; Luo et al., 2005), heart (Liu et al., 1997; Murphy et al., 1991; Wang et al., 2003), liver (Gores et al., 1989), and lungs (Rios et al., 2005). Here we will review recent findings implicating NHE-1 activation as a critical event in the pathogenesis of cellular dysfunction after cerebral ischemia, and the growing evidence supporting the use of NHE inhibitors as neuroprotective agents following cerebral ischemia.

2. Na$^+$/H$^+$ Exchanger isoform-1 (NHE-1) in cerebral ischemia

Ischemia and reperfusion injury is a complex and incompletely understood phenomenon. Ischemia deprives the cell of the energy required for normal cell function and leads to loss of ionic homeostasis within the cell due to opening of ionotropic glutamate receptors (Nishizawa, 2001) and acid sensing non-glutamate-dependent channels (Xiong et al., 2004), as well as activation of ion transport proteins such as NHE-1, Na$^+$/K$^+$/Cl$^-$ cotransporter (NKCCl) (Chen et al., 2005), and the Na$^+$/Ca^{2+} exchanger (NCXs) (Hoyt et al., 1998). Reperfusion triggers a cascade of intracellular events including release of reactive oxygen species (ROS) and inflammatory mediators, which exacerbate injury and promote cell death. Ischemia and reperfusion induces intracellular acidosis due to a shift from aerobic to anaerobic glycolysis, and leads to an increase in $[Na^+]_i$ and $[Ca^{2+}]_i$ by mechanisms that include the activation of acid responsive ion transporters (Yao & Haddad, 2004). Recent findings from our group and others highlight the important role of NHE-1 in pH$_i$ regulation after cerebral ischemia and reperfusion.

2.1 NHE-1 mediated intracellular pH regulation

To regulate and maintain constant pH$_i$, eukaryotic cells express plasma membrane ion transporters such as NHE-1 that protect cells from internal acidification by exchanging extracellular Na$^+$ for intracellular H$^+$ (Luo et al., 2005). At physiological pH$_i$, NHE-1 is essentially inactive, despite the large inward Na$^+$ gradient established by Na$^+$/K$^+$- ATPase. However, upon exposure to intracellular acidification, NHE-1 is rapidly activated and uses the electrochemical gradient of Na$^+$ to pump H$^+$ out of the cell and restore pH$_i$. Upon restoration of pH$_i$, NHE-1 activity returns to steady state levels (Pedersen, 2006). Extracellular acidification (low pH$_o$) or removal of extracellular sodium suppresses this gradient-driven Na$^+$/H$^+$ exchange (Bobulescu et al., 2005). While NHE-1 serves to maintain homeostasis in the face of normal pH$_i$ fluctuations (which result from changes in metabolic activity), profound acidosis after anoxia can induce a NHE-1 mediated parodoxic alkalinization, a so-called "overshoot" of pH$_i$ restoration. We reported that post-anoxia alkalinization is ablated by pharmacological inhibition of NHE-1 and removal of extracellular sodium (Kintner et al., 2005). Protein kinase inhibitors attenuate this alkalinization, suggesting that activation of NHE-1 involves protein phosphorylation and multiple up-stream regulatory pathways such as extracellular signal-regulated kinases (ERK 1/2), protein kinase A (PKA), and protein kinase C (PKC) (Kintner et al., 2005; Luo et al., 2007; Yao et al., 2001).

2.2 Ionic homeostasis and brain cell function

Secondary active ion transport proteins are important in maintaining steady-state intracellular ion concentrations. NHE-1 plays an important role in regulation of many cellular processes in addition to pH_i and cell volume regulation, such as cell growth, proliferation and differentiation, cell migration and adhesion, cellular immunity, and as cytoskeletal scaffolding for the assembly of intracellular signaling complexes (De Vito, 2006; Luo & Sun, 2007; Luo et al., 2005; Meima et al., 2007; Orlowski & Grinstein, 2004; Pedersen et al., 2006; Xue & Haddad, 2010). Due to their high metabolic rate and rapid changes in metabolic demand, neurons are exposed to frequent fluctuations in pH_i, making efficient acid extrusion mechanisms essential for normal neuronal function. Neurons and astrocytes from mice deficient in the NHE-1 protein (NHE-1⁻/⁻) demonstrate decreased basal pH_i and are unable to recover from an acid load (Luo et al., 2005). NHE-1 is the predominant NHE isoform in the CNS (Ma & Haddad, 1997; Orlowski et al., 1992), and as evidence of its importance in normal neurologic function, NHE-1⁻/⁻ mice exhibit severe neurologic defects and seizures (Bell et al., 1999; Gu et al., 2001).

2.3 Role of NHE-1 in cellular dysfunction and cerebral injury during *in vivo* ischemia

Results from *in vivo* experimental studies support the importance of ion transport proteins in ischemia-mediated loss of ion homeostasis. NHE-1 activity in astrocytes (Cengiz et al., 2010), neurons (Manhas et al., 2010), and microglia (Shi et al., 2011) is stimulated following cerebral ischemia. Excessive stimulation of NHE-1 leads to intracellular Na⁺ overload, and in turn causes a rise in intracellular Ca^{2+} due to increased Ca^{2+} influx via reversal of the Na/Ca exchanger. Thus, NHE-1 activity contributes to cerebral ischemic damage in part by disruption of intracellular Na⁺ and Ca^{2+} homeostasis, an event which is characterized by rapid influx of Ca^{2+} and subsequent cell death.

2.3.1 Global ischemia

Global cerebral ischemia entails diminution in cerebral blood flow (CBF) over the entire brain, and is encountered clinically in cardiac arrest. On restoration of CBF, a secondary reperfusion brain injury may occur due to altered ionic homeostasis, increases in ROS, cerebral edema, and inflammatory cascades (Schaller & Graf, 2004). The contribution of NHE-1 activity to global cerebral ischemia has been reported in a number of animal models. In a gerbil model of transient forebrain ischemia, NHE-1 immunoreactivity was markedly increased in CA1 pyramidal neurons as well as in glial cells 4 days following injury, and inhibition of NHE protected CA1 pyramidal neurons and attenuated the activation of astrocytes and microglia (Hwang et al., 2008). Yorkshire-Duroc pigs treated with cariporide (HOE 642), a potent and selective inhibitor of NHE-1, at the onset of a 90 min deep hypothermic circulatory arrest demonstrated improved neurologic recovery (Castellá et al., 2005). Similarly, inhibition of NHE-1 with N-[aminoiminomethyl]-1-methyl-1H-indole-2-carboxamide methanesulfonate (SM-20220) improved neurologic function in a gerbil model of transient global cerebral ischemia (Kuribayashi et al., 2000). Administration of the NHE-1 inhibitor ethylisopropylamiloride (EIPA) prior to bilateral carotid artery occlusion in gerbils resulted in decreased hippocampal neuronal cell death and improved neurologic function (Phillis et al., 1999).

2.3.2 Focal ischemia

Unlike global cerebral ischemia, focal cerebral ischemia entails reduction in regional CBF in a specific vascular territory and is usually encountered clinically as an "ischemic stroke" due to thromboembolic or vaso-occlusive disease. An abundance of *in vivo* studies support the importance of NHE-1 in focal ischemia. The NHE-1 inhibitor SM-20220 reduces infarct size in both transient and permanent focal ischemia models (Kuribayashi et al., 1999). Another NHE inhibitor, Sabiporide, reduces infarct size and edema volume when administered before or after ischemia (Park et al., 2005).

Our investigations into the role of NHE-1 in cerebral ischemia have used both genetic and pharmacologic inhibition of NHE-1 in a mouse transient middle cerebral artery occlusion model (MCAO). Mice treated with HOE 642, a potent and selective inhibitor of NHE-1, prior to MCAO demonstrated a 35% reduction in infarct volume compared to vehicle treated controls. NHE-1 heterozygous mice (NHE-1$^{+/-}$), which demonstrate a ~ 70% reduction in NHE-1 protein expression, exhibited a similar reduction in infarct volumes, establishing the importance of NHE-1 over other NHE isoforms in the CNS (Luo et al., 2005; Wang et al., 2008). With T2-weighted and Diffusion Weighted MRI, we further confirmed that NHE-1$^{+/+}$ mice treated with HOE 642 immediately prior to reperfusion or 60 minutes post-reperfusiion, exhibited a significant reduction in infarct volume compared to NHE-1$^{+/+}$ vehicle control mice. NHE-1$^{+/-}$ mice demonstrated a significant reduction in infarct volume on T2 MRI at 72 hours after injury (Ferrazzano et al., 2011). These findings suggest that elevated NHE-1 activity contributes to neuronal injury following ischemia and reperfusion. We subsequently revealed that focal cerebral ischemia triggers a transient stimulation of the extracellular signal-regulated kinase/p90 ribosomal S6 kinase (ERK/p90^{RSK}) pathway that contributes to ischemic damage in part via phosphorylation of NHE-1 protein (Manhas et al., 2010). The NHE-1-mediated [Na$^+$]$_i$ overload causes reverse function of the Na$^+$/Ca^{2+} exchanger, elevating [Ca^{2+}]$_i$ and enhancing the p38 mitogen-activated protein kinase (MAPK) and/or nuclear factor kappa-light-chain-enhancer of activated B cells (NF-kB) (Liu et al., 2010). NHE-1 activity also plays a detrimental role in mitochondrial Ca^{2+} overload and mitochondrial dysfunction after ischemia as evidenced by attenuation of ischemia-induced cytochrome C release from mitochondria after NHE-1 inhibition (Wang et al., 2008). Interestingly, when NHE-1 activity is blocked either pharmacologically or by genetic knockdown, microglia activation and proinflammatory cytokine formation is significantly reduced in ischemic brains after MCAO (Shi et al., 2011). Taken together, these results strongly support that NHE-1 is activated after cerebral ischemia and worsens ischemic brain injury.

2.3.3 Hypoxia/Ischemia

Hypoxia-ischemia (HI) is a common cause of brain injury in neonates (Ferriero, 2004). We recently investigated the role of NHE-1 using a mouse model of neonatal hypoxia-ischemia as described by Vannucci (Vannucci & Vannucci, 2005). In these studies, post-natal day 9 mice (P9) underwent unilateral carotid artery ligation and subsequent exposure to 55 minutes of 8% O$_2$. Following carotid ligation, mice were treated with HOE 642 either immediately before or 10 minutes following exposure to hypoxia (Cengiz et al., 2010). Following HI, vehicle-treated control brains exhibited astrogliosis in the ipsilateral hippocampus, and reactive astrocytes expressed an abundant level of NHE-1. Inhibition of NHE-1 before or after HI resulted in decreased neurodegeneration in striatum, thalamus and hippocampus and improved performance on tests of motor learning and memory (Cengiz et al., 2010). These findings suggest that NHE-1 mediated disruption of ionic homeostasis can contribute to CA1 pyramidal neuronal injury after neonatal HI. Moreover, T2 weighted and Diffusion Tensor (DTI) MRI revealed that NHE-1 inhibition with HOE 642 after HI resulted in improved white matter injury in the corpus callosum, which correlated with improvements in memory and learning (Cengiz et al., 2011).

2.4 Role of NHE-1 in cellular dysfunction during *in vitro* ischemia

Extensive *in vitro* studies have established that ischemia stimulates NHE-1 by reduction in pH_i or via signaling pathways such as ERK-p90^{rsk}, PKA or PKC (Dunbar & Caplan, 2001; Herrera et al., 1994; Kintner et al., 2007a; Li et al., 2004). The role of NHE-1 in cerebral ischemia has been mainly examined in two types of *in vitro* ischemic models, oxygen glucose deprivation/reoxygenation (OGD/REOX) or the hypoxic, acidic, ion-shifted Ringers's solution (HAIR). Superfused brain slices also represent a useful preparation to study acid-base disturbance that occurs in the mammalian brain during *in vitro* ischemic conditions.

2.4.1 Cell cultures

NHE-1 activity is stimulated during *in vitro* ischemia and subsequent reoxygenation and contributes substantially to neuronal and glial cell injury. Acutely isolated CA1 neurons exhibit a tri-phasic response to 5 minutes of anoxia. During anoxia, an initial acidification progresses to alkalinization that is followed by further alkalinization on exposure to reoxygenation. This alkalinization is attenuated by reduction of external pH, removal of extracellular sodium, or inhibition of NHE-1 (Sheldon & Church, 2002; Yao et al., 2001). Additionally, inhibition of PKA can block post-anoxia alkalinization, suggesting cAMP-dependent signaling pathways for NHE-1 activation (Sheldon & Church, 2002).

We have demonstrated that NHE-1 is essential in pH_i regulation using an internal acid load in cultured cortical neurons (Luo et al., 2005). Additionally, we found that activation of NHE-1 after OGD/REOX results in a significant increase in neuronal $[Na^+]_i$. This rise in $[Na^+]_i$ following OGD is significantly attenuated in HOE 642-treated or NHE-1$^{-/-}$ neurons, and cell death is reduced (Luo et al., 2005). In a separate study, we demonstrated that NHE-1-mediated Na^+ entry leads to reverse activation of the Na^+/Ca^{2+} exchanger (NCX_{rev}) and rise in $[Ca^{2+}]_i$, which contribute to the selective dendritic vulnerability to *in vitro* ischemia (Kintner et al., 2010). Taken together, our studies suggest that NHE-1 activity in neurons is significantly stimulated in response to the metabolic acidification associated with an ischemic insult. This ischemia-induced increase in NHE-1 activity causes intracellular Na^+ and Ca^{2+} overload, and eventually leads to cell death.

In another series of studies, we examined the role of NHE-1 in ischemic astrocyte damage using OGD/REOX in cultured cortical astrocytes and found that NHE-1 is the primary pH regulatory mechanism after ischemia. Astrocyte NHE-1 activity is increased by ~ 1.8 fold during REOX (Kintner et al., 2004), and depends on ERK1/2 signaling pathways (Kintner et al., 2005). OGD/REOX results in a drop in pH_i by 0.29 pH units (Kintner et al., 2004), and inhibition of NHE-1 results in a further decrease of pH_i. Additionally, we observed that OGD/REOX triggers a ~5-fold increase in $[Na^+]_i$ and 26% increase in astrocyte cell volume. This increase in $[Na^+]_i$ and cell swelling are significantly reduced either with HOE 642 treatment or in NHE-1$^{-/-}$ astrocytes (Kintner et al., 2004). Using the HAIR model in astrocytes, we found a similar increase in $[Na^+]_i$ which could be abolished by the NHE-1 inhibitor HOE 642 (Kintner et al., 2007b). It has been reported that the expected rise in $[Ca^{2+}]_i$ after HAIR exposure is inhibited by NHE-1 inhibition with HOE 694 (Bondarenko et al., 2005). Taken together, these results indicate that NHE-1 activity raises $[Na^+]_i$ which fosters reversal of the Na^+/Ca^+ exchanger leading to increased intracellular Ca^{2+} and astrocyte cell death.

More recently, new evidence supports a role of NHE-1 in microglial pH_i regulation. Microglia activation by lipopolysaccharide (LPS), phorbol myristate acetate (PMA), or OGD/REOX triggers a concurrent stimulation of NHE-1 and NADPH oxidase (Liu et al., 2010). The elevation in NHE-1-mediated H^+ extrusion prevents intracellular acidosis, allowing for sustained NADPH oxidase function (Liu et al., 2010). Moreover, the coupling of NHE-1 activation with NCX_{rev} activates $[Na^+]_i$ and $[Ca^{2+}]_i$ dependent signaling, which promotes the microglial respiratory burst and production of proinflammatory cytokines (Liu et al., 2010).

2.4.2 Brain slice

Few studies have used brain slice preparations to examine acid-base homeostatic disturbances during ischemia. In hippocampal slices, hypoxia induces a significant drop in both pH_i and pH_o, and a brief alkaline peak is also occasionally observed (Fujiwara et al., 1992; Melzian et al., 1996; Roberts & Chih, 1997). In slice preparations from various brain regions, hypoxia causes acidosis with an approximately 0.8-1.2 pH_i unit drop (Ballanyi et al, 1996; Knopfel et al., 1998; Pirttila & Kauppinen, 1994). Cytosolic calcium changes are observed during ischemia in cortical brain slices that can be only partially inhibited by combined blockade of ion channels (Bickler and Hansen, 1994). Only one report shows a direct involvement of NHE mediated pH_i regulation in slice preparations. In brainstem slices from neonatal rats exposed to 10 minutes of anoxia, intracellular pH drops by 0.1-0.3 pH units in neurons. Inhibition of NHE with amiloride increases this anoxia-induced intracellular acidification (Chambers-Kersh et al., 2000).

2.5 NHE-1 inhibitors and potential therapies

Despite decades of research, the effective treatment and prevention of cerebral ischemic injury remains challenging. Inhibition of NHE-1 with either pharmacological agents or genetic ablation has been demonstrated to significantly reduce brain damage after ischemic insult, in both *in vitro* and *in vivo* models. These encouraging findings suggest the potential use of NHE inhibitors as neuroprotective therapies after cerebral ischemia.

2.5.1 Pharmacological approach

Two major classes of pharmacological agents are currently used to inhibit NHE-1 activity (Putney et al., 2002). The first class of drugs includes amiloride and its 5' alkyl-substituted derivatives (Counillon et al., 1993; Yu et al., 1993), such as ethylisopropylamiloride (EIPA), dimethylamiloride (DMA), 5-N (methylpropyl)amiloride (MPA), 5-(N-methyl-N-isobutyl)-amiloride (MIBA), and 5-(N, N-hexamethylene) amiloride (HMA). These agents are more effective inhibitors of NHE-1 than amiloride but have relatively weak selectivity toward NHE-1. The simultaneous replacement of the pyrazine ring by a phenyl and of the 6-chloro by sulfomethyl leads to another class of inhibitors that includes the benzoylguanidines and derivatives such as HOE 694 (Counillon et al., 1993) and HOE 642 (cariporide) (Scholz et al.,

1995). Both classes are more specific for NHE-1 than NHE-3, with the amiloride compounds demonstrating $\sim 10^2$-fold increased specificity and the HOE compounds $\sim 10^3$- to 10^5-fold more NHE-1 specificity. The HOE compounds are viewed as the most promising agents for treatment of ischemia-reperfusion injury due to their selectivity for NHE-1, and excellent solubility, resorption, and bioavailability profiles (Scholz et al., 1999; Baumgarth et al., 1997; Xue & Haddad, 2010). HOE compounds are competitive inhibitors of Na⁺ binding at the extracellular cation-binding site (Baumgarth et al., 1997; Counillon et al., 1993; Kinsella & Aronson, 1981; Mahnensmith & Aronson, 1985), while the amiloride derivatives also act non-competitively (Warnock et al., 1988). More recently, several new molecules have been designed as potential NHE blockers based on the bicyclic template, including SM-20220, SM-20550, BMS-284640, T-162559, and TY-12533, which have also shown promising results in *in vivo* studies of cerebral ischemia (Kitayama et al., 2001). The IC_{50} for the human NHE-1 are as follows: Amiloride = 10.7 μM, Cariporide = 0.08 μM, T-165229 = 13 nM. Importantly, the NHE inhibitors HOE 642 and SM-20220 not only reduce cell death and edema, but also improve neurological function in *in vivo* ischemia models, and have demonstrated benefits when administered after ischemia (Kintner et al., 2007b; Kuribayashi et al., 2000).

2.5.2 Transgenic approach
While pharmacological studies indicate that NHE-1 plays a central role in cerebral ischemia-reperfusion injury, the use of pharmacologic inhibitors to study ion transport function raises questions regarding dosing, absorption, species specific T1/2, and non-specific effects. For this reason, confirmation by an alternative method using NHE-1 knockdown mice is warranted. NHE 1⁻/⁻ mice exhibit neurologic abnormalities, seizures, ataxia, and growth retardation, and do not survive into adulthood (Bell et al., 1999; Gu et al., 2001). Therefore, NHE-1⁻/⁻ mice are useful for cultures of NHE-1 null neurons, astrocytes and microglia, but cannot be used for *in vivo* studies. NHE-1⁺/⁻ mice express <50% of NHE-1 protein levels, and are useful for *in vivo* studies of the role of NHE function after cerebral ischemia. A marked decrease of infarct volume, microglial activation and proinflammatory cytokine formation is found in NHE-1⁺/⁻ mice after MCAO (Luo et al., 2005). NHE-1 ⁺/⁻ and NHE-1 ⁻/⁻ cortical neurons and astrocytes demonstrate decreased cell death after OGD/REOX (Luo et al., 2005).
The fact that NHE-1 inhibitors applied during or after cerebral ischemia protect the brain against ischemic damage is now well established in animal studies. Despite the uniformity of results from animal models, a number of challenges remain before NHE-1 inhibitors can be translated into clinical use. Questions regarding safety, optimal dose, and timing of administration remain to be addressed, and large animal studies demonstrating improved functional outcomes are still lacking.

3. Conclusion

NHE-1 plays a pivotal role in maintaining tissue ionic homeostasis under normal physiological conditions. However, excessive stimulation of NHE-1 appears to be a major contributor to cellular damage in ischemic conditions. The proposed mechanism for injury induced by NHE-1 activation includes accumulation of $[Na^+]_i$, subsequent $[Ca^{2+}]_i$ overload via reverse activation of the Na^+/Ca^{2+} exchanger, and eventual cell death. Additionally, activation of MAPKs, and release of excitatory amino acids and ROS also contribute to cell damage and death after ischemia. NHE-1 inhibitors have been demonstrated to be neuroprotective in both *in vitro* and *in vivo* ischemia models, making NHE-1 an attractive therapeutic target for cerebral ischemia. Thus, mechanisms of NHE-1 activation in ischemia continue to present an interesting focus for future research in this field.

4. Acknowledgment

This work was supported by NIH grants R01NS48216 and R01NS38118 (D. Sun), 1UL1RR025011 from the Clinical and Translational Science Award (CTSA) program of the National Center for Research Resources (NCRR) (P. Ferrazzano), and P30HD03352 (Waisman Center).

5. References

Attaphitaya, S., Park, K. & Melvin, J.E. (1999). Molecular cloning and functional expression of a rat Na$^+$/H$^+$ exchanger (NHE5) highly expressed in brain. *Journal of Biological Chemistry*, 274, 4383-4388.

Ballanyi, K., Doutheil, J. & Brockhaus, J. (1996). Membrane potentials and microenvironment of rat dorsal vagal cells in vitro during energy depletion. *Journal of Physiology*, 495, 769–784.

Baumgarth, M., Beier, N. & Gericke, R. (1997). (2-Methyl-5-(methylsulfonyl)benzoyl) guanidine Na$^+$/H$^+$ antiporter inhibitors. *Journal of Medicinal Chemistry*, 40, 2017–2034.

Bell, S.M., Schreiner, C.M., Schultheis, P.J., Miller, M.L., Evans, R.L., Vorhees, C.V., Shull, G.E. & Scott, W.J. (1999). Targeted disruption of the murine *Nhe1* locus induces ataxia, growth retardation, and seizures. *American Journal of Physiology*, 276, C788 – C795.

Bickler, P.E. & Hansen, B.M. (1994). Causes of calcium accumulation in rat cortical brain slices during hypoxia and ischemia: role of ion channels and membrane damage. *Brain Research*, 665, 269-276.

Bobulescu, I.A., Di Sole, F. & Moe, O.W. (2005). Na$^+$/H$^+$ exchangers: physiology and link to hypertension and organ ischemia. *Current Opinion in Nephrology and Hypertension*, 14: 485-494.

Bondarenko, A., Svichar, N. & Chesler, M. (2005). Role of Na$^+$-H$^+$ and Na$^+$-Ca^{2+} exchange in hypoxia-related acute astrocyte death. *Glia*, 49, 143-152.

Bussolino, F., Wang, J.M., Turrini, F., Alessi, D., Ghigo, D., Costamagna, C., Pescarmona, G., Mantovani, A. & Bosia, A. (1989). Stimulation of the Na$^+$/H$^+$ exchanger in human endothelial cells activated by granulocyte- and granulocyte- macrophage-colony-stimulating factor. Evidence for a role in proliferation and migration. *Journal of Biological Chemistry*, 264, 18284–18287.

Castellá, M., Buckberg, G.D. & Tan, G. (2005). Neurologic preservation by Na$^+$-H$^+$ exchange inhibition prior to 90 minutes of hypothermic circulatory arrest. *The Annals of Thoracic Surgery*, 79, 646-654.

Cengiz, P., Kleman, N., Uluc, K., Kendigelen, P., Hagemann, T., Akture, E., Messing, A., Ferrazzano, P. & Sun, D. (2010). Inhibition of Na$^+$/H$^+$ exchanger isoform 1 is neuroprotective in neonatal hypoxic ischemic brain injury. *Anitoxidants and Redox Signaling,* 14, 1803-1813.

Cengiz, P., Uluc, K., Kendigelen, P., Akture, E., Hutchinson, E., Song, C., Zhang, L., Lee, J., Budoff, G., Meyerand, E., Sun, D. & Ferrazzano, P. (2011). Chronic neurological deficits in mice after perinatal hypoxia and ischemia correlate with hemispheric tissue loss and white matter inury detected by MRI. *Developmental Neuroscience,* (in press).

Chambers-Kersh, L., Ritucci, N.A., Dean, J.B. & Putnam, R.W. (2000). Response of intracellular pH to acute anoxia in individual neurons from chemosensitive and nonchemosensitive regions of the medulla. *Advances in Experimental Medicine and Biology,* 475, 453–464.

Chen, H., Luo, J., Kintner, D.B., Shull, G.E. & Sun, D. (2005). Na+-dependent chloride transporter (NKCC1)-null mice exhibit less gray and white matter damage after focal cerebral ischemia. *Journal of Cerebral Blood Flow and Metabolism,* 25, 54-66.

Counillon, L., Scholz, W., Lang, H.J. & Pouyssegur, J. (1993). Pharmacological characterization of stably transfected Na⁺/H⁺ antiporter isoforms using amiloride analogs and a new inhibitor exhibiting antiischemic properties. *Molecular Pharmacology,* 44, 1041-1045.

De Vito, P. (2006). The sodium/hydrogen exchanger: a possible mediator of immunity. *Cell Immunology,* 240, 69-85.

D'Souza, S., Garcia-Cabado, A., Yu, F., Teter, K., Lukacs, G., Skorecki, K., Moore, H.P., Orlowski, J. & Grinstein, S. (1998). The epithelial sodiumhydrogen antiporter Na⁺/H⁺ exchanger 3 accumulates and is functional in recycling endosomes. *Journal of Biological Chemistry,* 273, 2035-2043.

Dunbar, L.A. & Caplan, M.J. (2001). Ion pumps in polarized cells: sorting and regulation of the Na⁺, K⁺- and H⁺, K⁺-ATPases. *Journal of Biological Chemistry,* 276, 29617–29620.

Ferrazzano, P., Shi, Y., Manhas, N., Wang, Y., Hutchinson, B., Chen, X., Chanana, V., Gerdts, J., Meyerand, M.E. & Sun, D. (2011). Inhibiting the Na⁺/H⁺ exchanger reduces reperfusion injury: a small animal MRI study. *Frontiers in BioScience,* 3, 81-88.

Ferriero, D.M. (2004). Neonatal brain injury. *The New England Journal of Medicine,* 351, 1985-1995.

Fujiwara, N., Abe, T., Endoh, H., Warashina, A. & Shimoji, K. (1992). Changes in intracellular pH of mouse hippocampal slices responding to hypoxia and/or glucose depletion. *Brain Research,* 572, 335-339.

Gores, G.J., Nieminen, A.L., Wray, B.E., Herman, B. & Lemasters, J.J. (1989). Intracellular pH during "chemical hypoxia" in cultured rat hepatocytes. Protection by intracellular acidosis against the onset of cell death. *Journal of Clinical Investigation,* 83, 386-396.

Goyal, S., Heuvel, V.G. & Aronson, P.S. (2003). Renal expression of novel Na⁺/H⁺ exchanger isoform NHE8. *American Journal of Physiology Renal Physiology,* 284, F467-F473.

Gu, X.Q., Yao, H. & Haddad, G.G. (2001). Increased neuronal excitability and seizures in the Na⁺/H⁺ exchanger null mutant mouse. *American Journal of Physiology Cell Physiology,* 281, C496–C503.

Herrera, V.L., Cova, T., Sassoon, D. & Ruiz-Opazo, N. (1994). Developmental cell-specific regulation of $Na^{(+)}$-$K^{(+)}$-ATPase alpha 1-, alpha 2-, and alpha 3-isoform gene expression. *American Journal of Physiology*, 266, C1301–C1312.

Horikawa, N., Nishioka, M., Itoh, N., Kuribayashi, Y., Matsui, K. & Ohashi, N. (2001) The Na^+/H^+ exchanger SM-20220 attenuates ischemic injury in *in vitro* and *in vivo* models. *Pharmacology*, 63, 76–81.

Hoyt, K.R., Arden, S.R., Aizenman, E. & Reynolds, I.J. (1998). Reverse Na^+/Ca^{2+} exchange contributes to glutamate-induced intracellular Ca^{2+} concentration increases in cultured rat forebrain neurons. *Molecular Pharmacology*, 53, 742-749.

Hwang, I.K., Yoo, K.Y., An, S.J., Li, H., Lee, C.H., Choi, J.H., Lee, J.Y., Lee, B.H., Kim, Y.M., Kwon, Y.G. & Won, M.H. (2008). Late expression of Na^+/H^+ exchanger 1 (NHE1) and neuroprotective effects of NHE inhibitor in the gerbil hippocampal CA1 region induced by transient ischemia. *Experimental Neurology*, 212, 314-323.

Kinsella, J.L. & Aronson, P.S. (1981). Amiloride inhibition of the Na^+-H^+ exchanger in renal microvillus membrane vesicles. *American Journal of Physiology*, 241, F374–F379.

Kintner, D.B., G. Su, G., Lenart, B., Ballard, A.J., Meyer, J.W., Ng, L.L., Shull, G.E. & Sun, D. (2004). Increased tolerance to oxygen and glucose deprivation in astrocytes from Na^+/H^+ exchanger isoform 1 null mice. *American Journal of Physiology Cell Physiology*, 287, C12-C21.

Kintner, D.B., Look, A., Shull, G.E. & Sun, D. (2005). Stimulation of astrocyte Na^+/H^+ exchange activity in response to *in vitro* ischemia in part depends on activation of extracellular signal-regulatory kinase. *American Journal of Physiology Cell Physiology*, 289, C934-C945.

Kintner, D.B., Luo, J., Gerdts, J., Ballard, A.J., Shull, G.E. & Sun, D. (2007a). Role of Na^+-K^+-Cl^- cotransport and Na^+/Ca^{2+} exchange in mitochondrial dysfunction in astrocytes following *in vitro* ischemia. *American Journal of Physiology Cell Physiology*, 292, C1113-C1122.

Kintner, D.B., Wang, Y. & Sun, D. (2007b). The role of membrane ion transport proteins in cerebral ischemic damage. *Frontiers in Bioscience*, 12, 762-770.

Kintner, D.B., Chen, X., Currie, J., Chanana, V., Ferrazzano, P., Baba, A., Matsuda, T., Cohen, M., Orlowski, J., Chiu, S.Y., Taunton, J. & Sun, D. (2010). Excessive Na^+/H^+ exchange in disruption of dendritic Na^+ and Ca^{2+} homeostasis and mitochondrial dysfunction following *in vitro* ischemia. *Journal of Biological Chemistry*, 285, 35155-35168.

Kitayama, J., Kitazono, T., Yao, H., Ooboshi, H., Takaba, H., Ago, T., Fujishima, M. & Ibayashi, S. (2001). Inhibition of Na^+/H^+ exchanger reduces infarct volume of focal cerebral ischemia in rats. *Brain Research*, 922, 223-228.

Knopfel, T. Tozzi, A., Pisani, A., Calabresi, P. & Bernardi, G. (1998). Hypoxic and hypoglycaemic changes of intracellular pH in cerebral cortical pyramidal neurons. *Neuroreport*, 9, 1447-1450.

Kuribayashi, Y., Horikawa, N., Itoh, N., Kitano, M. & Ohashi, N. (1999). Delayed treatment of Na^+/H^+ exchange inhibitor SM-20220 reduces infarct size in both transient and permanent middle cerebral artery occlusion in rats. *International Journal of Tissue Reactions*, 21, 29-33.

Kuribayashi, Y., Itoh, N., Horikawa, N. & Ohashi, N. (2000). SM-20220, a potent Na^+/H^+ exchange inhibitor, improves consciousness recovery and neurological outcome following transient cerebral ischaemia in gerbils. *Journal of Pharmacy and Pharmacology*, 52, 441-444.

Li, C., Grosdidier, A., Crambert, G., Horisberger, J.D., Michielin, O. & Geering, K. (2004). Structural and functional interaction sites between Na,K-ATPase and FXYD proteins. *Journal of Biological Chemistry*, 279, 38895–38902.

Liu, H., Cala, P.M. & Anderson, S.E. (1997). Ethylisopropylamiloride diminishes changes in intracellular Na, Ca and pH in ischemic newborn myocardium. *Journal of Molecular and Cellular Cardiology*, 29, 2077–2086.

Liu, Y., Kintner, D.B., Chanana, V., Algharabli, J., Chen, X., Gao, Y., Chen, J., Ferrazzano, P., Olson, J.K. & Sun, D. (2010). Activation of microglia depends on Na $^+$ /H^+ exchange-mediated H^+ homeostasis. *Journal of Neuroscience*, 30, 15210–15220.

Luo, J. & Sun, D. (2007). Physiology and Pathophysiology of Na^+/H^+ Exchange Isoform 1 in the Central Nervous System. *Current Neurovascular Research*, 4, 205-215.

Luo, J., Chen, H., Kintner, D.B., Shull, G.E. & Sun, D. (2005). Decreased neuronal death in Na^+/H^+ exchanger isoform 1-null mice after *in vitro* and *in vivo* ischemia. *Journal of Neuroscience*, 25, 11256-11268.

Luo, J., Kintner, D.B., Shull, G.E. & Sun, D. (2007). ERK1/2-p90[RSK]-mediated Phosphorylation of Na+/H+ Exchanger Isoform 1, a role in ishcemic neuronal death. *Journal of Biological Chemistry*, 282, 28274-28284.

Ma, E. & Haddad, G.G. (1997). Expression and localization of Na^+/H^+exchangers in rat central nervous system. *Neuroscience*, 79, 591–603.

Mahnensmith, R.L. & Aronson, P.S. (1985). Interrelationships among quinidine, amiloride, and lithium as inhibitors of the renal Na^+-H^+ exchanger. *Journal of Biological Chemistry*, 260, 586–592.

Manhas, N., Shi, Y., Taunton, J. & Sun, D. (2010). p90[(RSK)] activation contributes to cerebral ischemic damage via phosphorylation of $Na^{(+)}/H^{(+)}$ exchanger isoform 1. *Journal of Neurochemistry*, 114, 1476-1486.

Meima, M.E., Mackley, J.R. & Barber, D.L. (2007). Beyond ion translocation: structural functionsof the sodium-hydrogen exchanger isoform-1. *Current Opinion in Nephrology and Hypertension*, 16, 365–372.

Melzian, D., Scheufler, E., Grieshaber, M. & Tegtmeier, F. (1996). Tissue swelling and intracellular pH in the CA1 region of anoxic rat hippocampus. *Journal of Neuroscience Methods*, 65, 183–187.

Murphy, E., Perlman, M., London, R.E. & Steenbergen, C. (1991). Amiloride delays the ischemia-induced rise in cytosolic free calcium. *Circulation Research*, 68, 1250-1258.

Nakamura, N., Tanaka, S., Teko, Y., Mitsui, K. & Kanazawa, H. (2005). Four Na^+/H^+ exchanger isoforms are distributed to golgi and post-golgi compartments and are involved in organelle pH regulation. *Journal of Biological Chemistry*, 280, 1561-1572.

Nishizawa, Y. (2001). Glutamate release and neuronal damage in ischemia. *Life Sciences*, 69, 369-381.

Numata, M. & Orlowski, J. (2001). Molecular cloning and characterization of a novel $(Na^+,K^+)/H^+$ exchanger localized to the trans-Golgi network. *Journal of Biological Chemistry*, 276, 17387-17394.

Orlowski, J. & Grinstein, S. (2004). Diversity of the mammalian sodium/proton exchanger SLC9 gene family. *Pflugers Arch- European Journal of Physiology*, 447, 549-565.

Orlowski, J., Kandasamy, R.A. and Shull, G.E. (1992). Molecular cloning of putative members of the Na/H exchanger gene family. cDNA cloning, deduced amino acid sequence, and mRNA tissue expression of the rat Na/H exchanger NHE-1 and two structurally related proteins. *Journal of Biological Chemistry*, 267, 9331-9339.

Park, H.S., Lee, B.K., Park, S., Kim, S.U., Lee, S.H., Baik, E.J., Lee, S., Yi, K.Y., Yoo, S.E., Moon, C.H. & Jung, Y.S. (2005). Effects of sabiporide, a specific Na^+/H^+ exchanger inhibitor, on neuronal cell death and brain ischemia. *Brain Research*, 1061, 67-71.

Pedersen, S.F. (2006). The Na^+/H^+ exchanger NHE1 in stress-induced signal transduction: implications for cell proliferation and cell death. *Pflugers Archiv - European Journal of Physiology*, 452, 249-259.

Pedersen, S.F., O'Donnell, M.E., Anderson, S.E. & Cala, P.M. (2006). Physiology and pathophysiology of Na^+/H^+ exchange and Na^+-K^+-$2Cl^-$ cotransport in the heart, brain, and blood. *American Journal of Physiology-Regulatory, Integrative and Comparative Physiology*, 291, R1-R25.

Phillis, J.W., Estevez, A.Y., Guyot, L.L. & O'Regan, M.H. (1999). 5-(N-Ethyl-N-isopropyl)-amiloride, an Na^+-H^+ exchange inhibitor, protects gerbil hippocampal neurons from ischemic injury. *Brain Research*, 839, 199-202.

Pirttila, T.R. & Kauppinen, R.A. (1994). Regulation of intracellular pH in guinea pig cerebral cortex ex vivo studied by ^{31}P and ^1H nuclear magnetic resonance spectroscopy: role of extracellular bicarbonate and chloride. *Journal of Neurochemistry*, 62, 656-664.

Putney, L.K., Denker, S.P. & Barber, DL. (2002). The changing face of the Na^+/H^+ exchanger, NHE1: structure, regulation, and cellular actions. *Annual Reviw of Pharmacology and Toxicology*, 42, 527-552.

Rios, E.J., Fallon, M., Wang, J. & Shimoda, L.A. (2005). Chronic hypoxia elevates intracellular pH and activates Na^+/H^+ exchange in pulmonary arterial smooth muscle cells. *American Journal of Physiology Lung Cellular and Molecular Physiology*, 289, L867-L874.

Roberts Jr., E.L. & Chih, C.P. (1997). The influence of age of pH regulation in hippocampal slices before, during, and after anoxia. *Journal of Cerebral Blood Flow and Metabolism*, 17, 560-566.

Sardet, C., Franchi, A. & Pouyssegur, J. (1989). Molecular cloning, primary structure, and expression of the human growth factor-activatable Na^+/H^+ antiporter. *Cell*, 56, 271-280.

Schaller, B. & Graf, R. (2004). Cerebral ischemia and reperfusion: The pathophysiologic concept as a basis for clinical therapy. *Journal of Cerebral Blood Flow & Metabolism,* 24, 351-371.

Scholz, W., Albus, U., Counillon, L., Gogelein, H., Lang, H.J. , Linz, W., Weichert, A. & Scholkens, B.A. (1995). Protective effects of HOE642, a selective sodium-hydrogen exchange subtype 1 inhibitor, on cardiac ischaemia and reperfusion. *Cardiovascular Research,* 29, 260-268.

Scholz, W., Jessel, A. & Albus, U. (1999). Development of the Na⁺/H⁺ exchange inhibitor cariporide as a cardioprotective drug: from the laboratory to the GUARDIAN trial. *Journal of Thrombosis and Thrombolysis,* 8, 61-70.

Sheldon, C. & Church, J. (2002). Intracellular pH response to anoxia in acutely dissociated adult rat hippocampal CA1 neurons. *Journal of Neurophysiology,* 87, 2209-2224.

Shi, Y., Chanana, V., Watters, J.J., Ferrazzano, P. & Sun, D. (2011). Role of sodium/hydrogen exchanger isoform 1 in microglial activation and proinflammatory responses in ischemic brains. *Journal of Neurochemistry,* (in press).

Szaszi, K., Paulsen, A., Szabo, E.Z., Numata, M., Grinstein, S. & Orlowski, J. (2002). Clathrin-mediated endocytosis and recycling of the neuronspecific Na⁺/H⁺ exchanger NHE5 isoform. Regulation by phosphatidylinositol 3'-kinase and the actin cytoskeleton. *Journal of Biological Chemistry,* 277, 42623-42632.

Vannucci, R.C. & Vannucci, S.J. (2005). Perinatal hypoxic-ischemic brain damage: evolution of an animal model. *Developmental Neuroscience,* 27, 81-86.

Wang, Y., Meyer, J.W., Ashraf, M. & Shull, G.E. (2003). Mice with a null mutation in the NHE1 Na⁺/H⁺ exchanger are resistant to cardiac ischemia-reperfusion injury. *Circulation Research,* 93, 776-782.

Wang, Y., Luo, J., Chen, X., Chen, H., Cramer, S.W. and Sun, D. (2008). Gene inactivation of Na⁺/H⁺ exchanger isoform 1 attenuates apoptosis and mitochondrial damage following transient focal cerebral ischemia. *European Journal of Neuroscience,* 28, 51-61.

Warnock, D.G., Yang, W.C., Huang, Z.Q. & Cragoe, E.J. Jr. (1988). Interactions of chloride and amiloride with the renal Na⁺/H⁺ antiporter. *Journal of Biological Chemistry,*263, 7216-7221.

Xiong, Z.G., Zhu, X.M., Chu, X.P., Minami, M., Hey, J., Wei, W.L., MacDonald, J.F., Wemmie, J.A., Price, M.P., Welsh, M.J. & Simon, R.P. (2004). Neuroprotection in ischemia: blocking calcium-permeable acid-sensing ion channels. *Cell,* 118, 687-698.

Xue, J. & Haddad, G.G. (2010). The Na⁺/H⁺ exchanger: A target for therapeutic intervention in cerebral ischemia, In: *New strategies in stroke intervention: Ionic transporters, pumps, and new channels,* Annunziato, L. pp. (113-128), Human press, a part of Springer Science, ISBN 978-1-60761-279-7, New York, USA

Yao, H. & Haddad, G.G. (2004). Calcium and pH homeostasis in neurons during hypoxia and ischemia. *Cell Calcium,* 36, 247-255.

Yao, H., Gu, X.Q., Douglas, R.M. & Haddad, G.G. (2001). Role of Na⁺/H⁺ exchanger during O_2 deprivation in mouse CA1 neurons. *American Journal of Physiology Cell Physiology,* 281, C1205-C1210.

Yu, F.H., Shull, G.E. & Orlowski, J. (1993). Functional properties of the rat Na/H exchanger NHE-2 isoform expressed in Na/H exchanger-deficient Chinese hamster ovary cells. *Journal of Biological Chemistry*, 268, 25536–25541.

8

Time-Window of Progesterone Neuroprotection After Stroke and Its Underlying Molecular Mechanisms

Weiyan Cai[1], Masahiro Sokabe[2] and Ling Chen[1,2]
[1]Department of Physiology, Nanjing Medical University, Jiangsu,
[2]Department of Physiology, Nagoya University Graduate School of Medicine,
Tsurumai, Nagoya,
[1]China,
[2]Japan

1. Introduction

Evidence exists for a gender difference in the vulnerability to either stroke or traumatic brain injury (TBI) in humans. For example, pre-menopausal women with the high serum levels of ovarian hormones estrogen (E2) and progesterone (P4) have a lower risk of stroke (Karmel et al., 1994; Sacco et al., 1997) and a better outcome following stroke (Thorvaldsen et al., 1995) or TBI (Groswasser et al., 1998) relative to men of the same age. After menopause, incidence of stroke in women increases abruptly (Wenger et al., 1993) coincident with decreases in the circulating levels of the ovarian steroid hormones, estrogen (E2) and progesterone (P4). Although clinical trial for TBI with P4 treatment has been well tolerated and giving improved outcomes (Wright et al., 2007; Stein et al., 2008), clinical trial with P4 treatment after cerebral stroke has yet to be initiated. There is increasing evidence that P4 exerts a potent neuroprotective effect against ischemia-induced brain injury in experimental models (Chen et al., 1999; Kumon et al., 2000; Morali et al., 2005; Sayeed et al., 2006) when administered either before insult or after the onset of reperfusion (Murphy et al., 2002; Sayeed et al., 2007). Furthermore, the administration of P4 promotes functional recovery after cerebral ischemia (Gibson & Murphy, 2004; Sayeed et al., 2007). Important enough, a single injection of P4 (4 mg/kg) conducted even 2 h after transient focal brain ischemia reduced cortical infarct volumes (Jiang et al., 1996). Our recent study (Cai et al., 2008) has demonstrated that in male rats a single injection of P4 (4 mg/kg) at 1 h or 48 h prior to an experimental stroke shows protective effects against the ischemia-induced neuronal death and the deficits in spatial cognition and LTP induction. However, to date no systematic study has conducted concerning the effects of P4 against brain injury beyond 6 h following the onset of ischemia (Gibson et al., 2008). Therefore, the present study focused on the effective time-window of neuroprotection by P4 treatment, which would give useful information in treating stroke.

Effects of P4 on the brain generally involve three principle mechanisms, including regulation of gene expression, activation of intracellular signal cascades and modulation of neurotransmitter systems. P4 has been well known to affect transcription processes through the action on the classical nuclear progesterone's receptor (P4R) followed by multiple interactions with DNA and sequence-specific transcription factors (Beato et al., 1995; Guerra-Araiza et al., 2003). The activation of P4R regulates the expression of anti-apoptotic proteins such as bcl-2, and pro-apoptotic genes including bax and bad and caspase-3 (Schlesinger and Saito, 2006). On the transcriptional level, P4 reduces both the nuclear concentration of NFκB and expression of NFκB target genes. P4 has been found to influence the activity of many signaling pathways so-called "nongenomic mechanisms" *via* a membrane-associated P4R (mP4R) that lacks functional DNA-binding domain (Guerra-Araiza et al., 2009). Increasing evidence indicates that P4R activates Src-ERK signaling pathway which serves as an indicator of growth factor activity in mammalian breast cancer cells (Boonyaratanakornkit et al., 2008; Faivre and Lange, 2007). Cai et al. (2008) has demonstrated that P4 triggers P4R-mediated long-lasting (> 48 h) phosphorylation of ERK1/2 and enhances the translocation of phosphorelated ERK2 into the nucleus. In addition, rapid effects of P4 is suggested to be mediated by membrane-associated P4-binding protein 25-Dx (Meffre et al., 2005) to increase the level of phosphorylated Akt in neuronal cells (Singh et al., 2001). The membrane-associated P4R component 1 (PGRMC1) has been reported to elevate the level of Akt phosphorylation in breast cancer (Neubauer et al., 2008). P4 increases the phosphorylation of ERK and Akt, and the expression of the regulatory (p85) subunits of phosphoinositide-3 kinase (PI3K) in the brain (Guerra-Araiza et al., 2009). Furthermore, the P4's metabolite allopregnanolone (ALLO) potentiates the GABAergic synapse activity (Ardeshiri et al., 2006). Finally, much attention has recently been attracted to the antagonizing effects of P4 on sigma-1 (σ_1) receptor (Maurice et al., 2006; Monnet & Maurice, 2006).

The objective of the present study was to determine the P4-neuroprotective effect and its effective therapeutic time-window after transient cerebral ischemia. To this end, male animals subjected to 60 min middle cerebral artery occlusion (MCAO) were given a pair of intraperitoneal injections of P4 (4 mg/kg) separated by 8 h starting at 1, 24, 48, 72 or 96 h after the initiation of cerebral ischemia by middle cerebral artery occlusion (MCAO), and the size of brain infarct, loss of pyramidal neurons in the hippocampal CA1 and cognitive performance of the animals were assessed on 7th day after MCAO. Using pharmacologic tools and western blot analysis, molecular mechanisms underlying the P4-neuroprotective effects against ischemia-induced cerebral injury were also investigated.

2. Materials and methods

2.1 Experimental animals

The present studies were approved by Animal Care and Ethical Committee of Nanjing Medical University. All procedures were in accordance with the guidelines of Institute for Laboratory Animal Research of Nanjing Medical University. Male Sprague-Dawley rats (200-250g, Oriental Bio Service Inc., Nanjing, China) before experiments were used throughout the study. We chose to use only adult male rats in the present study to avoide influence of the E2 effects (Nilsen and Brinton, 2003). Animal rooms were maintained on a 12:12 light-dark cycle starting at AM 7:00 and kept at a temperature of 22-23°C. The animals were permitted free access to food and tap water. All efforts were made to minimize animal suffering and to reduce the number of animals used.

2.2 Preparation of focal cerebral ischemia model

Focal cerebral ischemia was induced by middle cerebral artery occlusion (MCAO). Rats were anesthetized with a mixture of 70% N_2O and 30% O_2 containing 2.5% isoflurane, and were maintained by the inhalation of 1.5% isoflurane during the operation. Briefly, a heat-blunted black monofilament surgical suture (4/0 G) was inserted into the internal carotid artery to occlude the origin of MCA. Adequacy of vascular occlusion and reperfusion was monitored in the front parietal cortex of the occluded side with a multi-channel laser Doppler flow-meter (PF5050 Q4, Perimed, Jarfalla, Sweden). Body and head temperatures were controlled at 37±0.5°C using a water pads. Arterial blood pressure and gases were monitored through a femoral catheter. After 60 min of occlusion, the filament was withdrawn to allow for reperfusion. Sham-operated (sham-op) animals were treated identically, except that MCAs were not occluded.

2.3 Drug administration

P4 was dissolved in dimethylsulfoxide (DMSO), then in sesame oil to a final concentration of 1% DMSO. P4 (4 mg/kg) was intraperitonealy (i.p.) injected. Two injections of P4 with 8 h interval were given starting at 1, 24, 48, 72 or 96 h after the initiation of MCAO (post-MCAO). We selected this low dosage because P4 at this dosage is reported to significantly reduce the ischemic damage and regulate anti-apoptotic gene expression following TBI in rats (Stein, 2008). In addition, our study (Cai et al., 2008) determined that the treatment with the same dosage of P4 increases ERK1/2 phosphorylation.

To analyze the molecular mechanisms underlying the P4-actions, the P4R antagonist RU486 (3 mg/kg) and the 5α-reductase inhibitor finasteride (20 mg/kg) (Finn et al., 2006) were given by intraperitoneal injection (i.p.) at 30 min before each administration of P4. The MEK inhibitor U0126 (0.5 nmol) and the PI3K inhibitor LY294002 (0.3 nmol) were injected into the cerebroventricle (i.c.v.) at 30 min before each injections of P4. For i.c.v. implantation, rats were anaesthetized with ketamine (80 mg/kg i.p.). A guide cannula (10 mm length, 22 gauge) aiming above the right lateral ventricle was implanted. The inhibitors or vehicle were injected with a stepper-motorized micro-syringe (Stoelting, Wood Dale, IL, USA) at a rate of 0.5 µl/min. The drugs were prepared freshly on the day of experiment (final volume = 5µl/rat). Control rats were given an equal volume of vehicle.

2.4 Histological examination
2.4.1 Infarct volume measuring

Brains were removed on 7th day post-MCAO, sectioned into 5 equidistant slices (2.0-mm-thick), and incubated in a 2% 2,3,5-triphenyle-tetrazoliumchloride (TTC) solution (15 min) to visualize infarcted tissue. Measurements were performed by manually outlining the margins of the infarcted areas. Unstained areas of brain sections were defined as infarcted using the image analysis software NIH-Image 3.12. Briefly, the infarcted area on the ipsilateral side was indirectly measured by subtracting the noninfarcted area in the ipsilateral hemisphere from the total nonischaemic area of the contralateral (nonischaemic) hemisphere. Hemispheric infarcted areas were calculated separately on each coronal slice and scored from 1 to 5, and each such area was defined as a percentage of the affected hemisphere. The infarction volume did not differ significantly across the samples in MCAO-groups (P > 0.05).

2.4.2 Pyramidal cells counting

Rats were deeply anesthetized with pentobarbital (50 mg/kg), transcardially perfused with 4% paraformaldehyde at 7th day post-MCAO. The brains were removed, post-fixed for 24 h, and then processed for paraffin embedding. Coronal sections (4-µm-thick) including the dorsal hippocampus were cut and stained with toluidine blue. Healthy pyramidal cells showing a round cell body with a plainly stained nucleus were counted by eye using a conventional light microscope (PD70) with a 100×objective. The number of surviving CA1 pyramidal cells per 1 mm length along the extent of pyramidal layer were counted as neuronal density (cells/mm) (Cai et al., 2008). We also made supplemental examinations on several slices stained with trypan blue that stains dead cells, and obtained essentially the same result as that determined by eye with hematoxylin and eosin (HE) stained slices.

2.5 Behavioral analysis
2.5.1 Rota rod test

The Rota rod test was used to assess the sensorimotor coordination of rodent on 7th day post-MCAO (see Figure 1A) using an accelerating treadmill (TSE Systems, Germany; 3 cm diameter). For Rota rod training sessions, animals were habituated to the Rota rod and trained to remain on the rotating drum (constant speed 6 rpm) for a minimum of 90 s to provide a preoperative baseline. Animals not achieving baseline criteria were excluded from further study. In the testing sessions, animals were placed on the Rota rod, and the rotational speed was set to accelerate from 6 to 19 rpm over 180 s. The latency time to fall (time on rod), namely the time when the animal first fell off the drum, was recorded.

2.5.2 Morris Water Maze (MWM) test

Morris water maze test was performed from 4th day post-MCAO for consecutive 4 days (see Figure 2A) using a swimming pool (diameter: 180 cm; height: 30 cm) filled with water (20°C) to a depth of 15 cm. A transparent plexiglass platform (7 cm in diameter) was submerged with the top located 1 cm below the water surface. Swimming paths were analyzed by a computer system with a video camera (AXIS-90 Target/2; Neuroscience). After reaching the platform, rat was allowed to remain on it for 30 sec. If the rat did not find the platform within 90 sec, the rat was put on the platform for 30 sec. The escape-latency to reach hidden-platform was measured from three trials to provide a single value for each rat.

2.6 Western blot analysis

Rats were decapitated under deep anesthesia with ethyl ether. The hippocampus in ischemic hemisphere was taken quickly, then homogenized in a lysis buffer containing 50 mM TriseHCl (pH 7.5), 150 mM NaCl, 5 mM EDTA, 10 mM NaF, 1 mM sodium orthovanadate, 1% Triton X-100, 0.5% sodium deoxycholate, 1 mM phenylmethylsulfonyl fluoride and protease inhibitor cocktail (Complete; Roche, Mannheim, Germany). Protein concentration was determined with BCA Protein Assay Kit (Pierce, Rochford, IL, USA). Total proteins (20 µg) were separated by SDS-polyacrylamide gel electrophoresis (SDS-PAGE) and transferred to a polyphorylated difluoride (PVDF) membrane. The membranes were incubated with 5% bovine serum albumin or 5% nonfat dried milk in tris-buffered saline containing 0.1% Tween 20 (TBST) for 60 min at room temperature, and then were incubated with a mouse monoclonal anti-phospho-ERK1/2 antibody (diluted 1:2500, Cell Signaling, Beverly, MA) at 4°C overnight. After being washed with TBST for three times, the membranes were incubated with an HRP-labeled secondary antibody, and developed using the ECL detection Kit (Amersham Biosciences, Piscataway, NJ). Following visualization, the blots were stripped by incubation in stripping buffer (Restore, Pierce Chemical Co, Rockford IL) for 5 min, re-blocked for 60 min with 5% nonfat dried milk at room temperature, then incubated with anti-total ERK1/2 (diluted 1:5000, Cell Signaling, Beverly, MA). In each experiment, levels of both ERK1/2 and phosphorelated ERK1/2 (phospho-ERK1/2) were measured in the hippocampus of ischemic hemisphere in MCAO-rats and sham-op rats (control). For each animal, phospho-ERK1/2 was normalized by respective ERK1/2 protein. Each experimental group contained 12 rats. The Western blot bands were scanned and analyzed with the image analysis software package, NIH Image.

2.7 Data analysis/statistics
Data were retrieved and processed with the software Microcal Origin 6.1. The group data are expressed as the means ± standard error (SE). For comparison between two groups the 2-sided student t-test was used. For comparison between more than 2 groups one-way analysis of variance (ANOVA) followed by the Bonferroni's post hoc test was performed. Statistical analysis was performed using the software State7 (STATA Corporation, USA). For the analysis of Morris water maze test, statistical differences were determined by an ANOVA with repeated measures, followed by the Bonferroni post hoc test. Statistical analysis was performed using the State7 software (Stata Corporation, USA). Differences at P<0.05 were considered statistically significant.

3. Results

3.1 Effective time-window of P4 against ischemic brain infarct and motor dysfunction
To examine the effects of P4 on ischemia-induced brain infarction, a pair of injections (i.p.) of P4 (4 mg/kg) with an 8 h interval were given starting at 1, 24, 48, 72 or 96 h post-MCAO (Figure 1A). On 7th day post-MCAO the results of TTC staining showed that the 60 min MCAO caused approximately 34% brain infarction mainly in the striatum and the frontoparietal cortex (Figure 1B). In comparison with vehicle-treated MCAO-rats, infarct volumes were significantly decreased by the administration of P4 at 1 and 24 h (P<0.01, n=12) or 48 and 72 h post-MCAO (P<0.05, n=12), but not at 96 h (P>0.05, n=12). Similarly, the performance of rota rod test on 7th day post-MCAO perfectly restored in MCAO-rats treated with P4 at 1, 24, 48 (P<0.01, n=12) and 72 h post-MCAO (P<0.05, n=12; Figure 1C) compared to vehicle-treated MCAO-rats. By contrast, P4 when administered at 96 h post-MCAO had no effect on the ischemia-induced motor impairment (P>0.05, n=12). The results indicate that the administration of P4 after stroke exerts a powerful neuroprotection against ischemia-induced brain damages with a wide effective time-window up to 72 h.

3.2 Effective time-window of P4 against ischemic death of neuronal cells and cognitive impairment
Consistent with the previous report (Cai et al., 2008), the number of hippocampal CA1 pyramidal neurons in ischemic hemisphere decreased to approximately 50% of sham-op hemisphere on 7th day post-MCAO (P<0.01, n=8; Figure 2B). To examine the effects of P4 on ischemia-induced death of pyramidal neurons and impairment of spatial memory, a pair of injections (i.p.) of P4 (4 mg/kg) with an 8 h interval was given at 1, 24, 48, 72 or 96 h

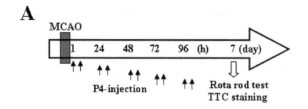

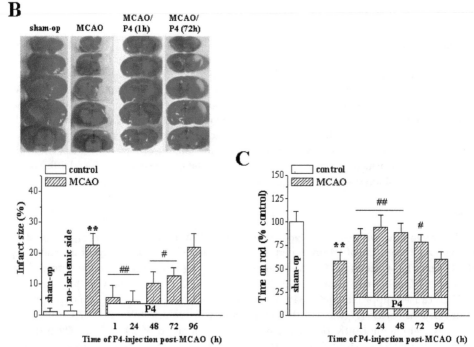

Fig. 1. Effects of P4 on ischemia-induced brain infarct and motor dysfunction. (**A**) Time chart of experimental procedure in Figure 1B&C. Two injections (i.p.) of P4 (4 mg/kg) with 8 h interval (black arrows) were given starting at 1, 24, 48, 72 or 96 h post-MCAO. (**B**) Time-window of P4-effect against MCAO-induced brain infarct. Representative pictures of TTC-staining in sham-op rats, MCAO-rats, P4-treated MCAO-rats (upper panels). Bar graph shows the size of brain infarct that was expressed as percentage of the non-infarcted hemisphere on 7th day post-MCAO. Horizontal hollow bar: P4 administration. (**C**) Time-window of P4-effect against ischemic motor dysfunction. Bar graph shows time on rod in sham-op (open bar) and MCAO-rats (hatched bars) on 7th day post-MCAO. **P<0.01 vs. sham-op rats; #P<0.05 and ##P<0.01 vs. MCAO-rats.

post-MCAO. The number of dead pyramidal cells was significantly reduced by the treatment with P4 at 1, 24 and 48 h (P<0.01, n=8) or 72 h post-MCAO (P<0.05, n=8) compared to vehicle-treated MCAO-rats. However, the administration of P4 at 96 h post-MCAO exerted no significant effect in reducing the number of ischemia-induced loss of

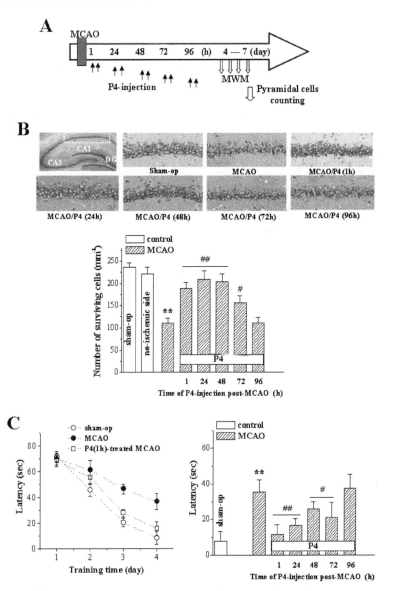

Fig. 2. Effects of P4 on ischemia-induced neuronal cell death and cognitive impairment.
(A) Time chart of experimental procedure in Figure 2B&C. Two injections (i.p.) of P4
(4 mg/kg) with 8 h interval (black arrows) were given starting at 1, 24, 48, 72 or 96 h post-
MCAO. (B) Time-window of P4-effect against MCAO-induced neuronal cell death.
Representative pictures of hippocampal CA1 region in sham-op rats, MCAO-rats, P4-treated
MCAO-rats (upper panels). Scale bar=100µm. Bar graph shows density of surviving neurons
in the hippocampal CA1 on 7th day post-MCAO. Horizontal hollow bar: P4 administration.
(C) Time-window of P4-effect against MCAO-induced deficits in spatial memory. Typical

trials of "Morris" water maze test (left panel) show latency (sec) to reach the hidden-platform against training time (day, day 4-7 post-MCAO) in sham-op rats, MCAO-rats, P4 (1h post-MCAO)-treated MCAO-rats. Bar graph shows the mean latency (±SEM) to reach the hidden-platform on 4th day post-training. **P<0.01 vs. sham-op rats; #P<0.05 and ##P<0.01 vs. MCAO-rats.

pyramidal cells (P>0.05, n=8). The P4 administration per se caused no observable change in CA1 pyramidal neurons on 7th day after sham-op. Spatial learning and memory function was examined by the Morris water maze test from 4th day post-MCAO for consecutive 4 days (Figure 2A). In comparison with sham-op rats, the escape-latency to reach the hidden-platform on 7th day post-MCAO increased approximately 2-fold (P<0.01, n=8; Figure 2C). The behavior of acquisition performance coincided with the histological changes; the prolongation of escape-latency was perfectly improved by the treatment with P4 at 1, 24 and 48 h post-MCAO (P<0.01, n=8), while was partially reduced by the injection of P4 at 72 h post-MCAO (P<0.05, n=8). By contrast, the administration of P4 at 96 h post-MCAO failed to affect the prolonged escape-latency (P>0.05, n=8). Both the histological and behavioral examinations here strongly suggest that the effective time-window of the neuroprotection by the P4 treatment is spanning from 1 h to 72 h post-MCAO. In the following sections, we describe the results on the analyses of the molecular mechanisms underlying the P4 affording neuroprotective effects on ischemia-induced death of pyramidal cells.

3.3 P4-neuroprotection at 1 h post-MCAO is mediated by its metabolite ALLO
A recent study (Ciriza et al., 2006) has revealed that the neuroprotection by P4 after ischemic brain injury is abolished by finasteride, a 5α-reductase inhibitor that inhibits the conversion of P4 to allopregnanolone (ALLO). To determine whether P4 exerts neuroprotection through its metabolite ALLO, finasteride (20 mg/kg i.p.) was given at 30 min prior to every P4-injection. The results showed that the pre-treatment with finasteride partially attenuated the neuroprotection of P4 at 1 h post-MCAO against MCAO-induced neuronal death (P<0.05, n=8; Figure 3A) and prolongation of escape-latency (P<0.05, n=8; Figure 3B), but it did not

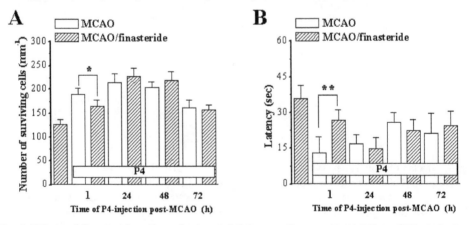

Fig. 3. Effects of finasteride, a 5α-reductase inhibitor, on the neuroprotection of P4 against MCAO-induced neuronal cell death (**A**) and cognitive impairment (**B**). Horizontal hollow bar: P4 administration. Animals were treated with finasteride at 30 min before every P4-injection. Note that the P4-neuroprotection at 1 h post-MCAO is partially blocked by

finasteride. *P<0.05 and *P<0.01 vs. P4-treated MCAO-rats at 1 h post-MCAO.
affect the neuroprotection by P4 at 24, 48 or 72 h post-MCAO (P>0.05, n=8). The results
indicate that the neuroprotection by P4 at 1 h post-MCAO is, if not all, caused by a
protective action of its metabolite ALLO against ischemia-induced brain damage.

3.4 P4-neuroprotection at 24 and 48 h post-MCAO is mediated by P4R activation

The neuroprotection by P4 administered at 48 h pre-MCAO has been known to depend on
P4R function (Faivre and Lange, 2007). To test this possibility in our case, the nuclear P4R
blocker RU486 (3 mg/kg, i.p.) was given at 30 min prior to each P4 injection. The results
showed that the pre-treatment with RU486 abolished the neuroprotective effects of P4 at 24
and 48 h post-MCAO against ischemia-induced neuronal death (P<0.01, n=8; Figure 4A) and
spatial memory impairment (P<0.01, n=8; Figure 4B), whereas it failed to affect the
neuroprotection by P4 at 1 or 72 h post-MCAO (P>0.05, n=8). Meanwhile, in the absence of
P4 the administration of RU486 at 24 or 48 h post-MCAO had no effect on either neuronal
death (P>0.05, n=8) or spatial cognitive function (P>0.05, n=8). These results suggest that the
neuroprotective effect of P4 administered at 24 and 48 h post-MCAO involves the P4R-
mediated mechanism.

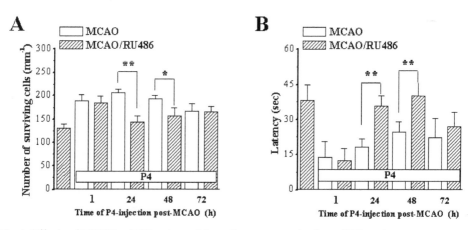

Fig. 4. Effects of RU486, a R4R antagonist, on the neuroprotection of P4 against
MCAO-induced neuronal cell death (**A**) and cognitive impairment (**B**). Horizontal hollow
bar: P4 administration. Animals were treated with RU486 at 30 min before every time
P4-injection. Note that the P4-neuroprotection at 24 and 48 h post-MCAO is blocked by
RU486. *P<0.05 and *P<0.01 vs. P4-treated MCAO-rats at 24 and 48 h post-MCAO.

3.5 P4-neuroprotection at 24 and 48 h post-MCAO depends on P4R-ERK signaling

As P4R-mediated ERK1/2 activation protects the ischemic brain damage (Cai et al., 2008),
the experiment was designed to explore the involvement of ERK1/2 in the P4R-dependent
neuroprotection after MCAO. Expectedly, the ERK kinase (MEK) inhibitor U0126 (0.3 nmol,
i.c.v.) blocked the neuroprotection by P4 at 24 and 48 h against MCAO-induced neuronal
death (P<0.01, n=8; Figure 5A) and spatial memory impairment (P4 at 24 h post-MCAO,
P<0.01, n=8; P4 at 48 h post-MCAO, P<0.05, n=8; Figure 5B), whereas it failed to affect the

P4R-independent neuroprotection exerted by P4 administered at 1 or 72 h post-MCAO (P>0.05, n=8). These results indicate that the P4R-mediated neuroprotection is highly coupled with ERK1/2 signaling pathway.

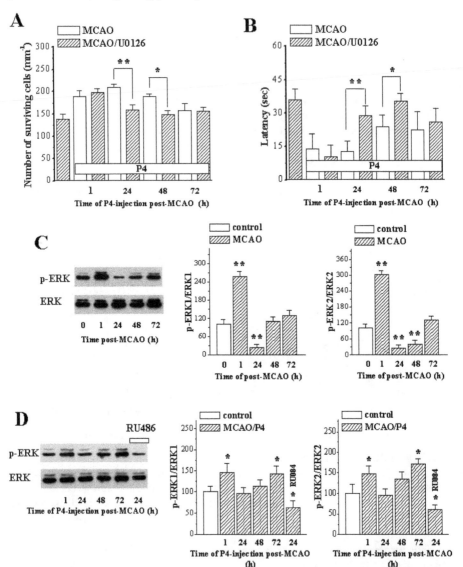

Fig. 5. Effects of U0126, a MEK inhibitor, on the neuroprotection of P4 against MCAO-induced neuronal cell death (**A**) and cognitive impairment (**B**). Horizontal hollow bar: P4 administration. Animals were treated with U0126 at 30 min before every time P4-injection. Note that the phospho-ERK1/2 at 24 and 48 h post-MCAO is blocked by U0126. *P<0.05 and *P<0.01 vs. P4-treated MCAO-rats at 24 and 48 h post-MCAO. (**C**) Kinetics of hippocampal

phospho-ERK1/2 at 1, 24, 48 and 72 h post-MCAO. Representative western blots represent ERK1/2 phosphorylation immunoreactivity obtained from whole-cell lysates. Level of phospho-ERK1/2 is expressed as a percentage of phospho-ERK1/2 in sham-op rats. (**D**) Effect of P4 on phospho-ERK1/2 at 1, 24, 48 and 72 h post-MCAO. P4 was given at 30 min before harvested hippocampus. Values of phospho-ERK1/2 were normalized by phospho-ERK1/2 in sham-op rats. *$P<0.05$ and **$P<0.01$ vs. sham-op group; #<0.05 vs. MCAO-rats treated with P4 at 24 h post-MCAO. Horizontal axis: Time of post-MCAO p4 injection.

Emerging evidence indicates that transient cerebral ischemia promotes the dephosphorylation of ERK1/2 (Jover-Mengual et al., 2007). To confirm this, kinetics of hippocampal ERK1/2 phosphorylation (phospho-ERK1/2) after MCAO was measured using Western blot analysis. In comparison with that before MCAO, the level of phospho-ERK1/2 was largely increased at 1 h post-MCAO ($P<0.05$, n=12; Figure 5C), followed by a persistent decrease at 24 h and 48 h post-MCAO ($P<0.05$, n=12), then returned to the basal level at 72 h post-MCAO ($P>0.05$, n=12). To investigate the effects of P4 on the changes in ERK1/2 phosphorylation after MCAO, the MCAO-rats were given a single injection of P4 at 1, 24, 48 or 72 h post-MCAO. Thirty minutes after the P4-injection hippocampal preparations were harvested to measure phospho-ERK1/2. As shown in Figure 5D, the treatment with P4 slightly attenuated the increased phospho-ERK1/2 at 1 h post-MCAO ($P<0.05$, n=12), perfectly rescued the reduction of phospho-ERK1/2 at 24 and 48 h post-MCAO ($P<0.01$, n=12), and elevated the level of phospho-ERK1/2 at 72 h post-MCAO ($P<0.05$, n=12). The P4R antagonist RU486 could block the protective effect of P4 on the reduction of phospho-ERK1/2 at 24 h post-MCAO ($P<0.05$ vs. P4-treated MCAO-rats, n=12). These observations clearly indicate that the P4R-dependent neuroprotection against ischemia-induced brain damage is mediated, at least in part, through the regulation of ERK1/2 activity.

3.6 P4-neuroprotection at 24–72 h post-MCAO requires PI3K signaling

As P4 increases the level of Akt-phosphorylation, a partial process of PI3K signaling (Guerra-Araiza et al., 2009), the specific PI3K inhibitor LY294002 (0.3 nmol) was injected into the cereboventricle (i.c.v.) at 30 min prior to P4 injection to examine the involvement of PI3K-Akt signaling pathway in the P4-neuroprotection. The results showed that the pre-treatment with LY294002 partially attenuated the neuroprotection of P4 at 24 and 48 h post-MCAO ($P<0.05$, n=8; Figure 6A) and completely abolished the neuroprotection of P4 at 72 h post-MCAO ($P<0.01$, n=8), whereas it had no effect on the neuroprotection of P4 at 1 h post-MCAO ($P>0.05$, n=8). Furthermore, the pre-treatment with LY294002 blocked the P4-improved impairment of spatial memory when administered at 24, 48 and 72 h post-MCAO ($P<0.05$, n=8; Figure 6B). The results indicate that the PI3K-Akt signaling is involved in the P4R-dependent and P4R-independent neuroprotections by P4, depending on the timing of P4 injection.

4. Discussion

The present study provides evidence that the treatment with P4 after transient brain ischemia exerts a powerful neuroprotection with a wide effective time-window up to 72 h post-MCAO. The neuroprotective effects of P4 were mediated by different molecular mechanisms depending on the timing of P4 administration after ischemia. The neuroprotection by P4 at 1 h post-MCAO appeared to be caused through P4's metabolite allopregnanolone (ALLO) because the protection was significantly attenuated by the 5α-reductase inhibitor finasteride. The neuroprotection of P4 at 24 and 48 h post-MCAO appeared to be P4R-dependent through rescuing the down-regulation of ERK1/2 phosphorylation after stroke. The neuroprotective effects of P4 at 72 h post-MCAO required PI3K activation in a P4R-independent way.

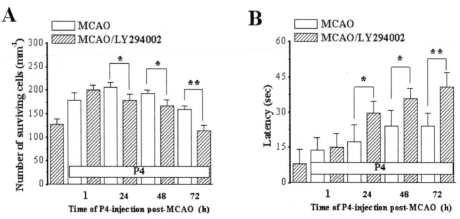

Fig. 6. Involvement of PI3K in P4-neuroprotection. Animals were treated with the specific PI3K inhibitor LY294002 (LY) at 30 min before administration of P4. Horizontal hollow bar: P4 administration. Note that the P4-neuroprotection at 24–72 hr post-MCAO requires PI3K signaling. *P<0.05 and **P<0.01 vs. MCAO-rats treated with P4 at 24, 48 and 72 hr post-MCAO.

4.1 Anti-excitotoxic effect of P4's metabolite ALLO at 1 h after MCAO

One recent report indicates that either P4 or ALLO when administered at 2 h post-MCAO is effective in reducing the infarct volume after focal brain ischemia, where ALLO shows more effective neuroprotection than its parent compound (Sayeed et al., 2007). Similarly, our results in the present study showed that the neuroprotection of P4 at 1 h post-MCAO was sensitive to the 5α-reductase inhibitor fenasteride. Thus, it is proposed that the acute neuroprotection of P4 within 1−2 h ischemia/reperfusion is caused by ALLO, a positive regulator of GABAA receptor (Belelli & Lambert, 2005). This notion is supported by an earlier study (Ardeshiri et al., 2006) showing that the GABAA receptor antagonist picrotoxin could prevent the neuroprotection afforded by P4. The P4 neuroprotection mainly focuses on some populations of neurons that are sensitive to excitotoxicty, including the pyramidal neurons in the hippocampus and cerebral cortex, Purkinje cells in the cerebellum, as well as the neurons in the dorsal striatum and the caudate nucleus (Monnet and Maurice, 2006; Schumacher et al., 2007). Immediately after ischemia, excessive presynaptic glutamate releases result in the accumulation of extracellular glutamate to reach concentrations that induce over-activation of glutamate receptors called excitotoxicity (Jabaudon et al., 2000; Phillis and O'Regan, 2003). The process of excitotoxicity has been demonstrated in several experimental models of cerebral ischemia (Butcher et al., 1990). Therefore, it is highly likely that P4 and ALLO at 1 h post-MCAO prevent the brain injury by suppressing over-excitation of pyramidal neurons through the activation of GABA$_A$ receptors.

However, we noted that the treatment with finasteride could not completely block the P4-neuroprotection at 1 h post-MCAO (see Figure 3A). Excessive presynaptic glutamate releases after cerebral ischemia lead to neuronal death mainly by excessive calcium entry through N-methyl-D-aspartate receptor (NMDAr). Our recent study (Cai et al., 2008) has revealed that P4, as a potential σ_1 receptor antagonist (Monnet and Maurice, 2006), reduces Ca^{2+} influx across NMDAr-channels to protect hippocampal neurons from ischemia-induced cell death. In addition, at 1 h after brain ischemia the activation of σ_1 receptor by PRE-084, a σ_1 receptor agonist, exacerbates ischemia-induced neuronal cell death in an NMDAr-dependent manner (Li et al., 2009). However, conflicting results have reported that the activation of σ_1 receptor enhances presynaptic glutamate release in the hippocampal CA1 (Meyer et al., 2002), and promotes the Ca^{2+} influx across NMDAr-channels (Monnet et al., 2003) and the Ca^{2+} efflux from calcium pools via inositol 1,4,5-trisphosphate receptors (Su and Hayashi, 2003). This discrepancy may be due to the difference in experimental condition or timing of P4 action. Further studies are required to directly observe the P4 effects on NMDAr-Ca^{2+} influx in an acute phase after stroke.

4.2 P4R-dependent ERK activation at 24—48 h after stroke

Our results revealed that the P4R-mediated ERK1/2 signaling was involved in the neuroprotection by P4 at 24−48 h post-MCAO. P4R ligand has been demonstrated to induce a transient (5−10 min after P4-application) activation of Src-Ras-ERK1/2 and a persistent (6−72 h) ERK1/2 activation (Faivre and Lange, 2007). Recently, Cai et al. (2008) provided in vivo evidence that P4 acts on P4R to trigger a long-lasting (> 48 hr) phosphorylation of ERK1/2, resulting in a promoted translocation of phosphorelated ERK2 into the nucleus. The translocation of ERK1/2 is a pivotal and necessary process for the activation of cAMP response element binding protein (CREB) (Nilsen and Brinton, 2003). The ERK1/2-CREB signaling has been implicated to play a critical role in the brain ischemic tolerance (Gonzalez-Zulueta et al., 2000) and neuronal cell survival (Singh, 2005; 2006). The CREB cascade can increase the expression of anti-apoptotic molecules such as Bcl-2 and Bcl-XL (Yao et al., 2005) and decrease the expression of pro-apoptotic molecules such as Bax, Bad and caspase-3 (Djebaili et al., 2004). Consistent with the results reported by Jover-Mengual et al. (2007), we in the present study showed a decreased activity of ERK1/2 at 24 and 48 h post-MCAO. More importantly, the activation of P4R at 24−48 h after ischemia could rescue the down-regulation of ERK1/2. Therefore, it is highly likely that the P4R-dependent neuroprotection is closely coupled with ERK1/2 signaling.

On the other hand, western blot analysis showed a transient elevation of ERK1/2 phosphorylation at 1 h post-MCAO. The elevation of ERK1/2 activity immediately after stroke has also been observed in humans (Slevin et al., 2000) and a rat model of cerebral ischemia (Wang et al., 2003), in which increased intracellular Ca^{2+} levels ($[Ca^{2+}]_i$) after ischemia seem to lead hyper-activation of ERK1/2. Alessandrini et al. (1999) and Namura et al. (2001) provided evidence for a neuroprotective role of MEK inhibitor following transient ischemia as manifested by the reduction of infarct size and improvement of functional outcome. The neuroprotection by MEK-inhibition in ischemic brain is associated with an activation of potential anti-apoptotic pathway that suppresses caspase-3 activation and apoptosis (Wang et al., 2003). To our surprise, we observed that the treatment with P4 could attenuate the elevation of ERK1/2 phosphorylation at 1 h post-MCAO. Because the neuroprotection by P4 at 1 h post-MCAO was P4R-independent, it is proposed that P4 prevents ischemia-increased $[Ca^{2+}]_i$ by antagonizing σ_1 receptor, which may stabilize the ERK1/2 activation.

4.3 PI3K signaling is required for P4R-independent and P4R-dependnet neuroprotections

P4 has been reported to enhance the phosphorylation of Akt/PKB (Singh et al., 2001; Kuolen et al., 2008) in the hippocampus and cerebellum (Guerra-Araiza et al., 2009). On the other hand, PI3K signaling is believed to suppress apoptotic cell death via its downstream effectors, such as Akt/PKB, to inhibit the Bcl2 family protein Bad (Noshita et al., 2001). Using the specific PI3K inhibitor LY294002, the present study provided in vivo evidence that the PI3K signaling is required for the P4-neuroprotection at 24−72 h post-MCAO against ischemia-induced brain damage. In human breast cancer cells, P4 induces rapid and transient activation of PI3K-Akt pathway in a P4R-dependent manner (Migliaccio et al., 1998; Castoria et al., 2001). It was reported that progestins rapidly activated PI3K-Akt pathway via P4R (Vallejo et al., 2005; Ballare et al., 2006). However, our results here showed that the PI3K-mediated neuroprotection by P4 administered at 72 h post-MCAO is P4R-independent. P4 is reportedly to regulate PI3K signaling pathway through its metabolites (Guerra-Araiza et al., 2009), but our data determined that the neuroprotection of P4 at 24−72 h post-MCAO was insensitive to the inhibition of 5α-reductase by fenasteride. P4-binding membrane protein 25-Dx (also known as PGRMC1) in the brain (Krebs et al., 2000; Sakamoto et al., 2004) is involved in the anti-apoptotic actions of P4 (Peluso et al., 2006, 2008). Further studies are needed to elucidate whether P4 cascades PI3K signaling after stroke through P4-binding 25-Dx mechanisms.

4.4 Clinical significance

P4 treatment after ischemia at relatively a low dose (4 mg/kg) exerts powerful neuroprotective effects with a wide, at least up to 72 h post ischemia, effective time-window, which would provide a great benefit in treating stroke. The present study provides evidence that the P4 neuroprotection has a wide effective time-window that is realized by a time dependent multiple neuroprotective mechanisms after ischemia. The results shown here not only help to understand the correlation between the declined level of P4 and the abruptly increasing incidence of stroke following the menopause, but also provide a novel the therapeutic opportunity of P4 against the ischemic brain injury.

5. Acknowledgments

This work was supported by grants for NSFC (30872725; 81071027; 31171440) to Chen L.
We declare that there is no competing financial that could be construed as influencing the results or interpretation of the reported study.

6. References

Alessandrini A, Namura S, Moskowitz MA & Bonventre JV. (1999). MEK1 protein kinase inhibition protects against damage resulting from focal cerebral ischemia. *Proc Natl Acad Sci USA*, vol. 96, pp. 12866−12869

Ardeshiri A, Kelley MH, Korner IP, Hurn PD & Herson PS. (2006). Mechanism of progesterone neuroprotection of rat cerebellar Purkinje cells following oxygen-glucose deprivation. *Eur J Neurosci*, vol. 24, pp. 2567–2574

Ballare C, Vallejo G ,Vicent GP, Saragüeta P & Beato M. (2006). Progesterone signaling in breast and endometrium. *J Steroid Biochem Mol Biol* vol. 102, pp. 2–10

Beato M, Herrlich P & Schutz G. (1995). Steroid hormone receptors: many actors in search of a plot. *Cell*, vol. 83, pp. 851–857

Belelli D & Lambert JJ. (2005). Neurosteroids: endogenous regulators of the GABA (A) receptor. *Nat Rev Neurosci vol.* 6, pp. 565–575

Boonyaratanakornkit V, Bi Y, Rudd M & Edwards DP. (2008). The role and mechanism of progesterone receptor activation of extra-nuclear signaling pathways in regulating gene transcription and cell cycle progression. *Steroids*, vol. 73, pp. 922–928

Butcher SP, Bullock R, Graham DI & McCulloch J. (1990). Correlation between amino acid release and neuropathologic outcome in rat brain following middle cerebral artery occlusion. *Stroke*, vol. 21, pp. 1727-1733

Cai W, Zhu Y, Furuya K, Li Z, Sokabe M & Chen L. (2008). Two different molecular mechanisms underlying progesterone neuroprotection against ischemic brain damage. *Neuropharmacology*, vol. 55, pp. 127–138

Castoria G, Migliaccio A, Bilancio A, Di Domenico M, de Falco A, Lombardi M, Fiorentino R, Varricchio L, Barone MV & Auricchio F. (2001). PI3-kinase in concert with Src promotes the S-phase entry of oestradiol-stimulated MCF-7 cells. *EMBO J*, vol. 20, pp. 6050–6059

Chen J, Chopp M & Li Y. (1999). Neuroprotective effects of progesterone after transient middle cerebral artery occlusion in rat. *J Neurol Sci*, vol. 171, pp. 24–30

Ciriza I, Carrero P, Frye CA & Garcia-Segura LM. (2006). Reduced metabolites mediate neuroprotective effects of progesterone in the adult rat hippocampus. The synthetic progestin medroxyprogesterone acetate (Provera) is not neuroprotective. *J Neurobiol*, vol. 66, pp. 916–928

Djebaili M, Hoffman SW & Stein DG. (2004). Allopregnanolone and progesterone decrease cell death and cognitive deficits after a contusion of the rat pre-frontal cortex. *Neuroscience*, vol. 123, pp. 349–359

Faivre EJ & Lange CA. (2007). Progesterone receptors upregulate Wnt-1 to induce epidermal growth factor receptor transactivation and c-Src-dependent sustained activation of Erk1/2 mitogen-activated protein kinase in breast cancer cells. *Mol Cell Biol*, vol. 27, pp. 466–480

Finn DA, Beadles-Bohling AS, Beckley HE, Ford MM, Gililland KR, Gorin-Meyer RE & Wiren KM. (2006). A new look at the 5alpha-reductase inhibitor finasteride. *J compilation* ,vol. 12, pp. 53–76

Gibson CL & Murphy SP. (2004). Progesterone enhances functional recovery after middle cerebral artery occlusion in male mice. *J Cereb Blood Flow Metab*, vol. 24, pp. 805–813

Gibson CL, Gray LJ, Bath PM & Murphy SP. (2008). Progesterone for the treatment of experimental brain injury; a systematic review. *Brain*, vol. 13, pp. 318-328

Gonzalez-Zulueta M, Feldman AB, Klesse LJ, Kalb RG, Dillman JF, Parada LF, Dawson TM & Dawson VL. (2000). Requirement for nitric oxide activation of p21(ras)/extracellular regulated kinase in neuronal ischemic preconditioning. *Proc Natl Acad Sci USA*, vol. 97, pp. 436–441

Groswasser Z, Cohen M & Keren O. (1998). Female TBI patients recover better than males. *Brain Inj*, vol. 12, pp. 805–808

Guerra-Araiza C, Amorim MA, Pinto-Almazán R, González-Arenas A, Campos MG & Garcia-Segura LM. (2009). Regulation of the phosphoinositide-3 kinase and mitogen-activated protein kinase signaling pathways by progesterone and its reduced metabolites in the rat brain. *J Neurosci Res*, vol. 87, pp. 470-481

Guerra-Araiza C, Villamar-Cruz O, González-Arenas A, Chavira R & Camacho-Arroyo I. (2003). Changes in progesterone receptor isoforms content in the rat brain during the oestrous cycle and after oestradiol and progesterone treatments. *J Neuroendocrinol*, vol. 15, pp. 984–990

Jabaudon D, Scanziani M, Gähwiler BH & Gerber U. (2000). Acute decrease in net glutamate uptake during energy deprivation. *Proc Natl Acad Sci U S A*, vol. 97, pp. 5610-5615

Jiang N, Chopp M, Stein D & Feit H. (1996). Progesterone is neuroprotective after transient middle cerebral artery occlusion in male rats. *Brain Res*, vol. 30, pp. 101–107

Jover-Mengual T, Zukin RS & Etgen AM. (2007). MAPK signaling is critical to estradiol protection of CA1 neurons in global ischemia. *Endocrinology*, vol. 148, pp. 1131–1143

Kannel WB, Ho K & Thom T. (1994). Changing epidemiological features of cardiac failure. *Br Heart J* , vol. 72, pp. 3–9

Koulen P, Madry C,Duncan RS, Hwang JY, Nixon E, McClung N, Gregg EV & Singh M. (2008). Progesterone potentiates IP(3)-mediated calcium signaling through Akt/PKB. *Cell Physiol Biochem*, vol. 21, pp. 161–172

Krebs CJ, Jarvis ED, Chan J, Lydon JP, Ogawa S & Pfaff DW. (2000). A membrane-associated progesterone-binding protein, 25-Dx, is regulated by progesterone in brain regions involved in female reproductive behaviors. *Proc Natl Acad Sci USA* , vol. 97, pp. 12816–12821

Kumon Y, Kim SC, Tompkins P, Stevens A, Sakaki S & Loftus CM. (2000). Neuroprotective effect of postischemic administration of progesterone in spontaneously hypertensive rats with focal cerebral ischemia. *J Neurosurg* , vol. 92, pp. 848–852

Li Z, Cui S, Zhang Z, Zhou R, Ge Y, Sokabe M & Chen L. (2009). DHEA-neuroprotection and -neurotoxicity after transient cerebral ischemia in rats. *J Cereb Blood Flow Metab*, vol. 29, pp. 287-296

Maurice T, Gregoire C & Espallergues J. (2006). Neuro(active)steroids actions at the neuromodulatory sigma(1) receptor: Biochemical and physiological evidences, consequences in neuroprotection. *Pharmacol Biochem Behav*, vol. 84, pp. 581–597

Meffre D, Delespierre B, Gouézou M, Leclerc P, Vinson GP, Schumacher M, Stein DG & Guennoun R. (2005). The membrane-associated progesterone-binding protein 25-Dx is expressed in brain regions involved in water homeostasis and is up-regulated after traumatic brain injury. *J Neurochem*, vol. 93, pp. 1314–1326

Meyer DA, Carta M, Partridge LD, Covey DF & Valenzuela CF. (2002). Neurosteroids enhance spontaneous glutamate release in hippocampal neurons. Possible role of metabotropic sigma1-like receptors. *J Biol Chem*, vol. 277, pp. 28725–28732

Migliaccio A, Piccolo D, Castoria G, Di Domenico M, Bilancio A, Lombardi M, Gong W, Beato M & Auricchio F. (1998). Activation of the Src/p21ras/Erk pathway by progesterone receptor via cross-talk with estrogen receptor. *EMBO J*, vol. 17, pp. 2008–2018

Monnet FP & Maurice T. (2006). The sigma1 protein as a target for the non-genomic effects of neruo(active)steroids: molecular, physiological, and behavioral aspects. *J Pharmacol Sci*, vol. 100, pp. 93−118

Monnet FP, Morin-Surun MP, Leger J & Combettes L. (2003). Protein kinase C-dependent potentiation of intracellular calcium influx by σ1 receptor agonists in rat hippocampal neurons. *J Pharmacol Exp Ther*, vol. 307, pp. 705−712

Morali G, Letechipia-Vallejo G, Lopez-Loeza E, Montes P, Hernández-Morales L & Cervantes M. (2005). Post-ischemic administration of progesterone in rats exerts neuroprotective effects on the hippocampus. *Neurosci Lett*, vol. 382, pp. 286−290

Murphy SJ, Littleton-Kearney MT & Hurn PD. (2002). Progesterone administration during reperfusion, but not preischemia alone, reduces injury in ovariectomized rats. *J Cereb Blood Flow Metab*, vol. 22, pp. 1181−1188

Namura S, Iihara K, Takami S, Nagata I, Kikuchi H, Matsushita K, Moskowitz MA, Bonventre JV & Alessandrini A. (2001). Intravenous administration of MEK inhibitor U0126 affords brain protection against forebrain ischemia and focal cerebral ischemia. *Proc Natl Acad Sci USA*, vol. 98, pp. 11569−11574

Neubauer H, Clare SE, Wozny W, Schwall GP, Poznanovic S, Stegmann W, Vogel U, Sotlar K, Wallwiener D, Kurek R, Fehm T & Cahill MA. (2008). Breast cancer proteomics reveals correlation between estrogen receptor status and differential phosphorylation of PGRMC1. *Breast Cancer Res*, vol. 15, pp. R85.

Nilsen J & Brinton RD. (2003). Divergent impact of progesterone and medroxyprogesterone acetate (Provera) on nuclear mitogen-activated protein kinase signaling. *Proc Natl Acad Sci USA*, vol. 100, pp. 10506−10511

Noshita N, Lewén A, Sugawara T & Chan PH. (2001). Evidence of phosphorylation of Akt and neuronal survival after transient focal cerebral ischemia in mice. *J Cereb Blood Flow Metab*, vol. 21, pp. 1442−1450

Peluso JJ, Pappalardo A, Losel R & Wehling M. (2006). Progesterone membrane receptor component 1 expression in the immature rat ovary and its role in mediating progesterone's antiapoptotic action. *Endocrinology*, vol.147, pp. 3133−3140

Peluso JJ, Romak J & Liu X. (2008). Progesterone receptor membrane component-1 (PGRMC1) is the mediator of progesterone's antiapoptotic action in spontaneously immortalized granulosa cells as revealed by PGRMC1 small interfering ribonucleic acid treatment and functional analysis of PGRMC1 mutations. *Endocrinology*, vol. 149, pp. 534−543

Phillis JW & O'Regan MH. (2003). Characterization of modes of release of amino acids in the ischemic/reperfused rat cerebral cortex. *Neurochem Int*, vol. 43, pp. 461-467.

Sacco RL. (1998). Identifying patient populations at high risk for stroke. *Neurology*, vol. 51, pp. 27−30

Sakamoto H, Ukena K, Takemori H, Okamoto M, Kawata M & Tsutsui K. (2004). Expression and localization of 25-Dx, a membraneassociated putative progesterone-binding protein, in the developing Purkinje cell. *Neuroscience*, vol. 126, pp. 325−334

Sayeed I, Guo Q, Hoffman SW & Stein DG. (2006). Allopregnanolone, a progesterone metabolite, is more effective than progesterone in reducing cortical infarct volume after transient middle cerebral artery occlusion. *Ann Emerg Med*, vol. 47, pp. 381−389

Sayeed I, Wali B & Stein DG. (2007). Progesterone inhibits ischemic brain injury in a rat model of permanent middle cerebral artery occlusion. *Restor Neurol Neurosci*, vol. 25, pp. 151–159

Schlesinger PH & Saito M. (2006). The Bax pore in liposomes, Biophysics. *Cell Death Differ*, vol. 13, pp. 1403–1408

Schumacher M, Guennoun R, Stein DG & De Nicola AF. (2007). Progesterone: therapeutic opportunities for neuroprotection and myelin repair. *Pharmacol Ther*, vol. 116, pp. 77–106

Singh M. (2001). Ovarian hormones elicit phosphorylation of Akt and extracellular-signal regulated kinase in explants of the cerebral cortex. *Endocrine*, vol. 14, pp. 407–415

Singh M. (2005). Mechanisms of progesterone-induced neuroprotection. *Ann NY Acad Sci USA*, vol. 1052, pp. 145–151

Singh M. (2006). Progesterone-induced neuroprotection. *Endocrinology*, vol. 29, pp. 271–274

Slevin M, Krupinski J, Slowik A, Rubio F, Szczudlik A & Gaffney J. (2000). Activation of MAP kinase (ERK-1/ERK-2), tyrosine kinase and VEGF in the human brain following acute ischaemic stroke. *Neuroreport*, vol. 11, pp. 2759–2764

Stein DG. (2008). Progesterone exerts neuroprotective effects after brain injury. *Brain Res Rev*, vol. 57, pp. 386-397.

Su TP & Hayashi T. (2003). Understanding the molecular mechanism of sigma-1 receptors: towards a hypothesis that sigma-1 receptors are intracellular amplifiers for signal transduction. *Curr Med Chem*, vol. 10, pp. 2073–2080

Thorvaldsen P, Asplund K, Kuulasmaa K, Rajakangas AM & Schroll M. (1995). Stroke incidence, case fatality, and mortality in the WHO MONICA project. *Stroke*, vol. 26, pp. 361–367

Vallejo G, Ballare C, Baranao JL, Beato M & Saragüeta P. (2005). Progestin activation of nongenomic pathways via cross talk of progesterone receptor with estrogen receptor-induces proliferation of endometrial stromal cells. *Mol Endocrinol*, vol. 19, pp. 3023–3037

Wang Z, Chen X, Zhou L, Wu D, Che X & Yang G. (2003). Effects of extracellular signal-regulated kinase (ERK) on focal cerebral ischemia. *Chin Med J (Engl)*, vol. 116, pp. 1497–503

Wenger NK, Speroff L & Packard B. (1993). Cardiovascular health and disease in women. *N Engl J Med*, vol. 329, pp. 247–256.

Wright DW, Kellermann AL, Hertzberg VS, Clark PL, Frankel M, Goldstein FC, Salomone JP, Dent LL, Harris OA, Ander DS, Lowery DW, Patel MM, Denson DD, Gordon AB, Wald MM, Gupta S, Hoffman SW & Stein DG. (2007). ProTECT: a randomized clinical trial of progesterone for acute traumatic brain injury. *Ann Emerg Med*, vol. 49, pp. 391–402

Yao XL, Liu J, Lee E, Ling GS & McCabe JT. (2005). Progesterone differentially regulates pro- and anti-apoptotic gene expression in cerebral cortex following traumatic brain injury in rats. *J Neurotrauma*, vol. 22, pp. 656–668

9

PPAR Agonism as New Pharmacological Approach to the Management of Acute Ischemic Stroke

Elisa Benetti[1], Nimesh Patel[2] and Massimo Collino[1]

[1]Dipartimento di Scienza e Tecnologia del Farmaco,
University of Turin, Turin,
[2]Centre for Translational Medicine and Therapeutics, Queen Mary University of London,
The William Harvey Research Institute, London,
[1]Italy
[2]UK

1. Introduction

Despite increasing knowledge of the biochemical mechanisms that occur in the brain following an ischemic insult and the availability of several diverse animal models of stroke, there are still no drugs that can be given to stroke patients soon after the onset of symptoms to minimize the subsequent neurological damage. To date, the thrombolytic compound recombinant tissue Plasminogen Activator (rt-PA) remains the only approved drug for the treatment of stroke. At present, intravenous administration of rt-PA is the only proven effective treatment to re-establish cerebral blood flow in the case of acute vessel occlusion, but unfortunately, only few patients with acute ischemic stroke are qualified to receive this drug. The failure of rt-PA to achieve rapid reperfusion in many patients and its bleeding risk have prompted the development of fibrinolytic agents with greater fibrin specificity and better risk-benefit profiles, such as tenecteplase or desmoteplase, which are now under active investigation. Early restoration of blood flow remains the treatment of choice for limiting brain injury following stroke, but a second fundamental goal of intervention is to protect neurons by interrupting or slowing the ischemic cascade. Current research is being done to develop neuroprotective agents that are able to block amino acid pathways and decrease neurotransmitter activity of injured tissue. Drugs blocking voltage-dependent calcium channels were effective in stroke rodent models but the results of clinical trials have been often discouraging. Overactivation of the N-methyl-D-aspartate receptor (NMDAR) is crucial for neuronal death after stroke. Several compounds that interfere with glutamate receptor activation have been developed and tested, in particular noncompetitive NMDA antagonists. However, their clinical use is limited by intolerable side effects, including some psycomimetic symptoms, as these blockers may also impair some key brain functions mediated by the same receptor. Accumulating evidence strongly suggests that apoptosis contributes to neuronal cell death in stroke injury and currently several caspase inhibitors are under investigation, but to date the efficacy of antiapoptotic agents in human stroke patients has not yet been tested. Anti-inflammatory approaches to stroke treatment intended to block cell-mediated inflammation with different strategies such as humanized antibodies against ICAM-1, inhibitors of interleukin-1 beta or a interleukin-1 receptor antagonist. However, there have been no successful clinical trials of these anti-inflammatory agents so far.

The complexity of events in cerebral ischemia and the disappointing results from human clinical stroke trials using a single agent suggest that perhaps to treat the stroke a new pleiotropic approach is required. In the pharmacological perspective, the evaluation of drugs with multiple effects on the ischemic cascade may be more effective in reducing infarct size and improving outcome in respect to single target strategy, because the ischemic cascade is diverse and it is likely that many different mechanisms of ischemia induced cell death occur simultaneously. Therefore, the development of neuroprotective drugs with multiple effects on the ischemic cascade is potentially more appealing than drugs acting on only one component of the cascade, if the safety profile is reasonable and the preclinical assessment package fulfils recent recommendations. Most recent discoveries portray Peroxisome Proliferator-Activated Receptors (PPARs) as promising pharmacological targets for the treatment of acute ischemic stroke, thanks to their ability to simultaneously interfere with several mechanisms that underlie the pathophysiology of brain ischemia, thus leading to an interesting protective strategy to counteract the multiple deleterious effects of ischemic injury.

2. PPAR

Peroxisome Proliferator-Activated Receptors (PPARs) are members of the nuclear hormone receptor (NHR) superfamily of ligand-activated transcription factors. There are three PPAR subtypes: α, β/δ and γ, named also NR1C1, NR1C2 and NR1C3, respectively, according to the unified nomenclature of nuclear receptors (Nuclear Receptors Nomenclature Committee, 1999). The three isoforms are the products of distinct genes: the human PPARα gene was mapped on chromosome 22 in the general region 22q12–q13.1, the PPARγ gene is located on chromosome 3 at position 3p25, whereas PPARβ/δ has been assigned to chromosome 6, at position 6p21.1–p21.2 (Sher, Yi et al. 1993; Greene, Blumberg et al. 1995; Yoshikawa, Brkanac et al. 1996). PPARs were originally identified by Isseman and Green (Issemann and Green 1990) after screening the rat liver cDNA library with a cDNA sequence located in the highly conserved C domain of NHRs. The name PPAR is derived from the fact that activation of PPARα, the first member of the PPAR family to be cloned, results in peroxisome proliferation in rodent hepatocytes (Desvergne and Wahli 1999). Activation of neither PPARβ/δ nor PPARγ, however, elicits this response and, interestingly, the phenomenon of peroxisome proliferation does not occur in humans. The molecular basis for this difference between species is not yet clear. With respect to the PPARγ isotype, alternative splicing and promoter use results in the formation of two further isoforms: PPARγ1 and PPARγ2. In particular, differential promoter usage and alternate splicing of the gene generates three mRNA isoforms. PPARγ1 and PPARγ3 mRNA both encode the PPARγ1 protein product which is expressed in most tissues, whereas PPARγ2 mRNA encodes the PPARγ2 protein, which contains an additional 28 amino acids at the amino terminus and is specific to adipocytes (Gurnell 2003). PPARβ/δ was initially reported as PPARβ in Xenopus laevis and NUC1 in humans (Schmidt, Endo et al. 1992). Subsequently, a similar transcript was cloned from mice and termed PPARδ (Amri, Bonino et al. 1995). Though now recognised as homologues for each other, it was not originally certain whether PPARβ from Xenopus was identical to murine PPARδ, hence the terminology PPARβ/δ.

All members of this superfamily share the typical domain organization of nuclear receptors (Figure 1). The N-terminal A/B domain contains a ligand-independent transactivation function. In the α and γ isotypes, the activity of this domain can be regulated by Mitogen-Activated Protein Kinase (MAPK) phosphorylation (Hu, Kim et al. 1996). The C domain is the DNA binding domain with its typical two zinc-finger-like motifs, as previously described for the steroid receptors, and the D domain is the co-factor docking domain (Schwabe, Neuhaus et al. 1990). The E/F domain is the ligand binding domain, it contains a ligand-dependent trans-activation function (AF)-2 (Fajas, Auboeuf et al. 1997), and is able to interact with transcriptional coactivators such as steroid receptor coactivator (SRC)-1 (Onate, Tsai et al. 1995) and CREB-binding protein (CBP) (Amri, Bonino et al. 1995).

PPAR DOMAIN STRUCTURE

ISOFORMS	ENCODING GENE	AMINO ACID IDENTITY (% vs α) DBD	AMINO ACID IDENTITY (% vs α) LBD	AMINO ACID NUMBER
α (NR1C1)	22q12-q13.1	-	-	468
β/δ (NR1C2)	6p21.1-p21.2	86%	70%	441
γ (NR1C3)	3p25	83%	68%	477

Fig. 1. Schematic representation of the domain organization of human PPAR isoforms. The A/B domain contains the Activation Function 1 (AF-1) which has a ligand-independent transcriptional activity. The C domain corresponds to the DNA Binding Domain (DBD). The D domain is the co-factor docking domain. The E/F domain contains the Ligand Binding Domain (LBD) and carries the Activation Function 2 (AF-2), which has a ligand-dependent transcriptional activity. The human chromosome regions in which disting genes encoding for PPAR isoforms are mapped, the percentage of amino acid sequence identity (in comparison with PPARα) and the amino acid number of different isoforms are reported in the Table.

The highest PPARα expression has been found in the liver and in tissues with high fatty acid catabolism, such as the kidney, heart, skeletal muscle, and brown fat (Lefebvre, Chinetti et al. 2006). PPARα mainly regulates energy homeostasis, activating fatty acid catabolism and stimulating gluconeogenesis (Kersten, Seydoux et al. 1999). This increased fatty acid oxidation in response to PPARα activation with a selective agonist, WY14643, results in lower circulating triglyceride levels and reduction of lipid storage in liver, muscle, and adipose tissue (Chou, Haluzik et al. 2002), which is associated with improved insulin sensitivity (Kim, Haluzik et al. 2003). Consequently, fibrates (fenofibrate, bezafibrate, gemfibrozil), which are synthetic agonists for PPARα, are in wide clinical use for the treatment of dyslipidaemias.

PPARγ is expressed in white and brown adipose tissue, gut, and immune cells (Feige, Gelman et al. 2006). It is involved in adipocyte differentiation and lipid storage in white adipose tissue (Rosen, Sarraf et al. 1999). Furthermore, PPARγ is involved in glucose metabolism via an improvement of insulin sensitivity (Hevener, He et al. 2003). Therefore, synthetic PPARγ agonists (thiazolidinediones) are in clinical use as insulin sensitizers to treat patients with type-2 diabetes.

PPARβ/δ remained an enigma for almost a decade after its cloning in 1992. It has been reported to be ubiquitously expressed in almost every tissue and, in the past, this widespread tissue expression has suggested a possible "general housekeeping" role for PPARβ/δ (Kliewer, Forman et al. 1994). More recently, the use of transgenic mouse models and the availability of high-affinity synthetic ligands has led researchers to a better understanding of its physiological role. Specifically, increasing evidence has shown a particular role for PPARβ/δ in insulin sensitivity regulation, lipid metabolism and the inflammation response. However, in contrast to PPARα and γ, PPARβ/δ agonists are not yet in clinical use.

2.1 Endogenous and synthetic PPAR ligands

Although many fatty acids are capable of activating all three PPAR isoforms, some fatty acids are also specific for a particular PPAR isoform. X-ray crystallography studies of PPARβ/δ revealed an exceptionally large ligand-binding pocket of approximately 1,300 Å3, similar to that of PPARγ but much larger than the pockets of other nuclear receptors (Xu, Lambert et al. 1999). The increased dimension is believed to accommodate the binding of various fatty acids or other amphipathic acids to PPARβ/δ via hydrogen bonds and hydrophobic interactions. The long-chain polyunsaturated fatty acids and their oxidized derivatives, especially eicosanoids such as 8-S-hydroxyeicosatetraenoic acid (8-S-HETE), leukotriene B4 (LTB4) and arachidonate monooxygenase metabolite epoxyeicosatrienoic acids have been shown to potently activate PPARα with high affinity (Theocharisa, Margeli et al. 2003; Feige, Gelman et al. 2006). PPARγ can be activated by several prostanoids, such as 15-deoxy-Δ12,14-prostaglandin J2 (15d-PGJ2) and 12- and 15-hydroxy-eicosatetraenoic acid (12- and 15-HETE), which are derivatives of arachidonic acid synthesized through the lipoxygenase pathway, as well as modified oxidised lipids, 9- and 13-hydroxyoctadecadienoic acids (9- and 13-HODE) (Willson, Brown et al. 2000; Theocharisa, Margeli et al. 2003). PPARβ/δ agonists include linoleic acid, oleic acid, arachidonic acid and eicosapentaenoic acid (EPA), which have been shown to co-crystallize within the ligand binding domain of this nuclear receptor (Xu, Lambert et al. 1999). A number of eicosanoids, including prostaglandin (PG)A1 and PGD2, and carbaprostacyclin, a semi-synthetic prostaglandin, have micromolar affinities for PPARβ/δ (Forman, Chen et al. 1997). Recently, cows milk, ice cream, butter, and yoghurt were described as activators of PPARβ/δ in reporter assays, but a specific common compound was not identified (Suhara, Koide et al. 2009).

With respect to the synthetic ligands, fibrates (e.g. fenofibrate, clofibrate), which are hypolipidaemic drugs, are well-known ligands for PPARα (Willson, Brown et al. 2000). Fibrates are capable of activating PPARα at pharmacological doses leading to increased expression of lipid metabolizing enzymes that effectively lower serum lipid levels in humans. In contrast to the well-documented therapeutic effect, there is also evidence of liver toxicity induced by activation of PPARα, mainly hepatocarcinogenesis. The most serious safety risk associated with fibrates, although rare, is myopathy and rhabdomyolysis. Studies suggest that the mechanism of myotoxicity through fibrates is not entirely clear, because complex and multifactorial mechanisms are involved, including genetic predisposition, pharmacokinetics, drug interactions, and dose. It is of interest to note that increased expression of lipoprotein lipase, which is a known PPARα target gene, in skeletal muscle leads to severe myopathy in mice.

The most widely used PPARγ agonists belong to the thiazolidinedione (TZD) or glitazone class of anti-diabetic drugs used in the treatment of type-2 diabetes. Troglitazone, the first TZD approved for this use, was withdrawn from the market in March 2000 following the emergence of a serious hepatotoxicity in some patients. Since troglitazone induces CYP3A4, it has been hypothesized that potentially toxic quinones derived from CYP3A4-dependent metabolism could cause liver damage (Yamamoto, Yamazaki et al. 2002). Rosiglitazone and pioglitazone are the only available thiazolidinediones in North America, but meta-analyses of randomised controlled trials have suggested an increased risk of ischaemic cardiovascular events with rosiglitazone (Nissen and Wolski ; Singh, Loke et al. 2007). In contrast, meta-analysis of trials of pioglitazone indicates the possibility of an ischaemic cardiovascular benefit (Lincoff, Wolski et al. 2007). Robust evidence also shows that both drugs increase the risk of congestive heart failure and fractures, but whether any meaningful difference exists in the magnitude of risk between the two thiazolidinediones is not known (Singh, Loke et al. 2007; Loke, Singh et al. 2009). The European Medicines Agency has recommended the suspension of marketing authorisation for rosiglitazone, whereas the US Food and Drug Administration has allowed the continued marketing of rosiglitazone with additional restrictions.

On the contrary, there are no PPARβ/δ drugs in clinical use yet. However several selective PPARβ/δ ligands have been recently designed, including GW0742, GW2433, GW9578, L-783483, L-165041, or GW501516 (Berger, Leibowitz et al. 1999; Lim and Dey 2000; Martens, Visseren et al. 2002). As yet only one selective PPARβ/δ antagonist has been described GSK0660. In skeletal muscle myoblast cells in culture, GSK0660 inhibited GW0742 induction of established PPARβ/δ target genes (carnitine palmitoyltransferase 1A, angiopoietin-like 4 protein and pyruvate dehydrogenase kinase-4)(Shearer, Steger et al. 2008).

2.2 Molecular mechanisms of PPAR activation
There are at least three primary mechanisms by which PPARs can regulate biological functions: transcriptional transactivation, transcriptional transrepression and ligand-independent transrepression (Figure 2).

2.2.1 Mechanism of transcriptional transactivation
PPARs function as heterodimers with their obligatory partner the Retinoid X Receptor (RXR). Like other NHRs, the PPAR/RXR heterodimer most likely recruits co-factor complexes - either co-activators or co-repressors - that modulate its transcriptional activity (Shi, Hon et al. 2002). The PPAR/RXR heterodimer then binds to sequence specific PPAR Response Elements (PPREs), located in the 5'-flanking region of target genes, thereby acting as a transcriptional regulator (Palmer, Hsu et al. 1995). The PPRE consists of two direct repeats of the consensus sequence AGGTCA separated by a single nucleotide, which constitutes a DR-1 motif. PPAR binds 5' of RXR on the DR-1 motif and the 5'-flanking

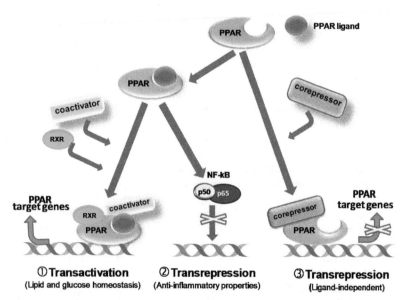

Fig. 2. Molecular mechanisms of PPAR activation. After ligand binding, PPAR undergoes conformational changes, which lead to recruitment of Retinoid X Receptor (RXR) and coactivators. The resultant heterodimer binds to specific DNA response elements called PPAR response elements, causing target gene transcription (Transactivation). A second mechanism (Transrepression) involves interfering with other transcription-factor pathways by negatively regulating the expression of pro-inflammatory genes. Lastly, PPAR may repress the transcription of direct target genes in the absence of ligands (ligand-independent Transrepression) recruiting corepressor complexes that mediate active repression.

sequence conveys the selectivity of binding between different PPAR isotypes (Juge-Aubry, Pernin et al. 1997). In the absence of a ligand, to prevent PPAR/RXR binding to DNA, high-affinity complexes are formed between the inactive PPAR/RXR heterodimers and co-repressor molecules, such as nuclear receptor co-repressor or silencing mediator for retinoic receptors. In response to ligand binding, PPAR undergoes a conformational change, leading to release of auxiliary proteins and co-repressors and recruitment of co-activators that contain histone acetylase activity. Acetylation of histones by co-activators bound to the ligand-PPAR complex leads to nucleosome remodelling, allowing for recruitment of RNA polymerase II causing target gene transcription. The search for PPAR target genes with identified PPREs has led to the identification of several genes involved in lipid metabolism, oxidative stress and inflammatory response, as widely documented in the literature.

2.2.2 Mechanism of transcriptional transrepression
PPARs can also negatively regulate gene expression in a ligand-dependent manner by inhibiting the activities of other transcription factors, such as Activated Protein-1 (AP-1), Nuclear Factor-κB (NF-κB) and Nuclear Factor of Activated T cells (NFAT) (ligand-dependent transrepression). In contrast to transcriptional activation, which usually involves the binding of PPARs to specific response elements in the promoter or enhancer regions of

target genes, transrepression does not involve binding to typical receptor specific response elements (Pascual and Glass 2006). Several lines of evidence suggest that PPARs may exert anti-inflammatory effects by negatively regulating the expression of pro-inflammatory genes. To date, several mechanisms have been suggested to account for this activity, but despite intensive investigation, unifying principles remain to be elucidated.

Firstly, competition for limited amounts of essential, shared transcriptional co-activators may play a role in transrepression. The activated PPAR/RXR heterodimer reduces the availability of co-activators required for gene induction by other transcriptional factors. Thus, without distinct co-factors, transcription factors cannot cause gene expression.

Secondly, PPAR/RXR complexes may cause a functional inhibition by directly binding to transcription factors, preventing them from inducing gene transcription or inducing the expression of inhibitory proteins, such as the protein inhibitor of kappa B (IκB)α, which sequesters the NF-κB subunits in the cytoplasm and consequently reduces their DNA binding activity (Delerive, Martin-Nizard et al. 1999).

Thirdly, PPAR/RXR heterodimers may also inhibit phosphorylation and activation of several members of the MAPK family. In general very little is known about the molecular mechanisms by which PPARs and their ligands modulate kinase activities.

Recent studies have suggested another mechanism based on co-repressor-dependent transrepression by PPARs. Evidence has been presented in which PPARβ/δ controls the inflammatory status of macrophages based on its association with the transcriptional repressor BCL-6 (Lee, Chawla et al. 2003). Free BCL-6 suppresses the expression of multiple proinflammatory cytokines and chemokines. PPARβ/δ, but not PPARα and PPARγ, exhibits BCL-6 binding ability (Barish, Atkins et al. 2008; Takata, Liu et al. 2008). In the absence of a ligand, PPARβ/δ sequesters BCL-6 from inflammatory response genes. In contrast, in the presence of a ligand, PPARβ/δ releases the repressor, which now distributes to NF-κB-dependent promoters and exerts anti-inflammatory effects by repressing transcription from these genes.

2.2.3 Mechanism of ligand-independent transrepression

PPARs may repress the transcription of direct target genes in the absence of ligands (ligand-independent repression). PPARs bind to response elements in the absence of any ligand and recruit co-repressor complexes that mediate active repression. The co-repressors are capable of fully repressing PPAR-mediated transactivation induced either by ligands or by cAMP-regulated signalling pathways. This suggests co-repressors as general antagonists of the various stimuli inducing PPAR-mediated transactivation. Co-repressors can display different ligand selectivity: the nuclear receptor co-repressor NCoR interacted strongly with the ligand-binding domain of PPARβ/δ, whereas interactions with the ligand-binding domains of PPARγ and PPARα were significantly weaker (Krogsdam, Nielsen et al. 2002).

Very recently, a team of Harvard Medical School researchers has shown that PPARγ is phosphorylated at Ser273 by cyclin dependent kinase 5 (CDK5) during obesity which results in deregulation of a subset of genes; including a number of key metabolic regulators, such as adipsin, the first fat cell-selective gene whose expression is altered in obesity and adiponectin, a central regulator of insulin sensitivity *in vivo* (Choi, Banks et al.). Ser273 phosphorylation did not alter the chromatin occupancy of PPARγ, suggesting that other mechanisms, such as differential recruitment of co-regulators, may cause these differences in target gene expression. PPARγ ligands inhibited Ser273 phosphorylation and reversed associated changes in gene expression. Critically, the extent to which PPARγ ligands inhibit CDK5-mediated phosphorylation of PPARγ is not correlated with the extent to which they exert PPAR agonism, suggesting that these compounds have two distinct and separable activities. Whether or not similar mechanisms of receptor phosphorylation lead to changes in gene expression also in the other two PPAR isoforms -α and β/δ is a very important question, so far not yet addressed.

3. PPAR in the brain

All three PPAR isotypes are co-expressed in the nervous system during late rat embryogenesis. Their expression peaks in the central nervous system at mid-gestation. Whereas PPARβ/δ remains highly expressed in this tissue, the expression of PPARα and PPARγ decreases postnatally in the brain (Braissant, Foufelle et al. 1996). While PPARβ/δ has been found in neurons of numerous brain areas of adult rodents, PPARα and PPARγ have been localized to more restricted areas of the brain (Moreno, Farioli-Vecchioli et al. 2004). The localization of PPARs has also been investigated in purified cultures of neural cells. PPARβ/δ is expressed in immature oligodendrocytes where its activation promotes differentiation, myelin maturation and turnover. The PPARγ isotype is the dominant isoform in microglia. Astrocytes possess all three PPAR isotypes, although to different degrees depending on the brain area and animal age (Cristiano, Bernardo et al. 2001). The role of PPARs in the CNS is mainly related to lipid metabolism; however, these receptors have been implicated in neural cell differentiation and death as well as in inflammation and neurodegeneration. The expression of PPARγ in the brain has been extensively studied in relation to inflammation and neurodegeneration. PPARα has been suggested to be involved in acetylcholine metabolism, excitatory amino acid neurotransmission and oxidative stress defence. PPARβ/δ seems to play a critical role in regulating myelinogenesis and differentiation of cells within the CNS (Peters, Lee et al. 2000).

4. PPARs and cerebral ischemia

4.1 Experimental data on the effects of PPAR ligands in ischemic stroke

Although the relevance of animal models to the development of therapies for acute stroke has been often questioned, evidence demonstrates that animal models of stroke do have clinical relevance and are useful in the development of drugs that attenuate the ischemic damage. The characteristics of brain injury depends on the severity and the duration of cerebral blood flow reduction but it can be significantly exacerbated by the following phase of reperfusion; for this reason several animal models of the so-called "cerebral ischemia/reperfusion injury (IRI)" have been developed, demonstrating that often reperfusion after a long ischemic period may cause a larger infarct than that associated with permanent vessel occlusion. In general, the role of neuroprotective agents is to interfere with one or more of the mechanisms involved in the "IRI cascade" and thereby limit the resultant tissue damage. It seem reasonable to assume that drugs that work on a specific biochemical mechanism must be given at the time that the mechanism is active, mainly during ischemia and/or reperfusion. Accordingly, in general, two different experimental paradigms can be identified: prophylactic administration, aimed to evaluate drug effects on stroke prevention, and therapeutic administration, when the drug is administered during reperfusion to test its potential beneficial effects on IRI after stroke had occurred. A role for PPARs in reducing IRI has been first established in animal models of acute myocardial infarction (Yue Tl, Chen et al. 2001). More recently, good evidence supporting the beneficial role of PPAR in stroke has been provided by several *in vivo* experimental models of cerebral IRI, evaluating the effects of both prophylactic and therapeutic administration of PPAR agonists. It has been demonstrated that a 14-day preventive treatment with fenofibrate reduced susceptibility to stroke in apolipoprotein E-deficient mice as well as decreased cerebral infarct volume in wild-type littermates (Deplanque, Gele et al. 2003). The authors demonstrated that fenofibrate administration was associated with a decrease in cerebral oxidative stress depending on the increase in activity of several anti-oxidant enzymes and with a reduced expression of adhesion molecules. In another study, it was confirmed that two different PPARα agonists, fenofibrate and WY14643, provided similar brain protection when administered 3 or 7 days, respectively, before the induction of cerebral ischemia (Inoue, Jiang et al. 2003). More recently, we have found that PPARα agonists may also reduce cerebral I/R injury when administered just before ischemia or during reperfusion (Collino, Aragno et al. 2006). We showed that the potential neuroprotective effects of PPARα agonists is manifested by modulation of protein S100B levels in the rat CNS. S100B is a calcium-binding protein, mainly expressed in the brain and recent preclinical and clinical studies indicate that increased S100B levels is a reliable indicator of infarct size in acute ischemic stroke (Buyukuysal 2005; Foerch, Singer et al. 2005). Pre-treatment of rats with the selective PPARα agonist, WY14643, prior to cerebral ischemia causes a marked reduction of S100B levels in the rat hippocampus. This protective effect is reversed by administration of the PPARα antagonist, MK886, thus confirming the involvement of PPARα activation in neuroprotection. Similarly, fenofibrate pretreatment for 14 days significantly reduced the cerebral infarct volume in an experimental model of Middle Cerebral Artery Occlusion (MCAO), although its withdrawal 3 days before induction of cerebral ischemia decreased the neuroprotective effect (Ouk, Laprais et al. 2009). Also prophylactic administration of gemfibrozil resulted in reduction of infarct size 24 h after MCAO and increased cortical blood flow in the ischemic hemisphere (Guo, Wang et al. 2009). However, the principal focus of studies of PPAR agonists has been on agonists of the PPARγ isoform. Emerging studies have reported the protective effects of PPARγ agonist administration in animal models of cerebral IRI (Sundararajan, Gamboa et al. 2005; Collino, Aragno et al. 2006; Allahtavakoli, Shabanzadeh et al. 2007) and in models of permanent ischemia (Sayan-Ozacmak, Ozacmak et al.; Zhang, Xu et al.). The effect of delayed post ischemia administration of a PPARγ agonist, rosiglitazone, has been recently evaluated, demonstrating that post-treatment with rosiglitazone, 24 h after stroke induction, may reduce ischemic injury, improve neurological outcome, and prevent neutrophilia, thus supporting an extended therapeutic window for the treatment of ischemic stroke (Allahtavakoli, Moloudi et al. 2009). Recent experimental data confirmed that PPARγ agonists are protective at clinically relevant doses, independent of any effects on systemic blood pressure or cerebral blood flow and, most notably, the timing of reperfusion relative to drug administration, may significantly influence the ability of PPARγ agonists to reduce infarction volume and improve neurologic function following ischemic injury (Gamboa, Blankenship et al.). The relevance of PPARγ as an endogenous protective factor was also shown by the fact that treatment with a PPARγ antagonist increased infarct size (Victor, Wanderi et al. 2006). Moreover, it was demonstrated that in primary cortical neurons of PPARγ KO mice exposed to ischemia there was a reduced expression of numerous key gene products (including superoxide dismutase-1, catalase, and glutathione S-transferase) along with an increased damage. PPARγ mRNA is up-regulated in ischemic brain, especially in the peri-infarct area. Increased PPARγ mRNA was detected in the infarcted brain as early as 6 h following focal ischemia (Ou, Zhao et al. 2006), and PPARγ immunopositive neurons were detected between 4 h and 14 days, whereas in neurons and microglia only transiently at 12 h in the post-ischemic brain (Zhao, Patzer et al. 2005; Victor, Wanderi et al. 2006). The beneficial role of PPARβ/δ in stroke has been demonstrated by two different studies in which PPARβ/δ knockout mice subjected to cerebral IRI showed significantly larger infarct size than wild-type littermates (Pialat, Cho et al. 2007). This finding is confirmed by another study demonstrating that intracerebroventricular administration of high affinity PPARβ/δ agonists such as L-165041 and GW501516 significantly decreased the infarct volume at 24 h of reperfusion after cerebral ischemia in rats (Iwashita, Muramatsu et al. 2007).

4.2 Clinical evidence of beneficial effects of PPAR ligands in ischemic stroke

Although various PPAR agonists applied before the onset of ischemia can effectively protect the brain in animal models of acute IRI, these treatments are seldom possible in the clinical setting of stroke because patients with stroke present after onset of the ischemic attack. Neuroprotective interventions applied after the onset of ischemia would thus seem to have greater clinical potential. Although some preclinical data provide evidence that administration of PPAR agonists during reperfusion decreases cerebral IRI, to date, there are no clinical data on the therapeutic efficacy of PPAR agonists administration after the onset of the ischemic event. Nevertheless, it must be noted that there may be subgroups of patients at high risk for stroke that could benefit from taking neuroprotective agents as prophylactic treatment. As already mentioned, pioglitazone and rosiglitazone (the TZD class of PPARγ agonists) have proven to be beneficial in type-2 diabetes mellitus patients. Diabetics are at an increased risk of stroke incidence and stroke causes more damage in diabetics compared to normoglycemic individuals. For this reason, such patients might benefit from taking an antidiabetic medication with neuroprotective properties, which might lessen the incidence and/or the severity of acute ischemic stroke. However, it's important to assess whether the potential benefits of taking an oral neuroprotective drug chronically outweighs the risks, including potential side effects. The use of a PPARγ agonist, specifically pioglitazone, as a preventive approach to ischemic brain injury has been recently addressed by two large clinical trials: the Prospective Pioglitazone Clinical Trial in Macrovascular Events (PROactive) and the Insulin Resistance Intervention after Stroke Trial (IRIS trial). The PROactive study has demonstrated that pioglitazone significantly reduces the combined risk of heart attacks, strokes and death by 16% in high risk patients with type-2 diabetes (Dormandy, Charbonnel et al. 2005). Enhanced functional recovery was also reported in a small group of stroke patients with type-2 diabetes treated with pioglitazone (Lee, Olson et al. 2006). However, it remain unclear whether the suggested beneficial effects of pioglitazone are mediated by insulin sensitization or by additional observed reductions in risk factors, such as hyperthension and dyslipidemia. This question and that related to the potential beneficial effects of pioglitazone in non-diabetic patients with stroke will be addressed by the IRIS trial, a randomized, double-blind, placebo-controlled trial on more than 3000 non-diabetic subjects who are insulin resistant and have had a recent transient ischemic attack or ischemic stroke. The IRIS study (ClinicalTrials.gov Identifier: NCT00091949) began on February 2005 and it is still recruiting patients. Interestingly, high plasma levels of 15d-PGJ2 (the natural ligand for PPARγ) have been associated with good neurological outcome and smaller infarct volume in patients with an acute atherothrombotic stroke (Blanco, Moro et al. 2005). Moreover, a recent report suggests that the Pro12Ala polymorphism of PPARγ2 is associated with a reduced risk for ischemic stroke (Lee, Olson et al. 2006), further supporting the importance of PPARs in cerebral ischemia. Nevertheless, as TZDs are hampered by adverse effects related to increased weight gain, fluid overload, and congestive heart failure, the risks associated with chronic TZD administration needs to be better elucidated.

Abnormal levels of serum lipids, including triglycerides, low density lipoprotein (LDL) and high density lipoprotein (HDL), are regarded as other important risk factors for cerebrovascular disease, including stroke. The association between hypercholesterolemia and stroke has become more apparent because of data from prospective cohort studies that show higher risks of ischemic stroke with increasing levels of total cholesterol in both men and women. Increased HDL cholesterol levels have a protective effect against the occurrence of ischemic stroke and elevated triglyceride levels have also been reported as a risk factor for stroke. Overall, elevated total cholesterol confers an approximately two-fold relative increase in stroke risk for men and women. As fibrates are used as lipid-lowering agents, it has been supposed that these PPARα agonists could also protect the brain against noxious biological reactions induced by cerebral IRI. A recent systematic meta-analysis of randomized clinical trials shows that fibrates do not significantly reduce the odds of stroke (Saha, Kizhakepunnur et al. 2007). However, data from large trials specifically investigating the role of fibrates in stroke event reduction are needed to conclusively elucidate their potential neuroprotective role. For instance, a large clinical trial, named Action to Control Cardiovascular Risk in Diabetes (ACCORD) is currently testing the ability of fenofibrate to decrease stroke incidence in high-risk patients with type-2 diabetes (ACCORD study group 2007).

5. Molecular mechanisms of beneficial effects of PPARs against cerebral ischemia

Cerebral IRI is known to induce generation of ROS, as well as the expression of cytokines, adhesion molecules and enzymes involved in the inflammatory response, and is known to be regulated by oxygen- or redox-sensitive mechanisms. Recent studies have confirmed the pivotal role of both oxidative stress and inflammatory response in the pathogenesis of acute ischemic stroke. Through various mechanisms PPARs can regulate both inflammatory and oxidative pathways and PPAR agonist-induced neuroprotection seems to be specific for injuries in which inflammation or free radical generation are the main causes of cell damage. For instance, PPARα activation can induce expression and activation of antioxidant enzymes, such as superoxide dismutase (SOD) and glutathione peroxidase (GSH). We have demonstrated that administration of a highly selective PPARα agonist, WY14643, 30 min prior to IRI, decreased ROS production and lipid peroxidation in rats subjected to IRI and, at the same time, offered protection against GSH depletion (Collino, Aragno et al. 2006). Similar results on oxidative stress modulation have been reported when another PPARα agonist, fenofibrate, was tested in a mouse model of middle cerebral artery occlusion (Deplanque, Gele et al. 2003). Interestingly, PPARγ KO mice have been found to exhibit significant increases in oxidative stress and lipid peroxidation much earlier in their life than wild-type littermates (Poynter and Daynes 1998). The PPAR-induced protective effect on oxidative stress could be related to a direct effect on antioxidant enzyme expression, as the catalase and SOD gene promoters contain the PPRE. In fact, rats that have been treated with a diet containing PPARα ligands, WY14643 or fenofibrate, have demonstrated an enhanced expression of antioxidant enzymes such as SOD and catalase (Toyama, Nakamura et al. 2004). Based on gene expression microarray experiments, Coleman and colleagues (Coleman, Prabhu et al. 2007) have demonstrated that PPARβ/δ activation increased mRNA for aldheyde dehydrogenase and glutathione-S-transferase, thus protecting the cell from oxidative damage. In normotensive and hypertensive animals treated with rosiglitazone, ischemic hemispheres showed increased catalase and Cu/Zn-SOD activity in the peri-infarct region (Tureyen, Kapadia et al. 2007) and the level of Cu/Zn-SOD was demonstrated to increase in the ischemic cortex of animals treated with pioglitazone for 4 days prior to focal cerebral ischemia (Shimazu, Inoue et al. 2005). As we have recently shown, treatment of rats with either pioglitazone or rosiglitazone before occlusion of the common carotid artery decreased the production of ROS and nitrite, decreased lipid peroxidation and reversed the depleted stores of glutathione in the hippocampus (Collino, Aragno et al. 2006). These findings are supported by data from an *in vitro* model demonstrating that pre-treatment with PPARγ agonists protected an immortalized mouse hippocampal cell line against oxidative stress induced by glutamate or hydrogen peroxide (Aoun, Watson et al. 2003). Moreover, PPARγ agonists attenuate the expression of iNOS in inflammatory cells, which is an important source of nitric oxide (NO). NO may react with ROS to produce peroxynitrites, with deleterious effects on neuronal survival. Thus, iNOS inhibition may represent a further mechanism for neuroprotection by PPAR agonists. Mitochondria are the major source of ROS, which are mainly generated at complexes I and III of the respiratory chain. There is now evidence indicating that rosiglitazone and pioglitazone exert direct and rapid effects on mitochondrial respiration, inhibiting complex I and complex III activity (Brunmair, Lest et al. 2004). As PPARγ agonists partially disrupt the mitochondrial respiratory chain, both electron transport and superoxide anion generation are affected. Moreover, a novel mitochondrial target protein for PPARγ agonists ("mitoNEET") has recently been identified (Colca, McDonald et al. 2004). MitoNEET was found associated with components of complex III, suggesting how binding of PPARγ agonists to mitoNEET could selectively block different mitochondrial targets. The ability of PPARγ agonists to influence mitochondrial function might contribute to their inhibitory effects on ROS generation that is evoked by IRI.

Another mechanism through which PPAR agonists may provide neuroprotection is by down-regulating the inflammatory response associated with IRI. Depending on the affected tissue and which PPAR isoforms are involved, PPAR agonists can differently modulate the intensity, duration and consequences of inflammatory events. For instance, ischemia-induced COX-2 overexpression is prevented by PPARγ agonists but not by PPARα agonists (Sundararajan, Gamboa et al. 2005; Collino, Aragno et al. 2006; Collino, Aragno et al. 2006). Activation of PPARγ attenuates the expression of matrix metalloproteinase (MMP)-9 and various inflammatory cytokines in ischemic brain tissue (Pereira, Hurtado et al. 2005). PPARγ is constitutively expressed in macrophages and microglial cells and the systemic treatment of rodents with rosiglitazone reduces the infiltration of these cells into peri-infarct brain regions. Both chronic and acute administration of PPARγ agonists has been demonstrated to prevent cerebral IRI-induced expression of vascular cell adhesion molecule-1 (VCAM-1) and ICAM-1 in two independent studies (Deplanque, Gele et al. 2003; Collino, Aragno et al. 2006). In the brain, the decreased expression of these adhesion molecules might contribute to inhibit the infiltration of the brain ischemic area by neutrophils. Studies addressing the molecular mechanisms of these anti-inflammatory actions demonstrated that the involvement of PPARs in the control of IRI-induced inflammation is mediated mainly through their transrepression capabilities. PPARs can suppress the activities of many distinct families of transcription factors. The range of transcription factors affected and the mechanisms involved may be different for each PPAR isotype, although a common mechanism of PPARα and PPARγ neuroprotection appears to involve inhibition of p38 MAPK activation and NF-κB nuclear translocation. A recent study confirms that PPARγ activation prevents the post-ischemic cerebral expression of pro-inflammatory transcription factors, such as Egr1, C/EBP and NF-κB, possibly by decreasing DNA binding (Tureyen, Kapadia et al. 2007). The inhibitory protein IκBα, which is an indicator of NF-κB transcriptional activity, is remarkably increased in the brain of rats that underwent cerebral ischemia and completely blocked by rosiglitazone and 15d-PGJ2 administration, thus further confirming that both endogenous and synthetic PPARγ ligands inhibit NF-κB signalling (Pereira, Hurtado et al. 2006). Similarly, p38 MAPK and NF-κB activation by cerebral IRI has been demonstrated to be inhibited by pre-treatment with the PPARα agonist WY14643 or the PPARγ agonist pioglitazone. However, as MAPK and NF-κB are functionally interconnected and do not act independently, we cannot rule out the possibility that PPARs affect NF-κB activation by interfering with the MAPK signalling cascade or vice versa.

The generation of ROS is known to be associated with the induction of apoptosis and, in neurons, inhibition of cell death is an important factor to prevent during IRI. PPAR activation may decrease the IRI-induced activation of apoptotic pathways depending on the increase in activity and expression of numerous anti-oxidant enzymes. Moreover, by their anti-inflammatory action on microglia and astrocytes, PPAR agonists prevent the release of neurotoxic agents, which induce neuronal apoptosis. PPARγ agonists may attenuate ischemia-induced reactive oxygen species and subsequently alleviate the post-ischemic degradation of Bcl-2, Bcl-xl, and Akt, by increasing SOD/catalase and decreasing nicotinamide adenine dinucleotide phosphate oxidase levels (Fong, Tsai et al.). Chu and colleagues (Chu, Lee et al. 2006) have demonstrated that rosiglitazone-fed rats had better neurological scores and reduced number of TUNEL-positive cells following transient focal ischemia. Interestingly, these authors also reported an increased vasculature in the rosiglitazone-treated group with increased number of endothelial cells positive for BrdU, suggesting there may be enhanced angiogenesis following PPARγ activation. Administration of a selective PPARγ agonist (L-796449) 10 min prior to permanent cerebral artery occlusion, resulted in decreased apoptosis, measured as reduction of caspase-3 activity (Pereira, Hurtado et al. 2005). Another study confirmed inhibition on caspase-3 activity by both exogenous and endogenous PPARγ agonists, rosiglitazone and 15d-PGJ2, in the ischemic cortex (Lin, Cheung et al. 2006). The same authors observed that rosiglitazone and 15d-PGJ2 exhibit a concentration-dependent paradoxical effect on cytotoxicity, when tested in an *in vitro* model of hydrogen peroxide induced neuronal apoptosis. The drugs induced pro-apoptotic effects when used at concentrations higher that 5 μmol/L but protect neurons from necrosis and apoptosis at concentrations lower than 1 μmol/L. The reason for this paradoxical action is unclear and further studies are needed to better clarify the effects of PPARs in IRI induced-apoptosis and necrosis.

Recently published data suggest that an increased uptake of cerebral extracellular glutamate levels after ischemia may represent an additional mechanism for the neuroprotection exerted by PPARγ activation (Romera, Hurtado et al. 2007). Both *in vivo* and *in vitro* experiments showed that rosiglitazone administration increased the expression of the GLT1/EAAT2 glutamate transporter in the brain, thus preventing the extracellular glutamate levels from rising to neurotoxic values.

6. Conclusion

Although clinical data are limited, a wide array of evidence obtained in animal models now shows that PPAR activation may be a rational and effective strategy against ischemic brain damage. The beneficial effects of PPAR agonists in experimental models of stroke are mediated by different mechanisms, as expected based on their pleiotropic pharmacological profile. The neuroprotective actions appear to be mainly related to the reduction in oxidative damage as well as anti-inflammatory and anti-apoptotic effects. These results have been essentially obtained with PPARα and PPARγ agonists, while the PPARβ/δ pathway remains largely unexplored, despite a significant interest in this target. Selective activation of different isoforms of PPARs may account for the difference in molecular pathways underlying neuroprotection and these different features still remain far from being completely understood. In conclusion, currently available management protocols for patients with stroke may benefit from the use of PPAR agonists that target detrimental processes associated with IRI. However, several critical issues still need to be resolved. For instance, well-structured clinical trials aimed at evaluating the effects of PPAR ligands on stroke recovery are needed before firm conclusions are drawn about their therapeutic efficacy. A more stringent approach regarding the concentration range of PPAR agonists, especially within the CNS, and the duration of exposure should be applied. Also acceptable water solubility with satisfactory blood-brain barrier penetrability is an important aspect of PPAR agonists that needs to be optimized.

7. References

Allahtavakoli, M., R. Moloudi, et al. (2009). "Delayed post ischemic treatment with Rosiglitazone attenuates infarct volume, neurological deficits and neutrophilia after embolic stroke in rat." *Brain Res* 1271: 121-7.

Allahtavakoli, M., A. Shabanzadeh, et al. (2007). "Combination therapy of rosiglitazone, a peroxisome proliferator-activated receptor-gamma ligand, and NMDA receptor antagonist (MK-801) on experimental embolic stroke in rats." *Basic Clin Pharmacol Toxicol* 101(5): 309-14.

Amri, E. Z., F. Bonino, et al. (1995). "Cloning of a protein that mediates transcriptional effects of fatty acids in preadipocytes. Homology to peroxisome proliferator-activated receptors." *J Biol Chem* 270(5): 2367-71.

Aoun, P., D. G. Watson, et al. (2003). "Neuroprotective effects of PPARgamma agonists against oxidative insults in HT-22 cells." *Eur J Pharmacol* 472(1-2): 65-71.

Barish, G. D., A. R. Atkins, et al. (2008). "PPARdelta regulates multiple proinflammatory pathways to suppress atherosclerosis." *Proc Natl Acad Sci U S A* 105(11): 4271-6.

Berger, J., M. D. Leibowitz, et al. (1999). "Novel peroxisome proliferator-activated receptor (PPAR) gamma and PPARdelta ligands produce distinct biological effects." *J Biol Chem* 274(10): 6718-25.

Blanco, M., M. A. Moro, et al. (2005). "Increased plasma levels of 15-deoxyDelta prostaglandin J2 are associated with good outcome in acute atherothrombotic ischemic stroke." *Stroke* 36(6): 1189-94.

Braissant, O., F. Foufelle, et al. (1996). "Differential expression of peroxisome proliferator-activated receptors (PPARs): tissue distribution of PPAR-alpha, -beta, and -gamma in the adult rat." *Endocrinology* 137(1): 354-66.

Brunmair, B., A. Lest, et al. (2004). "Fenofibrate impairs rat mitochondrial function by inhibition of respiratory complex I." *J Pharmacol Exp Ther* 311(1): 109-14.

Buyukuysal, R. L. (2005). "Protein S100B release from rat brain slices during and after ischemia: comparison with lactate dehydrogenase leakage." *Neurochem Int* 47(8): 580-8.

Choi, J. H., A. S. Banks, et al. (2010). "Anti-diabetic drugs inhibit obesity-linked phosphorylation of PPARgamma by Cdk5." *Nature* 466(7305): 451-6.

Chou, C. J., M. Haluzik, et al. (2002). "WY14,643, a peroxisome proliferator-activated receptor alpha (PPARalpha) agonist, improves hepatic and muscle steatosis and reverses insulin resistance in lipoatrophic A-ZIP/F-1 mice." *J Biol Chem* 277(27): 24484-9.

Chu, K., S. T. Lee, et al. (2006). "Peroxisome proliferator-activated receptor-gamma-agonist, rosiglitazone, promotes angiogenesis after focal cerebral ischemia." *Brain Res* 1093(1): 208-18.

Colca, J. R., W. G. McDonald, et al. (2004). "Identification of a novel mitochondrial protein ("mitoNEET") cross-linked specifically by a thiazolidinedione photoprobe." *Am J Physiol Endocrinol Metab* 286(2): E252-60.

Coleman, J. D., K. S. Prabhu, et al. (2007). "The oxidative stress mediator 4-hydroxynonenal is an intracellular agonist of the nuclear receptor peroxisome proliferator-activated receptor-beta/delta (PPARbeta/delta)." *Free Radic Biol Med* 42(8): 1155-64.

Collino, M., M. Aragno, et al. (2006). "Oxidative stress and inflammatory response evoked by transient cerebral ischemia/reperfusion: effects of the PPAR-alpha agonist WY14643." *Free Radic Biol Med* 41(4): 579-89.

Collino, M., M. Aragno, et al. (2006). "Modulation of the oxidative stress and inflammatory response by PPAR-gamma agonists in the hippocampus of rats exposed to cerebral ischemia/reperfusion." *Eur J Pharmacol* 530(1-2): 70-80.

Cristiano, L., A. Bernardo, et al. (2001). "Peroxisome proliferator-activated receptors (PPARs) and peroxisomes in rat cortical and cerebellar astrocytes." *J Neurocytol* 30(8): 671-83.

Delerive, P., F. Martin-Nizard, et al. (1999). "Peroxisome proliferator-activated receptor activators inhibit thrombin-induced endothelin-1 production in human vascular endothelial cells by inhibiting the activator protein-1 signaling pathway." *Circ Res* 85(5): 394-402.

Deplanque, D., P. Gele, et al. (2003). "Peroxisome proliferator-activated receptor-alpha activation as a mechanism of preventive neuroprotection induced by chronic fenofibrate treatment." *J Neurosci* 23(15): 6264-71.

Desvergne, B. and W. Wahli (1999). "Peroxisome proliferator-activated receptors: nuclear control of metabolism." *Endocr Rev* 20(5): 649-88.

Dormandy, J. A., B. Charbonnel, et al. (2005). "Secondary prevention of macrovascular events in patients with type 2 diabetes in the PROactive Study (PROspective pioglitAzone Clinical Trial In macroVascular Events): a randomised controlled trial." *Lancet* 366(9493): 1279-89.

Fajas, L., D. Auboeuf, et al. (1997). "The organization, promoter analysis, and expression of the human PPARgamma gene." *J Biol Chem* 272(30): 18779-89.

Feige, J. N., L. Gelman, et al. (2006). "From molecular action to physiological outputs: peroxisome proliferator-activated receptors are nuclear receptors at the crossroads of key cellular functions." *Prog Lipid Res* 45(2): 120-59.

Foerch, C., O. C. Singer, et al. (2005). "Evaluation of serum S100B as a surrogate marker for long-term outcome and infarct volume in acute middle cerebral artery infarction." *Arch Neurol* 62(7): 1130-4.

Fong, W. H., H. D. Tsai, et al. (2010). "Anti-apoptotic actions of PPAR-gamma against ischemic stroke." *Mol Neurobiol* 41(2-3): 180-6.

Forman, B. M., J. Chen, et al. (1997). "Hypolipidemic drugs, polyunsaturated fatty acids, and eicosanoids are ligands for peroxisome proliferator-activated receptors alpha and delta." *Proc Natl Acad Sci U S A* 94(9): 4312-7.

Gamboa, J., D. A. Blankenship, et al. (2010). "Extension of the neuroprotective time window for thiazolidinediones in ischemic stroke is dependent on time of reperfusion." *Neuroscience* 170(3): 846-57.

Greene, M. E., B. Blumberg, et al. (1995). "Isolation of the human peroxisome proliferator activated receptor gamma cDNA: expression in hematopoietic cells and chromosomal mapping." *Gene Expr* 4(4-5): 281-99.

Guo, Q., G. Wang, et al. (2009). "Effects of gemfibrozil on outcome after permanent middle cerebral artery occlusion in mice." *Brain Res* 1279: 121-30.

Gurnell, M. (2003). "PPARgamma and metabolism: insights from the study of human genetic variants." *Clin Endocrinol (Oxf)* 59(3): 267-77.

Hevener, A. L., W. He, et al. (2003). "Muscle-specific Pparg deletion causes insulin resistance." *Nat Med* 9(12): 1491-7.

Hu, E., J. B. Kim, et al. (1996). "Inhibition of adipogenesis through MAP kinase-mediated phosphorylation of PPARgamma." *Science* 274(5295): 2100-3.

Inoue, H., X. F. Jiang, et al. (2003). "Brain protection by resveratrol and fenofibrate against stroke requires peroxisome proliferator-activated receptor alpha in mice." *Neurosci Lett* 352(3): 203-6.

Issemann, I. and S. Green (1990). "Activation of a member of the steroid hormone receptor superfamily by peroxisome proliferators." *Nature* 347(6294): 645-50.

Iwashita, A., Y. Muramatsu, et al. (2007). "Neuroprotective efficacy of the peroxisome proliferator-activated receptor delta-selective agonists in vitro and in vivo." *J Pharmacol Exp Ther* 320(3): 1087-96.

Juge-Aubry, C., A. Pernin, et al. (1997). "DNA binding properties of peroxisome proliferator-activated receptor subtypes on various natural peroxisome proliferator response elements. Importance of the 5'-flanking region." *J Biol Chem* 272(40): 25252-9.

Kersten, S., J. Seydoux, et al. (1999). "Peroxisome proliferator-activated receptor alpha mediates the adaptive response to fasting." *J Clin Invest* 103(11): 1489-98.

Kim, H., M. Haluzik, et al. (2003). "Peroxisome proliferator-activated receptor-alpha agonist treatment in a transgenic model of type 2 diabetes reverses the lipotoxic state and improves glucose homeostasis." *Diabetes* 52(7): 1770-8.

Kliewer, S. A., B. M. Forman, et al. (1994). "Differential expression and activation of a family of murine peroxisome proliferator-activated receptors." *Proc Natl Acad Sci U S A* 91(15): 7355-9.

Krogsdam, A. M., C. A. Nielsen, et al. (2002). "Nuclear receptor corepressor-dependent repression of peroxisome-proliferator-activated receptor delta-mediated transactivation." *Biochem J* 363(Pt 1): 157-65.

Lee, C. H., A. Chawla, et al. (2003). "Transcriptional repression of atherogenic inflammation: modulation by PPARdelta." *Science* 302(5644): 453-7.

Lee, C. H., P. Olson, et al. (2006). "PPARdelta regulates glucose metabolism and insulin sensitivity." *Proc Natl Acad Sci U S A* 103(9): 3444-9.

Lefebvre, P., G. Chinetti, et al. (2006). "Sorting out the roles of PPAR alpha in energy metabolism and vascular homeostasis." *J Clin Invest* 116(3): 571-80.

Lim, H. and S. K. Dey (2000). "PPAR delta functions as a prostacyclin receptor in blastocyst implantation." *Trends Endocrinol Metab* 11(4): 137-42.

Lin, T. N., W. M. Cheung, et al. (2006). "15d-prostaglandin J2 protects brain from ischemia-reperfusion injury." *Arterioscler Thromb Vasc Biol* 26(3): 481-7.

Lincoff, A. M., K. Wolski, et al. (2007). "Pioglitazone and risk of cardiovascular events in patients with type 2 diabetes mellitus: a meta-analysis of randomized trials." *JAMA* 298(10): 1180-8.

Loke, Y. K., S. Singh, et al. (2009). "Long-term use of thiazolidinediones and fractures in type 2 diabetes: a meta-analysis." *CMAJ* 180(1): 32-9.

Martens, F. M., F. L. Visseren, et al. (2002). "Metabolic and additional vascular effects of thiazolidinediones." *Drugs* 62(10): 1463-80.

Moreno, S., S. Farioli-Vecchioli, et al. (2004). "Immunolocalization of peroxisome proliferator-activated receptors and retinoid X receptors in the adult rat CNS." *Neuroscience* 123(1): 131-45.

Nissen, S. E. and K. Wolski (2010). "Rosiglitazone revisited: an updated meta-analysis of risk for myocardial infarction and cardiovascular mortality." *Arch Intern Med* 170(14): 1191-1201.

Onate, S. A., S. Y. Tsai, et al. (1995). "Sequence and characterization of a coactivator for the steroid hormone receptor superfamily." *Science* 270(5240): 1354-7.

Ou, Z., X. Zhao, et al. (2006). "Neuronal expression of peroxisome proliferator-activated receptor-gamma (PPARgamma) and 15d-prostaglandin J2--mediated protection of brain after experimental cerebral ischemia in rat." *Brain Res* 1096(1): 196-203.

Ouk, T., M. Laprais, et al. (2009). "Withdrawal of fenofibrate treatment partially abrogates preventive neuroprotection in stroke via loss of vascular protection." *Vascul Pharmacol* 51(5-6): 323-30.

Palmer, C. N., M. H. Hsu, et al. (1995). "Novel sequence determinants in peroxisome proliferator signaling." *J Biol Chem* 270(27): 16114-21.

Pascual, G. and C. K. Glass (2006). "Nuclear receptors versus inflammation: mechanisms of transrepression." *Trends Endocrinol Metab* 17(8): 321-7.

Pereira, M. P., O. Hurtado, et al. (2005). "The nonthiazolidinedione PPARgamma agonist L-796,449 is neuroprotective in experimental stroke." *J Neuropathol Exp Neurol* 64(9): 797-805.

Pereira, M. P., O. Hurtado, et al. (2006). "Rosiglitazone and 15-deoxy-Delta12,14-prostaglandin J2 cause potent neuroprotection after experimental stroke through noncompletely overlapping mechanisms." *J Cereb Blood Flow Metab* 26(2): 218-29.

Peters, J. M., S. S. Lee, et al. (2000). "Growth, adipose, brain, and skin alterations resulting from targeted disruption of the mouse peroxisome proliferator-activated receptor beta(delta)." *Mol Cell Biol* 20(14): 5119-28.

Pialat, J. B., T. H. Cho, et al. (2007). "MRI monitoring of focal cerebral ischemia in peroxisome proliferator-activated receptor (PPAR)-deficient mice." *NMR Biomed* 20(3): 335-42.

Poynter, M. E. and R. A. Daynes (1998). "Peroxisome proliferator-activated receptor alpha activation modulates cellular redox status, represses nuclear factor-kappaB signaling, and reduces inflammatory cytokine production in aging." *J Biol Chem* 273(49): 32833-41.

Romera, C., O. Hurtado, et al. (2007). "Ischemic preconditioning reveals that GLT1/EAAT2 glutamate transporter is a novel PPARgamma target gene involved in neuroprotection." *J Cereb Blood Flow Metab* 27(7): 1327-38.

Rosen, E. D., P. Sarraf, et al. (1999). "PPAR gamma is required for the differentiation of adipose tissue in vivo and in vitro." *Mol Cell* 4(4): 611-7.

Saha, S. A., L. G. Kizhakepunnur, et al. (2007). "The role of fibrates in the prevention of cardiovascular disease--a pooled meta-analysis of long-term randomized placebo-controlled clinical trials." *Am Heart J* 154(5): 943-53.

Sayan-Ozacmak, H., V. H. Ozacmak, et al. (2011). "Neuroprotective Efficacy Of The Peroxisome Proliferator-Activated Receptor-g Ligand In Chronic Cerebral Hypoperfusion." *Curr Neurovasc Res.* 8 (3): 190-9.

Schmidt, A., N. Endo, et al. (1992). "Identification of a new member of the steroid hormone receptor superfamily that is activated by a peroxisome proliferator and fatty acids." *Mol Endocrinol* 6(10): 1634-41.

Schwabe, J. W., D. Neuhaus, et al. (1990). "Solution structure of the DNA-binding domain of the oestrogen receptor." *Nature* 348(6300): 458-61.

Shearer, B. G., D. J. Steger, et al. (2008). "Identification and characterization of a selective peroxisome proliferator-activated receptor beta/delta (NR1C2) antagonist." *Mol Endocrinol* 22(2): 523-9.

Sher, T., H. F. Yi, et al. (1993). "cDNA cloning, chromosomal mapping, and functional characterization of the human peroxisome proliferator activated receptor." *Biochemistry* 32(21): 5598-604.

Shi, Y., M. Hon, et al. (2002). "The peroxisome proliferator-activated receptor delta, an integrator of transcriptional repression and nuclear receptor signaling." *Proc Natl Acad Sci U S A* 99(5): 2613-8.

Shimazu, T., I. Inoue, et al. (2005). "A peroxisome proliferator-activated receptor-gamma agonist reduces infarct size in transient but not in permanent ischemia." *Stroke* 36(2): 353-9.

Singh, S., Y. K. Loke, et al. (2007). "Long-term risk of cardiovascular events with rosiglitazone: a meta-analysis." *JAMA* 298(10): 1189-95.

Suhara, W., H. Koide, et al. (2009). "Cow's milk increases the activities of human nuclear receptors peroxisome proliferator-activated receptors alpha and delta and retinoid X receptor alpha involved in the regulation of energy homeostasis, obesity, and inflammation." *J Dairy Sci* 92(9): 4180-7.

Sundararajan, S., J. L. Gamboa, et al. (2005). "Peroxisome proliferator-activated receptor-gamma ligands reduce inflammation and infarction size in transient focal ischemia." *Neuroscience* 130(3): 685-96.

Takata, Y., J. Liu, et al. (2008). "PPARdelta-mediated antiinflammatory mechanisms inhibit angiotensin II-accelerated atherosclerosis." *Proc Natl Acad Sci U S A* 105(11): 4277-82.

Theocharisa, S., A. Margeli, et al. (2003). "Peroxisome proliferator activated receptor-gamma ligands as potent antineoplastic agents." *Curr Med Chem Anticancer Agents* 3(3): 239-51.

Toyama, T., H. Nakamura, et al. (2004). "PPARalpha ligands activate antioxidant enzymes and suppress hepatic fibrosis in rats." *Biochem Biophys Res Commun* 324(2): 697-704.

Tureyen, K., R. Kapadia, et al. (2007). "Peroxisome proliferator-activated receptor-gamma agonists induce neuroprotection following transient focal ischemia in normotensive, normoglycemic as well as hypertensive and type-2 diabetic rodents." *J Neurochem* 101(1): 41-56.

Victor, N. A., E. W. Wanderi, et al. (2006). "Altered PPARgamma expression and activation after transient focal ischemia in rats." *Eur J Neurosci* 24(6): 1653-63.

Willson, T. M., P. J. Brown, et al. (2000). "The PPARs: from orphan receptors to drug discovery." *J Med Chem* 43(4): 527-50.

Xu, H. E., M. H. Lambert, et al. (1999). "Molecular recognition of fatty acids by peroxisome proliferator-activated receptors." *Mol Cell* 3(3): 397-403.

Yamamoto, Y., H. Yamazaki, et al. (2002). "Formation of a novel quinone epoxide metabolite of troglitazone with cytotoxicity to HepG2 cells." *Drug Metab Dispos* 30(2): 155-60.

Yoshikawa, T., Z. Brkanac, et al. (1996). "Assignment of the human nuclear hormone receptor, NUC1 (PPARD), to chromosome 6p21.1-p21.2." *Genomics* 35(3): 637-8.

Yue Tl, T. L., J. Chen, et al. (2001). "In vivo myocardial protection from ischemia/reperfusion injury by the peroxisome proliferator-activated receptor-gamma agonist rosiglitazone." *Circulation* 104(21): 2588-94.

Zhang, H. L., M. Xu, et al. (2011). "Neuroprotective effects of pioglitazone in a rat model of permanent focal cerebral ischemia are associated with peroxisome proliferator-activated receptor gamma-mediated suppression of nuclear factor-kappaB signaling pathway." *Neuroscience* 176: 381-95.
Zhao, Y., A. Patzer, et al. (2005). "The intracerebral application of the PPARgamma-ligand pioglitazone confers neuroprotection against focal ischaemia in the rat brain." *Eur J Neurosci* 22(1): 278-82.

Permissions

The contributors of this book come from diverse backgrounds, making this book a truly international effort. This book will bring forth new frontiers with its revolutionizing research information and detailed analysis of the nascent developments around the world.

We would like to thank Maurizio Balestrino, MD, for lending his expertise to make the book truly unique. He has played a crucial role in the development of this book. Without his invaluable contribution this book wouldn't have been possible. He has made vital efforts to compile up to date information on the varied aspects of this subject to make this book a valuable addition to the collection of many professionals and students.

This book was conceptualized with the vision of imparting up-to-date information and advanced data in this field. To ensure the same, a matchless editorial board was set up. Every individual on the board went through rigorous rounds of assessment to prove their worth. After which they invested a large part of their time researching and compiling the most relevant data for our readers. Conferences and sessions were held from time to time between the editorial board and the contributing authors to present the data in the most comprehensible form. The editorial team has worked tirelessly to provide valuable and valid information to help people across the globe.

Every chapter published in this book has been scrutinized by our experts. Their significance has been extensively debated. The topics covered herein carry significant findings which will fuel the growth of the discipline. They may even be implemented as practical applications or may be referred to as a beginning point for another development. Chapters in this book were first published by InTech; hereby published with permission under the Creative Commons Attribution License or equivalent.

The editorial board has been involved in producing this book since its inception. They have spent rigorous hours researching and exploring the diverse topics which have resulted in the successful publishing of this book. They have passed on their knowledge of decades through this book. To expedite this challenging task, the publisher supported the team at every step. A small team of assistant editors was also appointed to further simplify the editing procedure and attain best results for the readers.

Our editorial team has been hand-picked from every corner of the world. Their multi-ethnicity adds dynamic inputs to the discussions which result in innovative outcomes. These outcomes are then further discussed with the researchers and contributors who give their valuable feedback and opinion regarding the same. The feedback is then collaborated with the researches and they are edited in a comprehensive manner to aid the understanding of the subject.

Apart from the editorial board, the designing team has also invested a significant amount of their time in understanding the subject and creating the most relevant covers. They scrutinized every image to scout for the most suitable representation of the subject and create an appropriate cover for the book.

The publishing team has been involved in this book since its early stages. They were actively engaged in every process, be it collecting the data, connecting with the contributors or procuring relevant information. The team has been an ardent support to the editorial, designing and production team. Their endless efforts to recruit the best for this project, has resulted in the accomplishment of this book. They are a veteran in the field of academics and their pool of knowledge is as vast as their experience in printing. Their expertise and guidance has proved useful at every step. Their uncompromising quality standards have made this book an exceptional effort. Their encouragement from time to time has been an inspiration for everyone.

The publisher and the editorial board hope that this book will prove to be a valuable piece of knowledge for researchers, students, practitioners and scholars across the globe.

List of Contributors

Miguel Cervantes and Graciela Letechipía-Vallejo
Laboratorio de Neurociencias. Facultad de Ciencias Médicas y Biológicas, "Dr. Ignacio Chávez", Universidad Michoacana de San Nicolás de Hidalgo, Morelia, Michoacán, Mexico

Ignacio González-Burgos
Laboratorio de Psicobiología, División de Neurociencias, Centro de Investigación, Biomédica de Occidente, Instituto Mexicano del Seguro Social, Guadalajara, Jalisco, Mexico

María Esther Olvera-Cortés
Laboratorio de Neurofisiología Experimental, Centro de Investigación Biomédica de Michoacán, Instituto Mexicano del Seguro Social, Morelia, Michoacán, Mexico

Gabriela Moralí
Unidad de Investigación Médica en Farmacología, UMAE Hospital de Especialidades, CMN S XXI, Instituto Mexicano del Seguro Social, México, D.F., Mexico

Joseph T. McCabe
Department of Anatomy, Physiology & Genetics, and The Center for Neuroscience & Regenerative Medicine, Uniformed Services University of the Health Sciences, Bethesda, Maryland, USA

Michael W. Bentley and Joseph C. O'Sullivan
U.S. Army Graduate School of Anesthesia Nursing, Graduate School, AMEDD Center and School, Academy of Health Sciences, Fort Sam Houston, San Antonio, Texas, USA

Masato Shibuya, Kenko Meda and Akira Ikeda
Department of Neurosurgery, Chukyo Hospital, Nagoya, Japan

Maurizio Balestrino, Enrico Adriano and Patrizia Garbati
Department of Neuroscience, Ophtalmology and Genetics, University of Genova, Italy

Carlos Silva-Islas, Ricardo A. Santana, Ana L. Colín-González and Perla D. Maldonado
Patología Vascular Cerebral, Instituto Nacional de Neurología y Neurocirugía Manuel Velasco Suárez México

Ornella Piazza
Anestesiologia e Rianimazione, Università Degli Studi di Salerno, Italy

Giuliana Scarpati
Anestesiologia e Rianimazione, Università Degli Studi di Napoli Federico II, Italy

Vishal Chanana
Waisman Center, University of Wisconsin, Madison, WI, USA

Dandan Sun
Dept. of Neurology, University of Pittsburgh, Pittsburgh, PA, USA

Peter Ferrazzano
Waisman Center, University of Wisconsin, Madison, WI, USA
Dept. of Pediatrics, University of Wisconsin, Madison, WI, USA

Weiyan Cai
Department of Physiology, Nanjing Medical University, Jiangsu, China

Masahiro Sokabe
Department of Physiology, Nagoya University Graduate School of Medicine, Tsurumai, Nagoya, Japan

Ling Chen
Department of Physiology, Nanjing Medical University, Jiangsu, China
Department of Physiology, Nagoya University Graduate School of Medicine, Tsurumai, Nagoya, Japan

Elisa Benetti and Massimo Collino
Dipartimento di Scienza e Tecnologia del Farmaco, University of Turin, Turin, Italy

Nimesh Patel
Centre for Translational Medicine and Therapeutics, Queen Mary University of London, The William Harvey Research Institute, London, UK